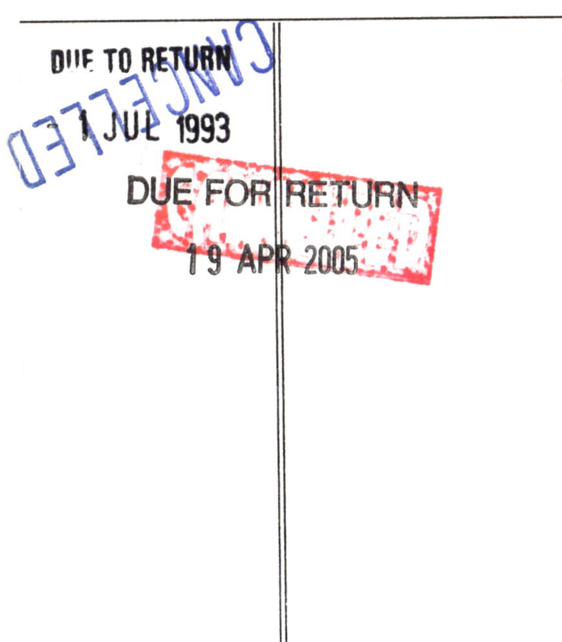
DUE TO RETURN
CANCELLED
1 JUL 1993
DUE FOR RETURN
19 APR 2005

# HISTOCOMPATIBILITY

# HISTOCOMPATIBILITY

## George D. Snell

Emeritus
The Jackson Laboratory
Bar Harbor, Maine

## Jean Dausset

Laboratoire d'Imuno-Hématologie
Institut de Recherches sur les Maladies du Sang
Université de Paris VII
Faculté de Médecine
Paris, France

## Stanley Nathenson

Departments of Microbiology and Immunology and of Cell Biology
Albert Einstein College of Medicine
Bronx, New York

ACADEMIC PRESS New York San Francisco London 1976

A Subsidiary of Harcourt Brace Jovanovich, Publishers

ACADEMIC PRESS, INC.
111 Fifth Avenue, New York, New York 10003

*United Kingdom Edition published by*
ACADEMIC PRESS, INC. (LONDON) LTD.
24/28 Oval Road, London NW1

Library of Congress Cataloging in Publication Data

Snell, George Davis, Date
Histocompatibility.

Includes bibliographies and index.
1. Histocompatibility. I. Dausset, Jean, joint author. II. Nathenson, Stanley G., joint author. III. Title.
QR184.3.S64 617′.95 75-32036
ISBN 0-12-653750-X

PRINTED IN THE UNITED STATES OF AMERICA

*To Rhoda, Rosa, and Susan*
*with love*

# CONTENTS

**Chapter 13 The Allogeneic Responses**

# PREFACE

At the beginning of the twentieth century, it had not as yet been established that allografts are rejected. Research studies with mice quickly demonstrated that they are. Students of histocompatibility then turned their attention to the causes of rejection, examining first the genetic, then the immunologic, and finally the chemical aspects of the rejection process. This volume presents the results of these investigations. How these studies relate to medicine, organ transplantation in man, basic immunology, cell membrane structures, and cancer research is also examined.

Transplantation studies have expanded enormously since the discovery in 1936 by Peter Gorer of *H-2*, the major histocompatibility system in the mouse. Dozens of other loci competent to engender transplantation reactions have been discovered, and *H-2* homologues have been found in man and a variety of other mammals and in birds. The picture that emerges is of a large family of genes whose common property is the determination of molecules that are localized in the plasma membrane and hence, at least in part, are exposed on the cell surface. Almost nothing is known about the function of these molecules, but it has become apparent that the end products of the major histocompatibility complex—*H-2* in the mouse and HLA in man—in some way play a fundamental role in the interactions of lymphocytes with one another, with foreign invaders whether in the form of allografts or microorganisms, and probably with potentially cancerous cells. HLA and *H-2* have emerged as important agents in the immune response and in the development of a variety of diseases, possibly autoimmune in nature. The volume of research in this area during 1974 and 1975 has been almost overwhelming.

In dealing with the resulting extensive literature, we have tried to be selective—to emphasize the forest and not the trees. But forests are complex systems—they cannot be understood without a good knowledge of their individual components—so we have not hesitated in presenting some information on aspects of a problem we consider important.

The research of the authors of this book, and of students of histocompatibility in general, has been generously supported by grants from the National Institutes of Health and other agencies. We are happy to express our gratitude to them.

Many people have assisted in one way or another in the preparation of this volume. The contribution of preprints by friends and colleagues has made it possible for us to incorporate the most up-to-date information. Joan Staats of the Jackson Laboratory has aided in various library searches. One part or another of the chapters written in Bar Harbor has been read and helpfully criticized by Drs. Bailey, Bennett, Cherry, Graff, Harrison, Kaliss, Heiniger, Mobraaten, Shultz, and Taylor. Dr. John Freed made a major contribution to the preparation of Chapter 11. We are greatly indebted to Lillian Runstuk, Barbara Dillon, Eleanor St Denis, Catherine Whelan, Annabel Somerset, and Annick Touboullic for typing. And finally, we want to express our appreciation to the staff of Academic Press for their help with the many technical details of preparing and publishing a book.

George D. Snell

# LIST OF ABBREVIATIONS

| | |
|---|---|
| A.B | Congenic resistant line produced by crossing inbred strains A and B |
| ALS | Anti-lymphocyte serum |
| ANAP | Agglutination-negative–absorption-positive |
| AS | Ankylosing spondylitis |
| BC | Backcross |
| B6 | Inbred mouse strain C57BL/6 |
| C | Inbred mouse strain BALB/c |
| cM | Centimorgan—the unit of crossing over |
| CMAD | Cell membrane alloantigen determining |
| CML | Cell-mediated lysis |
| CR | Congenic resistant |
| CREG | Cross-reacting group |
| CXB | RI strains produced by initial cross of strains BALB/c and C57BL/6 |
| CYNAP | Cytoxicity-negative–absorption-positive |
| $F_1$ | First filial generation following a cross |
| $F_2$ | Second filial generation following a cross |
| GVH | Graft-versus-host |
| II | Histocompatibility |
| LCM | Lymphocytic choriomeningitis |
| LD | Lymphocyte defined |
| MHC | Major histocompatibility complex |
| HHS | Major histocompatibility system |
| MLC | Mixed lymphocyte culture |
| MLR | Mixed lymphocyte reaction |
| MS | Multiple sclerosis |
| MST | Median survival time |

| | |
|---|---|
| NP-40 | Detergent used in solubilizing membrane alloantigens |
| N2 | Second of a series of matings to an inbred strain; corresponds to BC1 or the first backcross |
| PHA | Phytohemogglutinin |
| RI | Recombinant inbred |
| SD | Serologically defined |
| SLE | Systemic lupus erythematosus |

CHAPTER 1

# ISOGRAFTS SUCCEED, ALLOGRAFTS FAIL



The first principles of tissue and organ transplantation can be stated as two simple rules: autografts and isografts succeed, allografts fail. In the language of transplantation, *autografts* are grafts taken from and returned to a single donor; *isografts* are grafts exchanged between identical twins or between highly inbred and hence genetically identical animals; *allografts* are grafts exchanged between genetically dissimilar individuals. Isografts may also be referred to as *isogeneic* or *syngeneic* grafts, and allografts as *allogeneic* grafts. The terminology of histocompatibility is summarized in Table 1.1.

The compatibility of autografts and the incompatibility of allografts was suspected by at least one discerning surgeon nearly 400 years ago, and was sporadically but inadequately tested on numerous occasions over a period of three centuries. It was not, however, until the introduction of laboratory studies with inbred mice in the second quarter of this century that these principles were finally proved. It took only a few additional decades of intensive experimentation to show that the rejection of allografts is not an inviolable principle, and by appropriate means the rejection process can sometimes be circumvented. Organ transplantation in man thereby became a reality, and transplants of kidney

TABLE 1.1
TERMINOLOGY OF HISTOCOMPATIBILITY[a]

| Histogenetic relationship | Noun | Adjective | Serological counterparts |
|---|---|---|---|
| Graft taken from and returned to a single individual | Autograft | Autogeneic graft<br>Autogenous graft | Autoantigen<br>Autoantibody |
| Graft between twins or within inbred strains | Isograft | Isogeneic graft<br>Isogenic graft<br>Syngeneic graft | Autoantibody sometimes also applied here |
| Graft from parent to an $F_1$ between inbred strains | | Semiisogeneic<br>Semisyngeneic | |
| Graft between unlike individuals or inbred strains | Allograft<br>Homograft[b] | Allogeneic graft | Alloantigen<br>Alloantibody<br>Isoantibody[b] |
| Graft between different species | Xenograft<br>Heterograft | Xenogeneic graft | Xenoantigen<br>Xenoantibody |

[a] Preferred forms given first.
[b] Now rarely used.

and cornea standard procedures in the surgical armory. The same period saw an exponential growth in our understanding of the nature of tissue incompatibility and of the rejection process.

The first person who seems to have realized the importance of autografts was Tagliacozzi, an Italian, who, in 1596, described a technique of plastic surgery used to this day and known as the Tagliacozzi flap. This permitted the replacement of a lost nose with tissue taken from but left temporarily connected to the upper arm. Tagliacozzi's writings show a distrust of allografts that suggests the hard lessons of actual experience (Converse and Casson, 1968). The conviction that allografts are generally unsuccessful grew with the passage of time and the accumulation of medical experience. But allografts continued to be used, and the literature is full of murky reports of apparent but poorly documented successes.

## I. The Development and Value of Inbred Strains

The key to our understanding of the outcome of transplants was the development of inbred strains of laboratory animals. Information did come in from other sources. Experimental embryologists, although they could transplant between amphibian embryos—an observation that anticipated the concept of immunological self-tolerance—found that transplants between similarly paired adults were rejected. Also at the turn of the century, much work was done with tumors, which in some instances could be transplanted serially in noninbred animals. But the reproducibility and genetic uinformity, which only inbred strains can provide, was the requisite for really critical experimentation.

In 1912, and several subsequent years, H. S. Jennings published the first mathematical analyses of the effects of inbreeding. His demonstration that the outcome was genetic uniformity was perhaps the most important single stimulus to a wide variety of inbreeding experiments. Rats were inbred by Helen King and guinea pigs by Sewall Wright, but it was the inbreeding of mice by C. C. Little, and somewhat later by MacDowell, Strong, and others (Staats, 1966) that was to have the most profound effects on transplantation studies and, indeed, on the whole field of mammalian biology.

Between 1891, when Morau succeeded in serially transplanting a tumor of mice, and 1944, when Medawar reported the use of skin grafts in rabbits, transplantation researchers relied almost exclusively on transplantable tumors. The technique of transplantation was easy and rapid, and because tumors were less rigorous in their requirements for genetic compatibility than skin, a variety of experiments was feasible with only partially inbred strains. As a matter of fact, many of the mouse strains of this period in all probability were partly inbred. Wild mice live in small, interbreeding colonies, and the mice maintained by fancier and researcher had doubtless passed through genetic bottlenecks as new colonies were started from pairs or trios. It is not surprising, therefore, to find that an effective study of the genetics of transplantation was reported as early as 1916 by Little and Tyzzer. We shall confine our summary, however, to work of Little and co-workers carried out at The Jackson Laboratory between 1928 and 1935 using transplantable tumors and well-established inbred strains and to some later studies using skin grafts.

## II. Early Genetic Studies

The basic findings of both skin graft and tumor experiments are simply stated. Grafts were uniformly successful if made within inbred strains, and uniformly unsuccessful if made between inbred strains. Grafts made from either parent strain to first generation ($F_1$) hybrids grew in all animals. Most $F_2$ mice resisted parental generation grafts. These observa-

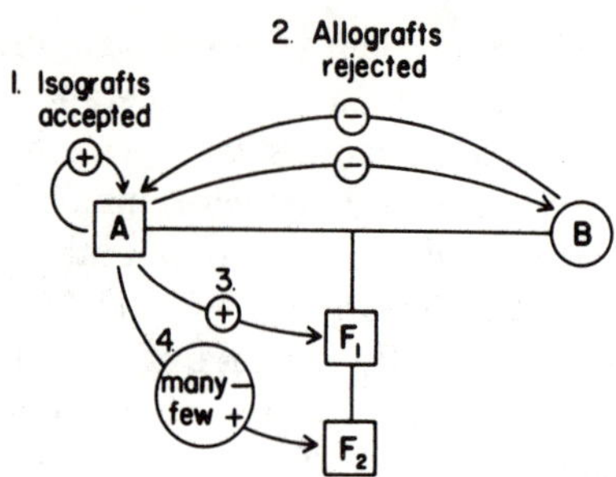


FIG. 1.1. Diagrammatic representation of the four laws of transplantation. A and B are two inbred strains, and $F_1$ and $F_2$ the first and second filial generations produced by crossing them. +, acceptance of grafts; —, rejection of grafts.

tions are summarized diagrammatically in Fig. 1.1. The results in a backcross (BC) derived by mating $F_1$ animals to one of the parent strains depended on which parent was the donor. When the parent used in the backcross was the donor, all BC mice were susceptible. When the opposite parent was the donor, most BC mice were resistant; in fact, even a higher proportion was resistant than in the $F_2$.

The actual results from an experiment by Cloudman (1932), using strains A and DBA, and a strain A tumor were

| | |
|---|---|
| Strain A | All susceptible (mice died) |
| Strain DBA | All resistant (mice survived) |
| $F_1$ | All susceptible |
| $F_2$ | 159 of 219 resistant |
| $F_1 \times A$ | All susceptible |
| $F_1 \times DBA$ | 106 of 116 resistant |

Prehn and Main (1958) carried out a comparable experiment using skin grafts. The strains employed were BALB/c and DBA/2; skin grafts were made from strain BALB/c; the grafts were scored for 200 days. The results were as follows:

| | |
|---|---|
| $F_2$ | 134 of 137 grafts rejected, |
| | 3 grafts survived > 200 days |
| BC to DBA/2 | 102 of 102 grafts rejected, |
| | 0 grafts survived > 200 days |

Most rejections occurred within the first few weeks, but 7 of the grafts to $F_2$ and 3 of the grafts to the backcross, which were ultimately rejected, survived more than 60 days. Parental and $F_1$ mice were not tested; by the time this experiment was performed the outcome was taken for granted. The very high proportion of resistant mice in the $F_2$ and BC generation in this skin graft study, as compared with the somewhat lower proportion in the tumor experiment, is typical. Tumors have a greater capacity than do skin grafts to overcome weak transplantation barriers.

One other recipient–donor combination requires mention. Grafts from $F_2$ or later generations are accepted by $F_1$ animals.

The success of transplants within inbred strains is paralleled by the success of transplants between identical twins, first reported by Bauer in 1927 (Converse and Casson, 1968) and since confirmed in numerous studies.

## III. The Laws of Transplantation

These results with mice and men can be condensed into five laws of transplantation. Laws is perhaps an overemphatic term, since, as we shall point out, there are exceptions, but the statements do have considerable generality. The reader should be reminded that the laws that follow apply to individuals of highly inbred strains or their derivative hybrid generations.

1. Isografts succeed.
2. Allografts fail.
3. Grafts from either parent strain to $F_1$ hybrids succeed.
4. Grafts made from a parent strain to $F_2$ hybrids, or to a backcross animals derived from a cross of $F_1$ individuals to the nondonor parent, succeed in only a fraction, and often a very small fraction, of recipients.
5. Grafts from $F_2$ or BC and subsequent generations made to $F_1$ individuals succeed.

While studies with tumor transplants and two thorough studies with skin transplants (Bailey and Mobraaten, 1969; Barnes and Cooper, 1969) all have given results in accord with law 5, one study in which skin grafts were employed yielded substantial numbers of rejections in the $F_2$ to $F_1$ and $F_3$ to $F_1$ combinations (Hildemann and Cooper, 1967), and a second study yielded a few such rejections (Rogers and Barnes, 1974). While the observations reported in these latter studies are not suspect, there are so many conflicts in the data, including conflicts where identical strain combinations were used, that a detailed summary at this time would appear pointless. Perhaps some unusual environmental factor was at work. It has, for example, been shown that certain virus infections can cause the rejection of normally compatible skin grafts

(Liozner *et al.*, 1970; Holtermann and Majde, 1971; Salaman *et al.*, 1972).

## IV. Histocompatibility Genes

The results summarized in the five laws of transplantation clearly point to a genetic basis for susceptibility and resistance. The success of transplants made between genetically identical individuals, their failure in genetically disparate pairs, the complete dominance of susceptibility, and the segregation of susceptibility and resistance in segregating generations are what might be expected of a trait determined by Mendelizing genes. Certainly more than one gene is involved, since susceptibility in the $F_2$ and backcross does not show simple 3:1 and 1:1 ratios. We may call the postulated genes *histocompatibility* or *H genes* (Snell, 1948).

If there are multiple *H* loci, symbols to designate separate loci are necessary. The standard convention is to append a hyphen and a number, e.g., *H-1*, *H-2*, *H-3*. Alleles are designated by small letter superscripts, e.g., $H\text{-}1^a$, $H\text{-}1^b$, $H\text{-}1^c$.

How do *H* genes act? A first clue is provided by a peculiarity of the ratios. With most inherited traits, a majority of $F_2$ individuals resemble the $F_1$. Here the situation is reversed; the $F_1$ is susceptible, but the majority of $F_2$ and backcross individuals are resistant. Evidently we are not dealing with a simple case of multifactorial inheritance. To get further clues, we turn again to some earlier transplantation studies.

It has been known since early in this century that animals in which a tumor allograft has temporarily grown and then regressed will more rapidly reject a second transplant of the same tumor. Usually the second transplant shows no detectable growth at all (Woglom, 1929). The engendered resistance shows a degree of specificity in that a second transplant may grow normally if it comes from a mouse unrelated to the donor of the first transplant (Andervont, 1933). In 1937, Gorer showed that the regression of a tumor allograft resulted in the development of antibodies demonstrable by their ability to agglutinate the red cells of the tumor donor. In 1944, Medawar duplicated the early tumor work with skin grafts, showing that the second of two successive skin grafts from the same donor was rejected more rapidly than the first. All these results pointed to an immunological basis for graft rejection.

If graft rejection is an immune process, then we have to assume that the histocompatibility gene product is an antigen. More specifically, it is an *alloantigen,* defined as an antigen capable of inciting an immune response when transferred within the species. (The term *isoantigen* was at one time used in this sense, but has been dropped, since the type of antigen we are talking about is detectable by *allografting,* but produces no effect when *isografted.*) It is at once apparent that there is a parallel with the blood groups, since these are families of red cell alloantigens revealed by the development of *alloantibodies,* following blood transfers between genetically different individuals.

If histocompatibility genes resemble, or in some cases perhaps are, blood group genes, we may assume that there is generally a rather simple relationship between gene and antigen. The adage, "one gene, one antigen," has been used in this connection, although more complex relationships are also known. We may also assume that, like the A, B, O blood groups where the A and B substances are both expressed in the heterozygote, the genes are *codominant.* This is not an essential assumption for present purposes, but was already plausible in the light of evidence available at the time of the early genetic studies. The assumption was in fact made by P. A. Gorer (personal communication). We shall present more specific evidence on these points in later chapters, but let us see what follows from these basic assumptions, which could reasonably be made on the basis of the evidence cited here.

We may designate as a *mismatch,* a donor possessing a histocompatibility allele and its derived alloantigen, and a recipient lacking them. The donor in a mismatch is a "have," the recipient a "have not." The histocompatibility differences between a mismatched donor and recipient may of course be multiple as well as single. Our basic postulate then becomes: mismatches lead to graft rejection, or the "have nots" reject the "haves." We shall see later that this postulate has to be qualified. It would be more accurate to say that mismatches lead to a reaction against the graft rather than always to graft rejection. Let us proceed for the time being with the simpler assumption.

From this assumption, it follows that the fraction of mismatches between a parent strain, used as donor, and its $F_2$ and backcross (BC) descendants increases exponentially with the number of *H* loci segregating in the cross. If parent A has the genotype $H^aH^a$ and parent B the genotype $H^bH^b$, then, in an $F_2$ challenged with a strain A ($H^aH^a$) graft, we may expect 1 $H^aH^a$ (susceptible), 2 $H^aH^b$ (susceptible), 1 $H^bH^b$ (resistant). The ratio of susceptible to resistant is 3:1. And in the backcross to strain B, we expect 1 $H^aH^b$ (susceptible), 1 $H^bH^b$ (resistant). The ratio of susceptible to resistant is 1:1.

If multiple *H* loci are segregating in a cross, a mismatch at any one locus can cause rejection. The chance of mismatch then increases with

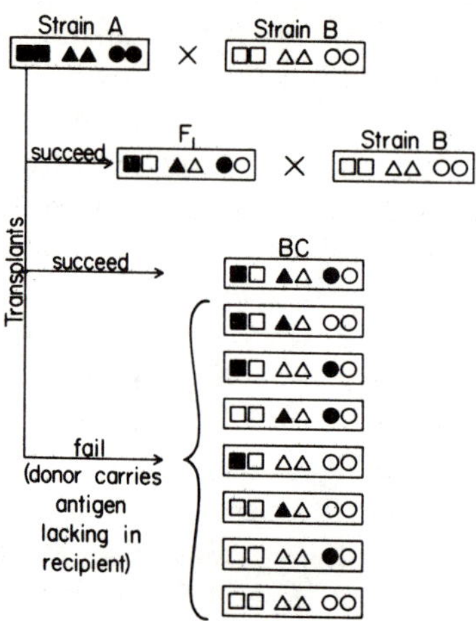


FIG. 1.2. Diagram showing the outcome of transplants made from strain A to $F_1$ and backcross generations derived from an A × B cross, where A and B differ one from the other at three histocompatibility loci.

the number of loci. The situation for a backcross involving a 3-locus difference is shown diagrammatically in Fig. 1.2. It will be seen that 1 out of 8 BC animals is matched with the strain A parent and hence is expected to accept a strain A graft, and 7 out of 8 animals are mismatched and hence are presumed rejectors. To generalize, if there is a difference at $n$ loci between the parent strain in a cross, the expected number of matches between parent and $F_2$ will be $(\frac{3}{4})^n$, and the expected number of mismatches $1-(\frac{3}{4})^n$. In the BC generation the figures will be $(\frac{1}{2})^n$ and $1-(\frac{1}{2})^n$, respectively. Thus the proportion of matches will decrease and the proportion of mismatches increase as the number of *H* locus differences in a cross goes up. The high proportion of rejectors actually observed in $F_2$ and BC generations is thereby explained simply by postulating the existence of many *H* loci.

We may then ask, how many histocompatibility loci are there? A postulate of four loci fits the Cloudman experiment in which a transplantable tumor was used. [Expected susceptible in $F_2 = (\frac{3}{4})^4 = 31.6\%$; observed = 27.4%. Expected susceptible in BC $= (\frac{1}{2})^4 = 6.2\%$; observed = 8.6%]. Some tests with tumors have led to estimates as high as nine loci. The experiment by Prehn and Main, performed with skin grafts, is fitted by a postulate of 13 loci. Other comparable experiments have indicated a slightly higher number. These are probably underestimates. Thus some loci probably would not segregate in any given cross, and linked loci would tend to appear as a single locus. In Chapter 3 we shall return to this subject again, with more data at our disposal.

## REFERENCES


Andervont, H. B. 1933. The specificity of immunity elicited by mouse sarcoma 180. *U S Public Health Rep* **48**:1472–1476.

Bailey, D. W., and L. E. Mobraaten. 1969. Histocompatibility of skin grafts from mice of $F_1$, $F_2$, and $F_3$ generations on $F_1$ generation hosts. *Transplantation* **7**:567–569.

Barnes, A. D., and B. T. Cooper. 1969. The genetic control of histocompatibility isoantigens. *Immunology* **17**:429–435.

Cloudman, A. M. 1932. A comparative study of transplantability of eight mammary gland tumors arising in inbred mice. *Am J Cancer* **16**:568–630.

Converse, J. M., and P. R. Casson. 1968. The historical background of transplantation. Pages 1–10 *in* F. T. Rapaport and J. Dausset, eds. Human transplantation. Grune & Stratton, New York.

Gorer, P. A. 1937. The genetic and antigenic basis of tumour transplantation. *J Pathol Bacteriol* **44**:691–697.

Hildemann, W. H., and E. L. Cooper. 1967. Transplantation genetics: Unexpected histoincompatibility associated with skin grafts from $F_2$ and $F_3$ hybrid donors to $F_1$ hybrid recipients. *Transplantation* **5**:707–720.

Holtermann, O. A., and J. A. Majde. 1971. An apparent histoincompatibility between mice chronically infected with lymphocytic choriomeningitis virus and their uninfected syngeneic counterparts. *Transplantation* **11**:20–29.

Liozner, A. L., G. J. Svet-Moldavasky, and D. M. Mkheidze. 1970. Tumor-induced skin heterogenization. III. Immunologic and immunogenetic mechanisms. *J Natl Cancer Inst* **45**:485–494.

Little, C. C., and E. E. Tyzzer. 1916. Further studies on inheritance of susceptibility to a transplantable tumor of Japanese waltzing mice. *J Med Res* **33**:393–425.

Medawar, P. B. 1944. The behavior and fate of skin autografts and skin homografts in rabbits. *J Anat* **78**:176–200.

Morau, H. 1891. Inoculation en série d'une tumeur épithéliale de la souris blanche. *C R Soc Biol (Paris)* **3**:289–290.

Prehn, R. T., and J. M. Main. 1958. Number of mouse histocompatibility genes involved in skin grafting from strain BALB/cAn to strain DBA/2. *J Natl Cancer Inst* **20**:207–209.

Rogers, K., and A. D. Barnes. 1974. A further study on the genetic rules of transplantation in the mouse. *Transplantation* **17**:435–436.

Salaman, M. H., N. Wedderburn, L. W. Poulter, and B. N. Dracott. 1972. Development of a new skin antigen and of tolerance to this antigen in mice infected with a lymphomagenic virus. *Transplantation* **14**:96–105.

Snell, G. D. 1948. Methods for the study of histocompatibility genes. *J Genet* **49**:87–108.

Staats, J. 1966. The laboratory mouse. Pages 1–9 *in* E. L. Green, ed. The biology of the laboratory mouse. McGraw-Hill, New York.

Woglom, L. W. 1929. Immunity to transplantable tumors. *Cancer Rev* **4**:129–214.

CHAPTER 2

# HISTOGENETIC METHODS



The evidence presented in Chapter 1 indicates that there are a dozen or more histocompatibility loci but does not in any way distinguish one locus from another. The loci certainly differ in their contribution to the economy of the cell, but the early transplantation studies were incompetent to reveal these differences. The loci, either alone or cumulatively, were capable, when mismatched, of causing graft rejection, and this was all we knew about them. Thus there was no basis, in these studies, for assigning individual symbols.

The methods of gene manipulation and transplantation, which permit identification of individual *H* loci, have been called *histogenetic methods*. We shall describe these methods in this chapter. Our purpose is to provide a sufficient background to allow the reader to understand experiments described subsequently. The reader interested in technical details should pursue the references listed at the end of this chapter.

## I. Types of Transplants Employed

Both transplantable tumors and normal tissues, especially skin, have been used as indicators of histoincompatibility. Since tumors are now rarely used in transplantation studies, we will omit any discussion of tumor transplant methods; information will be found in Snell (1953a). Billingham and Medawar (1951) have described a method of body skin grafting in mice that has been widely used. A graft, usually about 0.5 to 1.0 $cm^2$ (with the hair direction reversed), is secured with a plaster bandage until healing occurs. In interstrain grafts, rejection, indicated by loss of hair and sloughing, usually occurs in 10–12 days. More recently Bailey and Usama (1960) have described a method of tail skin grafting. Small slices of skin are removed from the tail with a scalpel, and placed, with hair direction reversed, on a similarly prepared bed. Up to 16 grafts can be placed on one tail. The grafts are protected initially by inserting the tail in glass tubing, held in place with tape. No bandage is necessary. The method of grafting is rapid, but scoring requires a little more time and skill than scoring body skin grafts. A variety of other normal tissue has been used. The continued survival of ovarian transplants in ovariectomized mice can be monitored by taking vaginal smears (Stevens, 1957; Krohn, 1965). Another tissue that has been used is heart muscle, transplanted to the ear. Survival can be determined by electrical recording of muscular contractions (Huff *et al.*, 1968). A feasible method of kidney transplantation has been developed in the rat (White and Hildemann, 1968). Some unique histocompatibility phenomena have been studied by Cudkowicz (1965) using marrow transplants in irradiated recipients; survival is demonstrated by the uptake of a radioactive label.

## II. Production of Congenic Resistant Strains

The genetic requirement for the identification of individual histocompatibility genes is the isolation of individual genes from a potpourri of loci, presumably functionally quite different but, as tested by histocompatibility, with essentially identical phenotypes. The method devised was the production of congenic resistant strains of mice (Snell, 1948).

A *congenic strain* is defined as a strain identical or almost identical with an inbred partner strain except for the presence of a foreign chromosome segment introduced by appropriate crosses from an unrelated stock. If the introduced chromosome segment carries a foreign histocompatibility gene, the strain is a *congenic resistant* or *CR strain* because grafts exchanged between it and the inbred partner will be resisted. A distinction is made between *congenic strains* and *coisogenic strains* (a term borrowed from *Drosophila* geneticists). The latter, in transplantation usage, are strains *identical* with an inbred partner except for a difference at a single locus. True coisogenic strains can arise only by mutation. However, congenic strains become approximately closer to the coisogenic state as the number of backcrosses or other matings used to introduce the foreign gene is increased.

The method originally employed for the production of CR strains was based on the use of transplantable tumors. This imposed the limitation that transplants could be made only from the inbred parent line in which a tumor was regularly carried, and not from mice of later, segregating generations. To recover resistant mice following an outcross, a "cross–intercross" system of matings had to be used (Green, 1966). The introduction by Bailey and Usama (1960) of the tail skin grafting technique removed this limitation, since any mouse could be used as a graft donor. This permitted the use of a backcross method that substantially reduced the number of generations required to produce adequate coisogenicity. We shall confine our discussion to the Bailey system.

The succession of matings and skin grafts used in the Bailey backcross system is shown in Fig. 2.1. We shall refer to the strain to which the backcrosses are made and which thereby becomes the inbred partner of the CR strain (strain A in the figure) as the *first parent,* and the strain from which the *H* gene is extracted (strain B in the figure) as the *second parent.* Since the two strains can be expected to differ by at least a dozen *H* loci, some alleles of the second parent should persist through several backcrosses to the first parent. It is therefore unnecessary to start testing for introduced *H* alleles until the third or fourth backcross generations. The third and fourth backcross (BC) generations we shall designate N4 and N5, where N1 corresponds to $F_1$ or the first filial generation and N2 to BC1 or the first backcross generation. (This is the standard usage at The Jackson Laboratory, but we should note that some authors equate N1 with BC1.) The test then consists of a graft from N4 or N5 mice to strain A. If an *H* allele foreign to strain A is still present, the graft will be resisted. Only incompatible donors are mated again to strain A; mice whose grafts are accepted are discarded. This process is repeated for a number of backcross generations, usually not less than 10. Since each backcross reduces the remaining strain B genes by half, only $(\frac{1}{2})^9$ of the genes of strain B should remain by N10, except for genes in the *H*-labeled chromosome segment. At this point brother–sister matings of tested mice are instituted. To pick out from N10F1, animals homozygous for the introduced $H^b$ allele, grafts

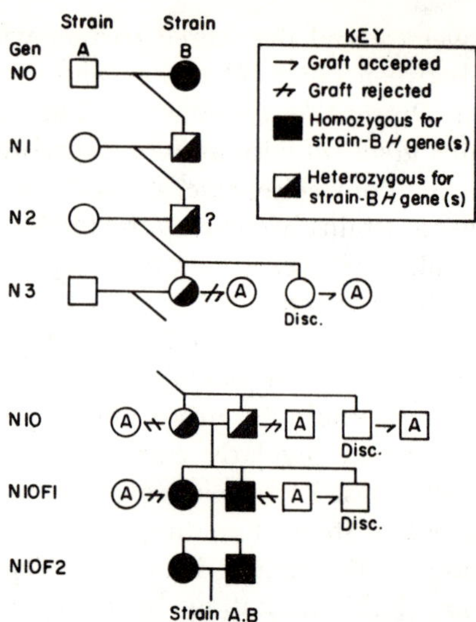


FIG. 2.1. System of crosses and skin transplants used for the production of congenic resistant lines in mice. N generations are generations derived from a mating to strain A; F generations are generations derived from brother × sister matings. Skin grafting may be started at N4 or N5 rather than at N3 as indicated in the figure. The choice of sexes indicated in the diagram will avoid the introduction of a Y chromosome from strain B, but many alternatives are possible. The end result of the procedures indicated is the production of a strain, A.B, identical with strain A except for the presence of an introduced strain B chromosome segment bearing a histocompatibility gene or genes foreign to strain A.

are made in the reverse direction, from strain A instead of to strain A. Only $H^bH^b$ mice, and not those of genotypes $H^aH^b$ or $H^aH^a$, will reject the strain A ($H^aH^a$) grafts. Rejectors are mated brother × sister, establishing a homozygous $H^bH^b$ line. Such a line, from an initial A × B cross, is given the designation A.B. The locus by which A and A.B differ and to which selection was applied in producing A.B is called the *defining locus* for this strain pair. Other loci introduced because of their linkage with the defining locus are called *passenger loci.*

In producing CR lines, it has been the usual practice to derive more than one line from any one initial cross. These lines are distinguished by appending a number, or a number and letter, in parentheses to the strain symbol. Also different crosses may be used. Thus there may be lines A.B(1), A.B(2), A.B(3), A.C(1), A.C(2), B.C(1), etc. If the defining locus of one of the lines, for example A.B(2), is shown to be $H\text{-}x$, with A having the allele $H\text{-}x^a$ and A.B(2) the allele $H\text{-}x^b$, then A.B(2) may be given the more informative designation A.B-$H\text{-}x^b$.

When several such lines are established, the information, and usually the only information, immediately at hand concerning them is that they are histoincompatible with their inbred partner. In some instances, however, it may have become apparent that some lines show rapid rejection of grafts exchanged with the inbred partner, and some lines show delayed rejection. Infrequently, a line may have received from the second parent strain a coat color gene, or a gene producing some other visible distinction from the congenic parent, suggesting a linkage of the visible marker and the introduced *H* gene. But while such information suggests that different *H* genes have been introduced into different CR lines, it does not prove it. Although *H* genes have been isolated, they still have not been identified. There are several methods by which such identification can be achieved. We now turn to a consideration of these methods.

## III. Analysis of Congenic Resistant Strains

### A. Linkage with Marker Genes

In the production of CR strains, the introduced *H* gene of necessity carries with it a foreign chromosome segment, probably many genes in length. Some, but not all, of the genes in the segment will be, like the *H* gene, foreign to the inbred partner. When any of these passenger genes are at known loci, they can be used as *marker genes* to aid in the identification of the *H* gene. Such markers are particularly convenient if they produce a visible effect, and they are particularly useful if their place on the linkage map is known. Any apparent association of an *H* gene with a marker requires checking, since it may be fortuitous owing to the presence of a contaminant chromosome segment. But once an association with a marker, already located, is proved, the linked *H* gene acquires an important index of individual identity. It itself can be placed on the linkage map, and it must be different from any other locus differently placed.

A variant of this linkage method has been exploited successfully by Bailey. Numerous lines that are congenic for visible marker genes have been produced by introducing the marker from one strain onto the genetic background of another. When the marker is dominant, this can be done by simple backcrossing. If the marker locus is linked to a histocompatibility locus, the *H* allele of the second parent may be introduced along with its marker. The introduced *H* gene can then be demonstrated simply by exchanging grafts between members of the congenic pair.

If grafts are rejected and if further tests confirm linkage with the marker, the existence of an *H* locus in the marked chromosome is established. Such a locus linked, for example, with the gene *go* may provisionally be designated *H*(*go*).

## B. Grafts between Congenic Resistant Strains

If two CR strains, A.B(1) and A.B(2), are derived from the same initial A $\times$ B cross, the identity or nonidentity of the introduced *H* gene can be determined by the simple expedient of grafting between them. Thus if strain A is $H\text{-}1^a$ (homozygous) and both A.B(1) and A.B(2) are $\text{H-1}^b$, grafts made between lines 1 and 2 will be accepted. But if A is $H\text{-}1^a$ $H\text{-}2^a$, A.B(1) is $H\text{-}1^b$ $H\text{-}2^a$, and A.B(2) is $H\text{-}1^a$ $H\text{-}2^b$, grafts between 1 and 2 will be rejected. The nonidentity of the loci by which the lines differ from A is established.

We refer to interstrain grafting as a simple expedient, and in theory it is; however where a substantial number of CR lines has been produced, the test can run to unmanageable proportions. Thus if there are 30 CR lines, grafts can be exchanged in $(30 \times 29)/2 = 435$ combinations. We shall find later that there is a time-saving alternative.

There are also other problems with the direct graft interchange method. In the case of two CR lines, A.B and A.C, derived from two different strains crossed to the same first parent, it may not work. In this situation there are three possibilities. If the grafts grow, we have firm evidence that A.B and A.C are identical. However failure to grow may mean either that A.B and A.C differ at different loci, or that they differ by different alleles at the same locus (e.g., A is $H\text{-}1^a$, A.B is $H\text{-}1^b$, and A.C is $H\text{-}1^c$). A negative outcome is therefore ambiguous. Some more discriminating method is necessary. The method appropriate for dealing with this situation is known as the $F_1$ or complementation test.

## C. The $F_1$ Test

The $F_1$ test involves three strains, a CR pair, A and A.B, differing at locus *H-x*, and an unknown, U. The test consists of a graft from A to an $(\text{A.B} \times \text{U})F_1$, or the reciprocal A.B to an $(\text{A} \times \text{U})F_1$. The graft constitutes a test for the *H-x* allele of U. If an A to (A.B $\times$ U) graft grows, it means that U shares with A the $H\text{-}x^a$ allele and can therefore complement A.B. If the graft does not grow, it means that U lacks the $H\text{-}x^a$ allele and cannot complement A.B.

To make this more explicit in terms of the genotypes of the three strains, we may write

$$\mathrm{A} = \frac{A\ H\text{-}x^a}{A\ H\text{-}x^a} \qquad \mathrm{A.B} = \frac{A\ H\text{-}x^b}{A\ H\text{-}x^b} \qquad U = \frac{U\ H\text{-}x^x}{U\ H\text{-}x^x}$$

where $A$ is the total genetic background of strain A other than the $H$-$x$ locus, and $U$ the total genetic background of strain U other than the $H$-$x$ locus. Because A and A.B are congenic, $A$ must also represent the genetic background of A.B. The test may then be written

$$\mathrm{A} \rightarrow (\mathrm{A.B} \times \mathrm{U})$$

or

$$\frac{A\ H\text{-}x^a}{A\ H\text{-}x^a} \rightarrow \frac{A\ H\text{-}x^b}{U\ H\text{-}x^x}$$

Because the common genetic background of A is represented in both recipient and donor, the graft will grow so far as background genes are concerned. Growth is contingent only on $H$-$x$. If $H$-$x^x$ = $H$-$x^a$, U supplies the missing element, and the graft is accepted. If $H$-$x^x$ = $H$-$x^b$ or $H$-$x^c$, U fails to provide the missing element, and the graft is rejected. The test thus types for $H$-$x^a$.

If the test is reversed, A.B → (A × U), it types U for $H$-$x^b$.

There is one necessary qualification to these statements. It is conceivable that two alleles, $H$-$x^b$ and $H$-$x^x$, will complement each other in such fashion that an $H$-$x^a$/$H$-$x^a$ graft is accepted by the hybrid $H$-$x^b$/$H$-$x^x$. What appeared to be a case of this sort was discovered early in the history of $H$-$2$. We now know, however, that $H$-$2$ is not one locus, but two and that the apparent exception involved recombinants and was not really an exception at all. No true exception is known, but we cannot say that one is not possible. This qualification should therefore be borne in mind in interpreting the $F_1$ test.

The $F_1$ test may, therefore, be used, with one possible but unlikely qualification, to type any strain for the two $H$ alleles by which the two members of any CR pair differ one from the other. It says that the unknown has or has not the *a* allele and has or has not the *b* allele. If the unknown has neither *a* nor *b*, it must have a third allele, *c*.

The application of the $F_1$ test to the typing of CR strains is simplest and most conclusive when the unknown and the test CR pair are on the same genetic background. This situation is illustrated in Fig. 2.2. If the graft grows, it proves that the two CR lines used in the test

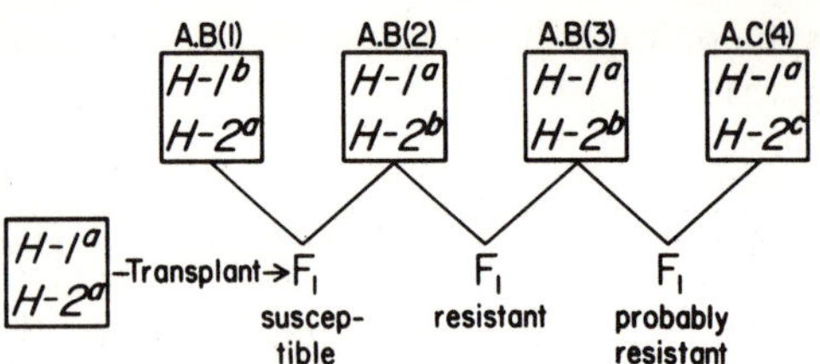


FIG. 2.2. Diagram illustrating the use of $F_1$ tests to determine the histocompatibility genotypes of four strains congenic with strain A.

differ from their common inbred partner at *different H* loci. The existence of two distinct loci is established, and we can assign corresponding symbols, e.g., *H-1* and *H-2*.

The situation is more complicated and may be less conclusive if the test is applied to congenic pairs derived from different parent strains, e.g., A, A.B, C, and C.D. Since in practice most CR strains have been put on a common background (strains C57BL/6 and C57BL/10), we need not pursue this particular case further.

## D. Recombinant Inbred Strains

*Recombinant inbred* (*RI*) *strains* are strains produced by crossing two inbred strains and inbreeding, brother × sister, multiple derivative lines (Bailey, 1971). The lines are separated at $F_2$, the first segregating generation, and inbreeding is continued for at least 20 generations. The result of this procedure, applied to an initial A × B cross, is the production of a group of lines, AXBA, AXBB, AXBC, etc., in which the segregating alleles of the two parent strains are fixed in a variety of patterns (Fig. 2.3). Any one line, AXBA, must have either the strain A allele or the strain B allele at any one segregating locus. A second line, AXBB, must likewise be fixed for the A or B allele. A *strain distribution pattern* is thus established, e.g., AABABBB for locus *x* as fixed in seven separate lines. An independent locus will in all probability have a different pattern, e.g., BAABBAA. However, a closely linked locus is likely to have a similar or identical pattern, e.g., BABABBB. For a single locus with two phenotypic expressions, the two expressions must show identical patterns.

A group of recombinant inbred strains can thus be thought of as a "frozen" segregated generation. Each segregant, represented by its own individual RI line, can be made available in quantity, and thus can be subjected to a diversity of tests over an extended period of time. Unlike backcross or $F_2$ individuals, each segregant line is *homozy-*

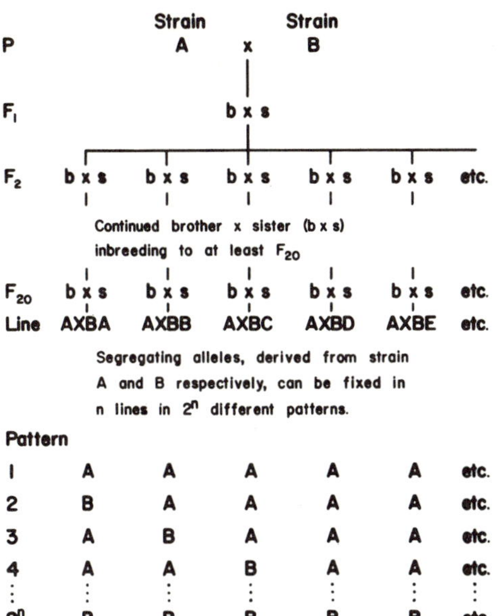


FIG. 2.3. Diagram illustrating the production of recombinant inbred strains from an initial cross between strains A and B and the way in which the alleles of loci at which A and B differ become fixed in a variety of patterns.

*gous* for one or the other allele at each segregating locus. There are no heterozygotes. This can be an important advantage when typing for a locus where the phenotypes of homozygote and heterozygote overlap. Thus over a period of time a group of RI strains can be typed for many loci, and a corresponding number of locus patterns established. If there are $n$ lines, $2^n$ patterns are possible. Identity or similarity of patterns establishes a presumption of linkage between the corresponding loci. Because recombination can occur not only in $F_2$ but also in subsequent generations for as long as either of two loci is segregating, recombination occurs more easily and linkage is less easily proved than in an $F_2$ or backcross. But if there are enough RI lines, close similarity of pattern can constitute virtual proof of linkage. And for proving nonidentity of loci, the increased chance or recombination is an advantage.

Recombinant inbred lines are particularly effective in the analysis of congenic resistant lines. They provide an immediate answer to the question, is the locus by which A.B(1) differs from A the same as the locus by which A.B(2) differs from A? Different patterns prove nonidentity, identical patterns establish a strong presumption of identity. However, to work in all instances, RI lines and CR lines should come from the same initial cross, so that the same loci and same alleles have segregated. Thus to test CR lines A.B(1), A.B(2), A.B(3), etc., AXB RI lines should be used.

The RI strain distribution of the defining locus of any CR line is provided by use of the $F_1$ test. The RI lines are crossed with A.B(1), A.B(2), etc., and the $F_1$ grafted with strain A skin. If, in the test with AXBA $\times$ A.B(1), the graft takes, AXBA is typed as having the A allele at the A.B(1) defining locus. If the graft is rejected, AXBA is typed as having the B allele. Repetition of the test with all AXB lines gives a strain distribution pattern for the A.B(1) defining locus.

The test is then repeated with A.B(2). If a different strain distribution pattern emerges, the defining locus of A.B(2) must be distinct from that of A.B(1). If the two lines give the same distribution pattern, they must have the same defining locus, barring the unlikely eventuality of identical patterns occurring by chance.

The use of recombinant inbred strains to type CR strains can involve an extensive crossing and grafting program. However, where there is a large battery of CR lines to type, it can be cheaper than the direct graft interchange method. It has the added advantage that it can provide evidence of linkage, either between different *H* loci or between *H* loci and any other loci for which there is an RI line strain distribution pattern.

## IV. The Use of Immunization

At an early stage in the production of congenic resistant lines, with transplantable tumors as the test agent, it became apparent that lines were being lost because the tumors were overriding some of the weaker histocompatibility barriers. Since it was already well established that resistance to a tumor could be increased by prior immunization, e.g., by giving the same tumor at a low dose level, the use of some sort of immunization procedure seemed indicated. Attempts to immunize with the tumor used for the final challenge resulted in complications, probably, as we now know, because immunity to tumor-specific antigens as well as to alloantigens was induced. A method of immunizing with normal tissues of the transplant donor strain was therefore developed. This method has less applicability when skin or other normal tissue grafts rather than tumors are used as the test agent, but can in some circumstances substantially increase the sensitivity even of skin graft histocompatibility typing.

The following relatively simple procedure was found to give effective immunization. A cell suspension of thymus, preferably from weanling mice, is prepared in the cytosieve* (Snell, 1953b) and injected intraperitoneally, $4 \times 10^6$ cells per mouse. The use of one weanling donor per 50 recipients has been found to give approximately this dose level, and cell counts are usually not necessary. One injection is often sufficient, but three injections at weekly intervals are more effective. The test graft is given 7 to 14 days after the last injection, with 8 to 10 days probably being the optimum.

## REFERENCES

Bailey, D. W. 1971. Recombinant-inbred strains. An aid to finding identity, linkage, and function of histocompatibility and other genes. *Transplantation* **11**:325–327.

Bailey, D. W., and B. Usama. 1960. A rapid method of grafting skin on tails of mice. *Transplant Bull* **7**:424–425.

Billingham, R. E., and P. B. Medawar. 1951. A technique of free skin grafting in mammals. *J Exp Biol* **28**:385–402.

Cudkowicz, G. 1965. The immunogenetic basis of hybrid resistance to parental marrow grafts. Pages 37–56 *in* J. Palm ed. Isoantigens and cell interactions. Wistar Institute Press, Philadelphia, Pennsylvania.

Green, E. L. 1966. Breeding systems. Pages 11–22 *in* E. L. Green, ed. Biology of the laboratory mouse. McGraw-Hill, New York.

Huff, R. W., A. G. Liebelt, and R. A. Liebelt. 1968. Implantation of allogeneic heart grafts in inbred mice. *Cardiovasc Res Cent Bull* **6**:127–139.

Krohn, P. L. 1965. Transplantation of endocrine organs, with special reference to the ovary. *Br Med Bull* **21**:157–161.

Snell, G. D. 1948. Methods for the study of histocompatibility genes. *J Genet* **49**:87–108.

Snell, G. D. 1953a. Transplantable tumors. Pages 338–391 *in* F. Homburger and H. Fishman, eds. The physiopathology of cancer. Harper (Hoeber), New York.

Snell, G. D. 1953b. A cytosieve permitting sterile preparation of suspensions of tumor cells for transplantation. *J Natl Cancer Inst* **13**:1511–1515.

Stevens, L. C. 1957. A modification of Robertson's technique of homoiotropic ovarian transplantation in mice. *Transplant Bull* **4**:106–107.

White, E., and W. H. Hildemann. 1968. Allografts in genetically defined rats: Difference in survival between kidney and skin. *Science* **162**:1293–1295.

* Cytosieves can be purchased from Anderson Glass Company, Old Turnpike Road, Fitzwilliam, New Hampshire.

CHAPTER 3

# THE NUMBER AND DIVERSITY OF HISTOCOMPATIBILITY LOCI

## I. The Production of CR Lines

Over 200 congenic resistant (CR) lines have been produced in mice and analyzed sufficiently to determine the histocompatibility locus and the histocompatibility allele by which each differs from its inbred partner. Most of these lines are still in existence. At present there is no substitute for CR lines in *H* gene analysis. Hence, since this genetic resource has not been duplicated in any other species, the mouse holds an altogether unique position in histocompatibility studies. For reviews, see Snell and Stimpfling (1966), Lengerová (1969), and Graff and Bailey (1973).

The congenic resistant (CR) strains of mice that have been produced for the study of histocompatibility genes may be divided into five groups.

1. A first group of lines was produced using transplantable tumors as the agent for selecting resistant animals (Snell, 1958). Numerous lines were lost because the tumors overrode the weak resistance engendered by some of the isolated *H* genes, but 38 lines were carried far enough for at least partial analysis. Thirty of these 38 turned out to differ from their inbred partner at a single locus, *H-2*. This locus had already been identified by Gorer by serological methods. The concentration of lines with this one difference was the first clue to the unique role played by *H-2* in transplantation phenomena. *H-2* is dealt with in detail in Chapter 6 where we shall see that it is actually a complex of linked loci with similar or interrelated effects. The two major histocompatibility loci in this complex are designated *H-2K* and *H-2D*.

2. A second group of 20 CR lines was produced using transplantable leukemias, which had been found to be more discriminating in their histocompatibility requirements than most other tumors, and prior immunization of the recipients with normal donor tissue (Snell and Bunker, 1965). These lines were all on a C57BL/10Sn (B10)* back-

* Since we shall make frequent reference to a number of specific inbred strains of mice, it may be helpful to the reader if we briefly describe the principles of strain nomenclature. For a detailed discussion the reader should consult Staats (1968). The symbol consists of two parts, a strain symbol and a substrain symbol, separated by a slant line. The strain symbol is typically a capital letter or letters, but may be or include a number. The substrain symbol always includes a capital letter or a capital and small letters, which are abbreviations for the name of the laboratory or person maintaining the stock (e.g., J for The Jackson Laboratory, Sn for Snell, By for Bailey). This may be preceded by a number or small letter indicative of a major subline difference. Where widely used strains have long symbols, standard abbreviations have been assigned, e.g., B10 for C57BL/10, B6 for C57BL/6, C for BALB/c).

ground, and all the second parents were chosen so as to have the same *H-2* allele as the B10 first parent, namely, *H-2*$^b$. Thus only non-*H-2* alleles could be isolated.

3. A third group of lines was established from the initial cross C57BL/6By × BALB/c, using skin grafts as the test agent for histoincompatibility (Bailey, 1971, 1975).

4. A fourth group of CR lines was produced by introducing visible or otherwise easily demonstrable marker genes, to which an *H* gene was linked, onto an inbred background. Such introduction is particularly easy if the marker gene is dominant, permitting introduction simply by repeated backcrossing without any special tests. In some cases the linkage of an *H* gene with the marker was known or suspected; in other cases it was a lucky accident. The background strain was usually B6 or B10.

5. A large family of CR lines has been produced specifically for the analysis of the *H-2* complex. The introduced *H* gene has usually been a recombinant between the two ends of *H-2*.

Klein (1973) has published a list of existing CR lines. This includes 104 lines which differ from their inbred partner at *H-2*, and 88 lines which differ at various non-*H-2* loci, or in a few cases at loci whose identity is undetermined. We shall be concerned in this chapter only with the non-*H-2* lines and with the histocompatibility loci whose identity they have served to establish.

## II. Histocompatibility Genes Revealed by CR Lines

### A. Identification by Linkage

In the first established group of CR lines, three lines were found to differ from their inbred partner by a locus producing a visible affect (Snell, 1958). One line, C3H.K, was albino, whereas its partner, C3H, has the agouti coat of the wild mouse. A second line, A.CA, had inherited the gene *Fu,* causing a kinky tail, from its CA ancestor; strain A has a straight tail. A third line, B10.LP, was agouti like the LP strain, whereas its partner, B10, is black. These relations are shown in Fig. 3.1. Appropriate tests in segregating generations showed that the histoincompatibility in each line accompanied the visible effect, proving linkage of the *H* gene and the marker gene. Since the albinism locus (*c*) is in chromosome 7, fused tail (*Fu*) in 17, and agouti (*A*) in 2, the linked *H* genes must be in distinct linkage groups and hence independent. This evidence,

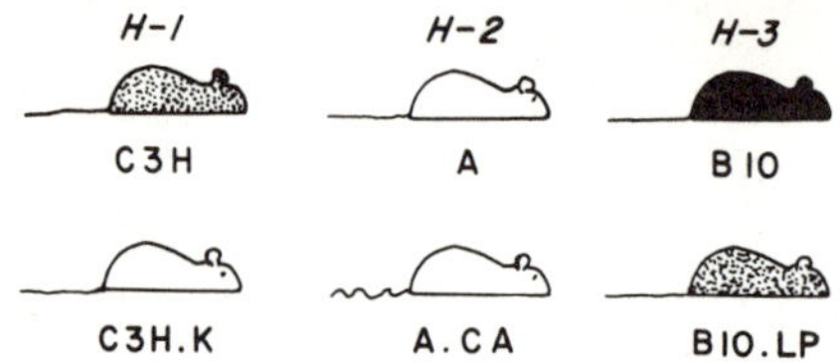


Fig. 3.1. Diagram illustrating the identification of histocompatibility loci through the introduction into congenic resistant lines of chromosome segments bearing markers as well as histocompatibility loci. Thus *H-1* was identified through the introduction into C3H.K of the gene for albinism, *H-2* through the introduction into A.CA of fused tail, and *H-3* through the introduction into B10.LP of agouti.

therefore, made it immediately possible to assign alleles $H\text{-}1^a$ and $H\text{-}1^b$ to C3H and C3H.K, respectively, $H\text{-}2^a$ and $H\text{-}2^f$ to A and A.CA, respectively, and $H\text{-}3^a$ and $H\text{-}3^b$ to B10 and B10.LP, respectively. As it happened, the *H-2* locus and its linkage with *Fu* was already known, but *H-1* and *H-3* were identified for the first time.

Among the second group of CR lines was one in which the linked genes albinism (*c*) and pink-eyed dilution (*p*) were introduced from strain 129 onto a B10 background. As expected, because of the already established linkage of *c* and *H-1*, this B10.129 line showed an *H-1* difference from B10. But when *c* and *p* were separated by crossing over, giving a B10.129-*c* and a B10.129-*p* line, both lines were found to be resistant to B10 grafts. The *H-1* incompatibility accompanied *c;* the B10.129-*p* line was shown by $F_1$ tests to have a previously unidentified incompatibility. The symbol *H-4* was assigned (Snell and Stevens, 1961). Crossover studies showed about 8% recombination between *c* and *H-1*, but failed to produce a separation between *p* and *H-4*. This might suggest that pink-eyed dilution itself was responsible for the histoincompatibility. However, two mutants to *p* were tested and found to be histocompatible with the line in which they originated (G. D. Snell and T. S. Hauschka, unpublished data).

By similar tests it was shown that B10.LP differs from B10 not only by *H-3*, but also by a second locus, *H-13*, both linked to agouti. The B6 × C cross, used by Bailey (1971, 1975) to produce a group of B6.C congenic resistant lines, segregated for a number of marker genes that turned out to be linked with histocompatibility loci (Bailey, 1975, and personal communication). Among the markers were the coat color genes *b* and *c*. Some of the B6.C lines carried the strain C alleles at the *b* and *c* loci. As expected, the histoincompatibility in the *c* or albino line was due to the introduction of an *H-1* allele. The *b* or brown line, following repeated backcrosses to B6, split into two lines, one brown and the other black, and both histoincompatible not only with B6 but with each other. These and other tests served to identify two loci, *H-15* and *H-16*, both like *b*, on chromosome 4. At least two other *H* loci have been located, by other methods, on this chromosome, and there are probably others. Additional linkages enabled Bailey to identify and map several other loci.

Numerous congenic lines have been produced by introducing visible marker genes onto a C57BL/6 background. Bailey has tested these by exchanged skin grafts and found a high proportion of histoincompatibilities. In the lines derived by minimum backcrossing, some of the histoincompatibilities were not linked to the marker. Other histoincompatibilities were very weak. But the lines have served to identify four new *H* loci linked, respectively, with *ln* in chromosome 1, *go* in chromosome 5, *js* on chromosome 11, and *ep* in chromosome 19; these have been given the provisional symbols *H*(*ln*), *H*(*go*), *H*(*js*), and *H*(*ep*), respectively.

Flaherty and Bennett (1973) and Flaherty and Wachtel (1975), using a quite different group of congenic strains, have reported evidence for seven additional *H* loci linked to marker genes. The markers employed in their study were *Ly-1, Ly-2, Ly-3, Tla,* and *Ea-2.* The first four of these determine alloantigens demonstrable, by appropriate alloantisera, on the surface of lymphocytes. Since *Ly-2* and *Ly-3* show complete linkage, they may represent allelic forms of one locus. *Tla* is closely linked to *H-2*. *Ea-2* determines an erythrocyte alloantigen. We will describe these loci in detail in Chapter 5.

Of the seven passenger *H* loci that Flaherty and co-workers have reported, only two have been separated from the defining locus in crossover experiments. These two are *H-32*, linked to *Tla,* and *H*(*Ly-2-N8*), linked to *Ly-2*. In a backcross, *H-32* and *Tla* showed 2.8% recombination. With respect to *H-2*, the order of the loci is *H-2–Tla–H-32*. *H*(*Ly-2-N8*) was separated from $Ly\text{-}2^a$ during repeated backcrosses to strain B6 at some point between generations N8 and N16. There is no information as to recombination percent.

The other five passenger *H* loci reported by Flaherty and co-workers have been designated *H-31*, *H*(*Ly-2-N16*), *H*(*Ly-1*), *H*(*Ly-2*, *Ly-3*), and *H*(*Ea-2*). The evidence that each of these is indeed a distinct passenger *H* locus and not a manifestation of the defining, serologically demonstrated locus of the respective congenic lines is indirect in each case. The following sorts of evidence are cited: (1) The histocompatibility effect and the serologically demonstrated antigen show different tissue distributions. (2) Skin grafts between the congenic pair do not give rise to antibody, although antibody is produced by injections of lymphoid tissue. (3) Epidermal cells separated by trypsination do not absorb the corresponding antibody. (4) The *H* locus and the serologically demonstrated locus show different directional effects.

The cumulative weight of these different lines of evidence is considerable, but proof of recombination that the histoincompatibilities are indeed due to passenger *H* loci would be highly desirable. This is especially so because all the histoincompatibilities are rather weak. Thus *H*(*Ea-2*) causes rejection only in mice immunized with bone marrow, although following such immunization rejection occurs regularly in about 10 days. It is fortunate, because of the great interest which is attached to the *H-2* complex, that the independence of at least one of the two *H* loci associated with *H-2* and *Tla* is particularly well established.

Figure 3.2 is a linkage map of the mouse showing those histocompatibility loci identified because of their association with a marker gene

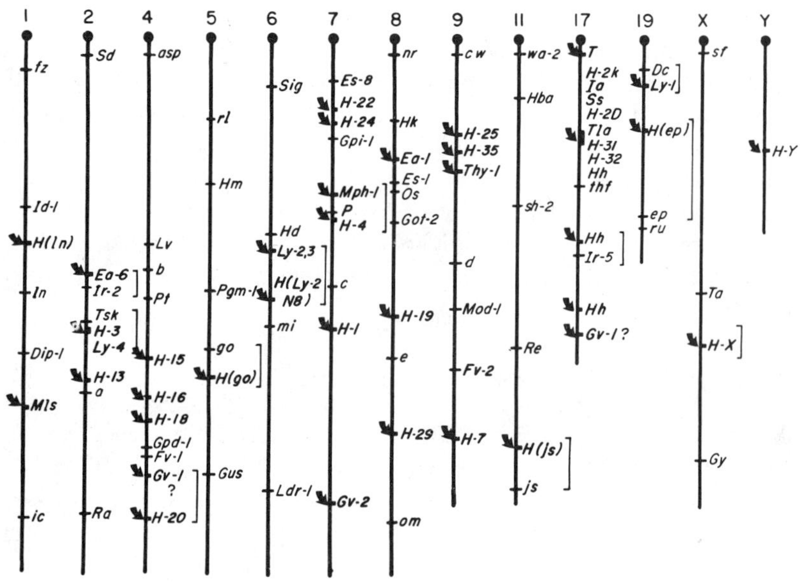


FIG. 3.2. Partial linkage map of the mouse. Of the 20 mouse chromosomes, only those that carry cell membrane alloantigen determining loci are shown. Centromeres are placed at the top of the figure. Histocompatibility loci and other loci determining alloantigens are indicated by arrows. A few nonalloantigen determining loci are included, in most cases because they have proved useful as markers. If loci are bracketed, their relative positions are not established. The *H-X* locus is known to be in the X chromosome; its position within the chromosome is unknown. (Based on chromosome map of the mouse prepared by Dr. Margaret Green. Dr. Donald Bailey has contributed much of the information concerning the position of histocompatibility loci. For sources of other infromation concerning cell membrane alloantigen determining loci, see text.)

plus a few located by other methods. Except for these loci, and other loci determining cell membrane alloantigens, only a selected group of genes is included. Twenty-six *H* loci are shown. These 26 include only three of the seven loci postulated by Flaherty and co-workers to account for linked histocompatibilities. The *Ly-1*-linked locus of these authors, not shown on the map, could be the same as Bailey's *H(ep)*, which is close to *Ly-1* on chromosome 19. The 26 *H* loci shown mark 11 of the 19 autosomes and both sex chromosomes.

### B. Identification by $F_1$ Test

In the CR lines of group 2, non-*H-2* histoincompatibilities from several different strains were introduced onto a B10 background and characterized as to identity or nonidentity by $F_1$ tests. Inevitably there were some duplications (*H-1* differences were found in a number of lines), but six new loci, assigned the symbols *H-7* through *H-12*, were identified (Snell and Bunker, 1965; Snell *et al.*, 1971). The symbols *H-5* and *H-6* were not used because these had been assigned to blood group loci.

### C. Identification by RI Strain Distribution Pattern

The 40 congenic resistant strains produced by Bailey (1971, 1975) all came from one initial cross, B6 × C. The same cross was the source of a group of 7 recombinant inbred (RI) lines. Each RI line was typed by an $F_1$ test to determine whether it carried the B6 or the C allele at the defining locus of each CR pair. The result was an RI strain distribution pattern for each CR line. Identity of patterns suggested identity or close linkage of the defining loci. Some representative patterns are shown in Table 3.1.

Three loci were shown by cross tests to be identical with the previously identified loci *H-1*, *H-2*, and *H-8*. As expected, these had distinct strain distribution patterns. Since *H-1* is closely linked to albinism (and was isolated in the same CR line) it is not surprising that the *H-1* and albinism (*c*) patterns are identical. We have already mentioned the linkage of *H-15* and *H-16* with *b* in chromosome 4 (Fig. 3.2). This shows up in Table 3.1 as similar but not identical patterns. *H-18*, also in chromosome 4, shows a quite different pattern from the adjacent *H-16*, but one similar to that of *Gpd-1*, adjacent to it on the other side. *H-22* and *H-24*, with patterns identical to *Gpi-1* (a marker in chromosome 7), are typical examples of loci easily located through their RI strain distribution patterns. Their nonidentity is proved by their

TABLE 3.1
STRAIN DISTRIBUTION PATTERNS, IN CXB RI LINES, OF C57BL/6 (B) AND BALB/c (C) ALLELES OF FOUR MARKER AND NINE HISTOCOMPATIBILITY LOCI[a]

| | Source of allele in RI strain | | | | | | |
|---|---|---|---|---|---|---|---|
| Locus | CXBD | CXBE | CXBG | CXBH | CXBI | CXBJ | CXBK |
| *c* [b] | B | B | C | B | C | B | B |
| *H-1* [b] | B | B | C | B | C | B | B |
| *H-2* | C | B | B | C | B | B | B |
| *H-8* | C | C | B | B | C | C | C |
| *b* [c] | B | B | C | C | C | C | B |
| *H-15* [c] | C | B | C | C | B | C | B |
| *H-16* [c] | C | B | C | C | C | B | B |
| *H-18* | C | C | C | C | C | B | C |
| *Gpd-1* | C | C | C | B | C | B | B |
| *H-21* | B | B | C | C | C | C | B |
| *H-22* [d] | B | C | B | C | C | C | B |
| *H-24* [d] | B | C | B | C | C | C | B |
| *Gpi-1* [d] | B | C | B | C | C | C | B |

[a] Bailey, 1971, 1975.

[b] *H-1* and *c* show identical strain distribution patterns and are linked.

[c] *H-15* and *H-16*, which show identical strain distribution patterns, are closely linked, and are also linked to *b* which shows a similar but not identical pattern.

[d] *H-22*, *H-24*, and *Gpi-1* show identical patterns and are linked.

mutual histoincompatibility. *H-21* (Table 3.1) is an example of a locus with a distinct strain distribution pattern that does not place it on the chromosome map.

Altogether Bailey's CR and RI lines have served to identify 21 new loci. These are numbered *H-15* through *H-38*, except that *H-31* and *H-32* used by Flaherty and Wachtel (1975), *H-33* assigned to Flaherty, and *H-14*, at one time were used for *Ea-2*, are omitted.

## III. Variations in Strength of Histocompatibility Alloantigens

As the production and testing of CR lines proceeded, it became apparent that the introduced histoincompatibilities varied greatly in strength (Counce *et al.*, 1956). Some prevented the growth of all tumor transplants and caused rapid rejection of skin grafts; others permitted the growth of a proportion of transplanted tumors and caused delayed rejection of skin. In general, the results with transplants of tumors and skin were congruent, but the skin data are more quantitative and reproducible. In Table 3.2 we give some representative skin graft data, mostly from a study by Graff *et al.* (1966a). A number of conclusions emerge.

1. Graft rejection time varies greatly from locus to locus. For unimmunized females with an *H-2K* difference, *median survival time* (MST) in studies by Graff and co-workers was 12 days. For other loci it ranged from 21 days (*H-3,* with B10 as the recipient), to 120 days (*H-4,* with B10 as the recipient), to a situation in which most grafts in unimmunized recipients were permanently accepted (*H-9*). It is noteworthy that all the loci in this group, including ones scarcely detectable by skin grafting, were isolated with transplantable leukemias plus prior immunization. Evidently transplantable tumors, properly used, can recognize some very weak histoincompatibilities. In general, histoincompatibilities that appear weak in one system appear weak also in the other (Graff *et al.*, 1966a).

2. Graft rejection times may vary substantially in reciprocal directions. Thus for *H-4,* grafts to B10 females showed an MST of 25 days; grafts in the opposite direction showed an MST of 120 days. For *H-1,* the corresponding figures were >250 days (all grafts survived) and 25 days. At loci with multiple alleles, each allelic pair may show its own characteristic rejection time.

3. Females usually reject grafts more rapidly than males. Thus for

TABLE 3.2
MEDIAN SURVIVAL TIMES (IN DAYS) OF SKIN GRAFTS MADE ACROSS SOME REPRESENTATIVE HISTOINCOMPATIBILITIES[a]

| | Unimmunized | | | | Immunized 3× | |
|---|---|---|---|---|---|---|
| | To B10 | | From B10 | | From B10 | |
| Locus | ♀ | ♂ | ♀ | ♂ | ♀ | ♂ |
| *H-2K* | 12 | | 12 | | | |
| *H-2D* | 16 | | 16 | | | |
| *H-7* | 33 | 47 | 23 | 25 | 10 | 11 |
| *H-3* | 52[b] | 46[b] | 21 | 30 | 10 | 11 |
| *H-1* | >250[d] | >250[d] | 25 | 26 | 11 | 10 |
| *H-4* | 25 | 24 | 120[b] | 119[b] | 22 | >250[c] |
| *H-10* | 71[b] | >300[c] | 91[b] | >250[c] | 45[c] | >250[c] |
| *H-9* | >300[c] | >300[d] | >400[c] | >300[c] | 23[b] | >250[c] |

[a] Graff *et al.*, 1966a; Graff and Bailey, 1973.
[b] Percent of grafts rejected <100, ≥50.
[c] Percent of grafts rejected <50, ≥12.
[d] Percent of grafts rejected <12, ≥0.

*H-7*, grafts to B10 females were rejected with an MST of 33 days, grafts to B10 males with an MST of 47 days. A glance at Table 3.2 will reveal other examples, and also a few exceptions, probably due to sampling error. Tumor grafts show the same phenomenon.

4. As the strength of the histoincompatibility decreases, the interval between the onset of the first symptoms of rejection and the occurrence of complete rejection increases (data not shown in table).

5. The weaker the histoincompatibility, the greater is the spread in the rejection time of individual grafts and the greater the chance of some grafts surviving permanently (data not shown in table).

6. Multiple histoincompatibilities exhibit additive or augmentative effects leading to curtailed allograft survival whenever the ratios between the constituent median survival times are of the order of 3:1 or less (Graff *et al.*, 1966b). Hildemann and Cohen (1967) have stressed the generality of rules 3, 4, 5, and 6.

7. Immunization can substantially shorten graft rejection time; with the weaker histoincompatibilities there may be no or few rejections in the absence of appropriate prior immunization. Thus (Table 3.2), for grafts from B10 donors with an *H-7* difference, immunization 3 times with $4 \times 10^6$ thymus cells reduced the MST from 23 to 10 days. For an *H-4* difference, the corresponding figures were 120 days (with 5 of 10 grafts not rejected) and 22 days. For an *H-9* difference, they were >400 days (11 of 19 grafts not rejected) and 23 days (3 of 8 grafts not rejected). Females with the weak *H-9* and *H-12* differences seemed to respond particularly well to immunization. Triple immunization was more effective than single immunization, especially with the weaker histoincompatibilities.

8. The weaker the histoincompatibility, the greater the difficulty of inducing immunity by prior injection of donor lymphoid cells and the greater the chance of inducing permanent survival (tolerance). The chance that tolerance will be induced increases both with the weakness of the histoincompatibility and the dose of cells used. For very weak histoincompatibilities, the dose margin may be very narrow (Graff, 1971).

9. Studies of *immune response genes*, described in Chapter 7, show that the survival of grafts is influenced not only by the histocompatibility genotype of donor and host but also, in the case of the host, by the presence or absence of particular alleles at loci which specifically influence rejection potential. The nonrejection of *H-1* grafts made with B10 as the donor (Table 3.2) may be largely an immune response gene effect. Thus rejection times cannot be interpreted solely in terms of the *H* genes themselves.

## IV. The *Sk* Locus

The murine *Sk* locus is a locus determining an alloantigen limited, so far as now known, to skin and brain. The first clues to its existence came from studies of self-tolerance in mice. The strain combination most commonly used by Medawar and his colleagues in their original tolerance studies was CBA and A. In this combination, neonatal inoculation of spleen cells from one strain into the other produced complete adult tolerance of donor skin grafts. Later investigations by many workers showed that this was not true in all strain combinations, and indeed that it was perhaps not true even though recipients remain permanently chimeric for donor lymphoid tissues. This suggested that skin and lymphocytes were antigenically different.

To test this possibility, Lance *et al.* (1971) produced lymphoid cell chimeras by injecting $(B6 \times A)F_1$ bone marrow and spleen into heavily irradiated adult B6 mice. Strain A skin grafts were applied 11 weeks later. Although tests of the recipients' red cells and lymphocytes showed that they had the $(B6 \times A)F_1$ *H-2* type, and hence that at least some donor antigens were present and tolerated, all A skin grafts were rejected with an MST of 26 days. If the skin grafts were made earlier than 11 weeks, there appeared to be greater tolerance of the skin.

The authors propose the following explanation. Skin has an alloantigen not present on lymphoid tissues. This exists in allelic forms in strains B6 and A. Freshly transferred $(B6 \times A)F_1$ lymphoid cells are tolerant to both allelic forms of this antigen as well as to their own lymphocyte antigens, but in the presence of only the B6 skin of the host, lose tolerance to the skin antigen of strain A. Hence A skin is rejected despite the blood cell chimerism. Loss of skin tolerance takes time; hence the requirement for a delay before skin grafting.

Subsequent studies added the following facts. Blood-cell-tolerant but skin-resistant chimeras form antibodies that are reactive with epidermal cells (Scheid *et al.*, 1972). In the strain B6–A combination, this is true irrespective of which direction the graft is made. Specificities Sk.1 of strain A and Sk.2 of strain B6 are thus identified. When A is the host and B6 is the skin donor, some grafts are not rejected, but antibody is still formed. The availability of antibody made it possible to determine, by absorption, the tissue distribution of the *Sk* antigen. It was found only on cells of epidermis and brain. In keeping with this, Steinmuller and Lofgreen (1974) showed that chimeras that rejected skin accepted heart tissue from the same donors.

Not only do skin-grafted chimeras form antibodies specific for epithelial cells, but, as shown by Gillette *et al.* (1972), their lymphocytes in culture react specifically with donor epithelial cells but not with donor lymphocytes.

The genetics of *Sk* has only been partly analyzed. Lance *et al.* (1971) transplanted skin from 40 backcross donors to radiation chimeras and found 22 rejections and 18 acceptances. This is a reasonable approximation to a 1:1 ratio, indicating that the skin-specific incompatibility is determined by a single locus. There was no association between rejection and *H-2*, which also segregated in the cross. Strains A and B6 clearly have different alleles. Since, in tolerance studies using strains A and CBA, skin grafts are permanently accepted, CBA presumably has the A allele. Other strain combinations besides B6 and A give rejections, but generally with a greater MST. Whether this means a diversity of alleles, or whether physiological factors are involved is not clear.

It is possible that *Sk* will turn out to be identical with one of the *H* loci identified by Bailey. This could be testable with Sk antibody. It cannot be identical with any of the two first groups of identified loci, since the tumors used to produce the corresponding CR lines presumably lack the Sk antigen.

## V. The Y-Linked Histocompatibility Locus

### A. Evidence for a Y-Borne Locus

Studies of sex determination and sex-linked inheritance in *Drosophila* gave rise to the dogma that the Y chromosome is genetically inert. The evidence showed that sex was determined by the balance between the number of X chromosomes and the number of autosomes, the Y playing no role. Hence when Eichwald and Silmser (1955) showed that, at least in some inbred strains of mice, male to female skin grafts were rejected, suggesting the existence of a Y chromosome histocompatibility locus, considerable interest was aroused. Perhaps the dogma did not apply to mammals.

In discussing this subject and the related X-linked histocompatibility locus, we shall use the following symbols. $X^A$ and $Y^A$ stand, respectively, for the X and Y chromosomes of strain A. Correspondingly for B, we use $X^B$ and $Y^B$. The postulated Y-determined rejection can then be represented as

$$X^A Y^A \rightarrow X^A X^A$$

According to the Y-locus hypotheses, $Y^A$ must determine some product foreign to the $X^A X^A$ female, leading to graft incompatibility. The Y-linked locus itself is designated *H-Y*.

The Y-linked hypothesis was strengthened when Eichwald *et al.* (1957) showed that the rejection of second male to female grafts was accelerated (MST of 13 versus 31 days), indicating that rejection was an immune process. But as various authors pointed out, other explanations were possible. Fox and Sei-Byung (1958) suggested three possibilities: (1) a Y-linked histocompatibility gene; (2) an autosomal gene turned on by the androgens of the male or turned off by the estrogens of the female; (3) an alloantigen whose production was regulated by autosomal–X-chromosomal balance, in the way in which sex in *Drosophila* is regulated.

The Y-linked hypothesis was strengthened when Celada and Welshons (1963) showed that, under certain circumstances, mice are born which lack a Y chromosome (XO mice), and that these mice are not males, as they would be in *Drosophila,* but females. Hypothesis (3) was thereby rendered improbable, and an essential role for the Y chromosome in male determination was indicated. But hormonal control of the male antigen was not ruled out. This hypothesis received a boost when Vojtíšková and Poláčková (1966) showed that skin from B6 males castrated at birth and used as donors at 10–11 weeks of age survived $50 \pm 6$ days on B6 females, whereas skin from normal B6 males survived only $27 \pm 1$ days. Absence of male hormone in some way reduced the strength of the male antigen.

This finding touched off a spate of research on possibly endocrine influences on the male antigen. Silvers and Billingham (1968), for example, investigated the effect of temporary residence of female skin on males before retransplantation to females, and Vojtíšková and Poláčková (1973, and earlier papers) investigated the effect of estrogens, androgens, and antiadrogenic steroids. The studies, in sum, showed that sex hormones can modify the male–female graft phenomenon but cannot eliminate or replace it.

That hormones are not the determining factor was indicated by experiments of Hildemann *et al.* (1974) using parent to $F_1$ male grafts. When grafts were made in the following combination

$$\text{B6} ♂ \rightarrow (\text{B6} ♀ \times \text{A} ♂)\text{F}_1 ♂$$

Which can be represented by the formula

$$X^B Y^B \rightarrow X^B Y^A$$

100% of the grafts were rejected. The authors emphasize that the use of small grafts and appropriate strain combinations was a factor in the high rejection frequency. These results would seem to prove not only the influence of the Y chromosome but also the existence of more than one *H-Y* allele.

While the rejection of male to male grafts, presumably histoincompatible only in the Y chromosome, rules out hormonal influence in this particular test, these rejections might be explained as due to hybrid resistance instead of *H-Y* incompatibility. Hybrid resistance, a curious exception to the laws of transplantation, is seen when grafts are made from *H-2* homozygous donors to *H-2* heterozygous recipients (Chapter 8, Section II,A). According to current dogma, it occurs only in the case of bone marrow or leukemia transplants, but it is perhaps significant that the combination of a small graft and the use of B6 both as donor and one parent of the recipient are particularly favorable for its manifestation. The substitution of strain A.BY for strain A in the tests used by Hildemann *et al.*, in order to eliminate the *H-2* heterozygosity of the recipient on which hybrid resistance depends, should permit a resolution of this question.

### B. Tissue Distribution of the Male Antigen

Results with male to female grafts of tissues other than skin point to a rather wide distribution of the male antigen. Tissues for which rejection of male grafts has been noted include thymus (Hirsch, 1957), lymph nodes (Feldman, 1958), spleen, liver, lung, salivary gland (Eichwald *et al.*, 1958), male mammary glands (Moretti and Blair, 1966), pituitary (Hoshino and Moore, 1968), thyroid, parathyroid, adrenal (Gittes and Russell, 1961), embryonic trophoblast (Borland *et al.*, 1970), and peritoneal exudate cells (Wickstrand and Haughton, 1974). Tolerance to male skin has been induced with disrupted cells from liver, kidney, and spleen (Kelly *et al.*, 1964).

An important step in the further analysis of the Y antigen was taken when Goldberg *et al.* (1971) showed that antiserum from female mice that have rejected a succession of male skin grafts is cytotoxic for sperm. The method used was similar to the dye exclusion test used to study lymphocytotoxicity (Chapter 4). Koo *et al.* (1973) have studied the male antigen by immunoelectron microscopy, using hybrid antibody and tobacco mosaic virus as the label. The use of these methods has shown that (1) the murine male antigen is present on and largely confined to the acrosomal region of sperm and (2) the proportion of sperm labeled, while usually over 50%, is substantially under 100%. Hausman and Palm (1973) have reported similar findings in the rat by the use of somewhat different labeling methods.

The authors speculate that the sperm that label are mostly Y-bearing, and the unlabeled ones X-bearing. This would imply the continued production of the male antigen in the late stages of spermatogenesis when only the haploid complement of chromosomes is present. The existence of antigenic differences between male-determining and female-determining sperm could afford a means of sex control, and indeed, Bennett and Boyse (1973), using anti-H-Y-treated sperm, have reported a reduction of male offspring from 53.4 to 45.4%.

### C. Genes Modifying the Expression of *H-Y*

Eichwald and Silmser (1955), in their original description of the male antigen, noted that, whereas all male to female grafts within strain C57BL were rejected, fewer than half were rejected within strain A. There have been numerous subsequent reports of similar strain differences. Results from different laboratories have shown inconsistencies, but one could perhaps single out strain C57BL as standing at one extreme and CBA, C3H, and DBA/2 at the other extreme. Several studies have indicated that the virtual inability of females of the latter strains to reject male grafts is not due to lack of the male antigen. Thus Goldberg *et al.* (1972) found that anti-male antibody was formed by grafted C3H and DBA/2 females even though the male grafts were retained.

Strains C57BL and CBA were selected by Klein and Linder (1961) for a genetic analysis of genes modifying the expression of *H*-Y. Results of male to female skin grafts for the various parental and hybrid generations, given as number rejected : number accepted, are shown in the following tabulation.

| | |
|---|---|
| C57 → C57 | 26:0 |
| CBA → CBA | 0:35 |
| CBA → $F_1$ | 20:0 |
| CBA → backcross ($F_1 \times$ CBA) | 85:25 |

The ability of C57 females to reject male skin showed dominance in the $F_1$. In the backcross somewhat more than 75% of the grafts were rejected, suggesting a difference between the parental strains of at least two factors modifying the rejection process. One of the two genes indicated may well have been the *H-2*-linked immune response gene (Chapter 7).

### D. Antigens of the Heterogametic Sex in Species Other Than the Mouse

The Y antigen was identifiable, in the mouse, only by virtue of the availability of highly inbred strains. There are several other species sufficiently inbred to warrant a search for the sex antigen. Silvers and Yang

(1973) among others, have found rejection of male to female grafts in the rat. As demonstrated by Chai (1973), rabbits also manifest the male antigen. Just as in mice, there are strain differences in the degree of its expression. In chickens, the female is the heterogametic sex (male ZZ, female ZW). Hence if chickens possess a locus similar to *H-Y* of mice, it should be revealed by the rejection of ♀ → ♂ grafts. Gilmore (1967) has reported rejections in this donor-recipient combination. In the guinea pig, where two inbred strains are available, Bauer (1960) failed to find male-to-female graft rejection. Observations of most grafts were terminated at 80 days. In the hamster, using incompletely inbred strains in which intrastrain grafts often showed a very prolonged, chronic type of rejection, Adams *et al.* (1956) could distinguish no difference in male-to-female and female-to-male grafts.

Wachtel *et al.* (1974) have used the cross-reactivity of mouse female anti-male spleen cell antiserum as a test for the presence of the male antigen in species other than the mouse. It was demonstrated that male but not female spleen cells of rats, rabbits, and guinea pigs, and blood leukocytes of humans, removed activity. The rat showed the strongest cross-reaction, but male cells of all four species absorbed substantially. It may well be, therefore, that the H-Y antigen is widely distributed.

## VI. The X-Linked Histocompatibility Locus

If there is an X-linked histocompatibility locus analogous to the Y-linked locus, it could not be demonstrated by simple female to male grafts within an inbred strain, since identical X's would be present in the recipient and donor. It might be demonstrated, however, in grafts made from female to male $F_1$ hybrids, where donor and recipient could have different X's, although otherwise compatible. Two potentially different types of male recipients could be produced by the use of reciprocal crosses. Thus

$$♀ \text{ A} \times ♂ \text{ B gives } ♂ \; X^A Y^B$$
$$♀ \text{ B} \times ♂ \text{ A gives } ♂ \; X^B Y^A$$

Using males thus derived, incompatibilities might be expected in the combinations

$$F_1 \; ♀ \; X^A X^B \rightarrow F_1 \; ♂ \; X^B Y^A$$
$$F_1 \; ♀ \; X^A X^B \rightarrow F_1 \; ♂ \; X^A Y^B$$
$$\text{Parental} \; ♀ \; X^A X^A \rightarrow F_1 \; ♂ \; X^B Y^A$$
$$\text{Parental} \; ♀ \; X^B X^B \rightarrow F_1 \; ♂ \; X^A Y^B$$

Bailey (1963), using hybrids derived from B6 by BALB/c crosses, in fact, found skin graft rejection in these combinations. Mullen and

Hildemann (1972) have reported similar results in rats, and there is a corresponding Z-linked locus in chickens (Bacon, 1970). Bauer (1960) failed to find evidence for an X-linked locus in guinea pigs. As in the case of the Y-linked locus, there are variations in rejection times of grafts bearing the X-linked histoincompatibility, so that modifying factors have to be postulated (Bailey, 1964).

## VII. Number of Alleles at Histocompatibility Loci

It is commonplace in genetics that most loci have multiple alleles. Despite the technical difficulties of studying histocompatibility loci, we can now say with confidence that they are no exception. Virtually all the evidence comes from work with mice.

Loci ordinarily are identifiable only because they exist in at least two allelic forms. The Y-linked locus is an exception because it is totally absent in the female. Thus the original studies proved only the existence of one allele. However, the studies of Mullen and Hildemann (1972) with rats and Hidemann *et al.* (1974) with mice, using the $X^AY^A \rightarrow X^AY^B$ combination described in Section V,A, would seem, with the possible qualification mentioned in that section, to prove that there are at least two alleles. Silvers and Yang (1973) have suggested other qualifications.

Three alleles of the X-linked histocompatibility locus of mice have been identified (D. W. Bailey and C. K. Chai, personal communication). Hildemann *et al.* (1974) have made the interesting observation that in the combination $X^BY^A \rightarrow X^AY^B$ or its reciprocal, which should have both *H-X* and *H-Y* incompatibilities, rejection is weaker than in the case of either one incompatibility acting alone. They attribute this to antigenic competition, but it should be noted that this double combination, since it employs an $F_1$ as donor as well as recipient, is the only combination of those used that could not show hybrid resistance.

The *H-2* complex presents a special situation in that it can be studied serologically. There are about 40 identified alleles at *H-2D* and the same number at *H-2K* (Chapter 6); there are probably as many as yet unidentified.

With the exception of *H-2* and the very few other *H* loci demonstrable serologically, the only way in which autosomal *H* loci and individual alleles at these loci can be identified is through the production of congenic resistant (CR) lines. Since this is a time-consuming process, efforts at allelic analysis have been limited. Because of the linkage of *H-1* with c (albinism), and of *H-3* and *H-13* with the linked markers *we* and *a*, which permits the production of CR lines simply by following a visual trait in a backcross, these loci were selected for intensive study. A number of CR lines were produced in which the markers were introduced onto a B10 background. Analysis of these lines has served to identify three *H-1* alleles, three *H-13* alleles, and five *H-3* alleles. Two CR lines differing from B10 at *H-8* establish three alleles at this locus. This is the extent of our firm information about multiple alleles (reviewed in Graff and Bailey, 1973).

There is, however, another source of information. In using CR pairs to type various inbred strains, by the $F_1$ test, for the two alleles by which each pair differs, it has frequently turned out that a particular strain has neither the *a* nor the *b* allele (Graff and Bailey, 1973). This establishes the existence of a third allele. Moreover, if only a small minority of typed strains are *a* or *b*, it is plausible to assume that there is more than one unknown allele among the "not-*a*, not-*b*" lines. Thus of 12 lines typed for *H-4*, three had the *a* allele, and one the *b* allele. If these are average frequencies, then we might expect four additional alleles among the remaining 8 lines. The frequencies of different alleles doubtlessly varies greatly and introduces a major source of error into such calculations, but in any group of calculations these errors would tend to average out. Using this method, Graff and Bailey (1973) have estimated the number of alleles at 8 *H* loci. The figures arrived at are *H-1*, 12 alleles; *H-3*, 5; *H-4*, 6; *H-7*, 4; *H-8*, 7; *H-9*, 3; *H-12*, 3; and *H-13*, 4. These figures, while clearly only approximations, probably give a reasonable picture of allelic diversity in the laboratory mouse. The diversity would probably appear greater if wild mice could be studied. We know, for example, that at the blood group locus, *Ea-1*, there is only one allele in laboratory mice, but actually three if wild mice are analyzed. A considerable degree of multiple allelism is, therefore, probably characteristic of histocompatibility loci.

## VIII. Number of Histocompatibility Loci

### A. Studies with Mice

Estimates of the number of histocompatibility loci have been made for several different vertebrate species, ranging from guinea pigs to a teleost fish. As with most histocompatibility phenomena, by all odds the most informative studies have been made with mice, and we shall confine any detailed descriptions to this species. Most estimates have been based on a single method—transplantation from one or both parent strains used in a cross to a segregating generation derived from the cross. A quite different approach, using mutation data (which we describe in Section IX,D,4) has yielded an estimate of the number of *mutational sites.* This must bear some relation to the number of loci, but it is not the same thing.

In Chapter 1 we noted that two early experiments, one using a transplantable tumor and the other skin as the test graft, gave estimates of 4 and 13 loci, respectively. A number of other studies gave estimates in the neighborhood of 13. The authors usually pointed out that these estimates were likely to be low rather than high.

Clearly they were low, since data presented in this chapter and in Chapter 6 on *H-2* show that 45 loci with an effect in histocompatibility have been described. A few of these loci may turn out to represent duplications, or possibly to be invalid, but the number is certainly not far wrong.

A defect in the method used in the earlier tests of the number of *H* loci is that so few acceptancies are expected, even in the $F_2$ where histoincompatibilities are fewer than in the backcross, that the number of mice grafted has been insufficient to give reliable results. Several experiments have overcome this problem by testing a generation so designed as to carry an increased proportion of donor genes. All have yielded higher estimates of gene number than the earlier studies. We shall confine our description to a study by Brambilla *et al.* (1970) which is particularly informative.

The mating system used by these authors is shown in Fig. 3.3. B6

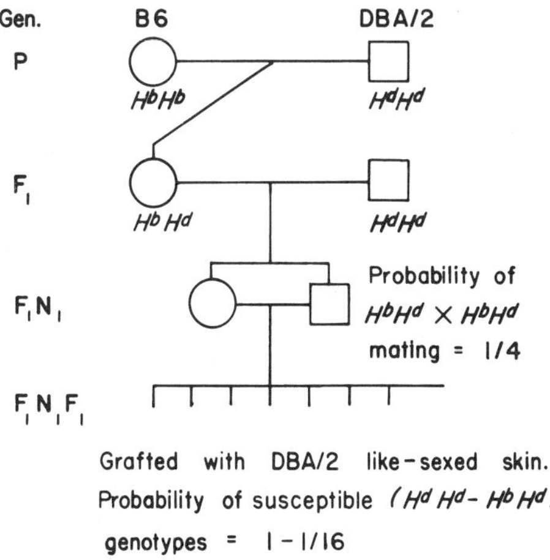


Fig. 3.3. Mating system used by Brambilla *et al.* (1970) in their analysis of the number of histocompatibility loci by which strains B6 and DBA/2 differ.

females were mated to DBA/2 males, and $F_1$ females backcrossed to DBA/2 to give an F1N1 generation. The F1N1 were mated brother × sister, and the F1N1F1 progeny were challenged with DBA/2 skin. The effect of this mating system was to reduce the proportion of B6 genes and hence to increase the proportion of histocompatible and hence susceptible animals. With respect to any one *H* locus, the chance that an animal would be susceptible was $1 - \frac{1}{16} = \frac{15}{16}$. If there were $n$ independently segregating and fully penetrant loci, the fraction of susceptible animals would be $(\frac{15}{16})^n$.

Sixty-three males and 120 females had grafts judged technically successful on the eighth postoperative day. These were followed to day 240. Grafts were judged to be rejected when the first definite signs of rejection appeared. The number of rejected grafts, and hence the estimate of locus number, increased steadily throughout the duration of the experiment. There was, in fact, a straight-line relationship between the estimated number of loci and the time after grafting. At the termination of the experiment, 10 grafts survived on males and 7 on females. The corresponding *H* locus estimates are 28 and 44. These estimates are much more in line with the number of actually identified loci than earlier estimates, but may for various reasons still be low.

## B. Factors Which May Lead to Underenumeration

The formula used for the estimation of *H*-locus number assumes that (1) the loci are fully penetrant, i.e., "incompatibility" always results in rejection, and (2) the loci segregate independently. In the typical interstrain cross, these assumptions are probably far from being realized. There are also other factors that tend to make an estimate of *H* gene number based on the segregating generation method an underestimate. While the exact weight to be attached to these various factors cannot be determined, it is important to examine them.

### *1. Loci with Incomplete Penetrance*

The studies cited earlier in this chapter show that *H* loci are not always fully penetrant. Loci vary in strength from *H-2K*, which consistently causes rejection in 9–12 days, to loci that are so weak that rejection is greatly delayed and may not occur in all animals. In a segregating generation, weak loci, if they cause rejection at all, may do so through some sort of cumulative effect rather than individually. If a rejection depends on the interaction of three loci, these will be enumerated in a calculation of locus number as something less than three loci, perhaps even as less than one locus, and the true locus number will be correspondingly underestimated.

The existence of weak *H* loci is probably an important source of underenumeration of *H* loci in all tests employing grafts made to a segregating generation. However, the study of Brambilla *et al.* (1970), because of the separation of data from the two sexes, the long period of observation, and the use of a sensitive test of rejection, was probably better than average in this respect.

### 2. *The Occurrence of Many Linked H Loci*

Another major source of underestimation of *H* locus number in studies of this type is their failure to adequately enumerate linked loci. Two closely linked genes would appear as one; two less closely linked genes could cause a frequency of rejection somewhat greater than that attributable to one locus, somewhat less than that attributable to two. With 45 reported loci and only 20 chromosome pairs, linkage is inevitable. And indeed, we already know of a number of linkages close enough to interfere with locus detection in a segregating generation, e.g., *H-3–H-13, H-15–H-16–H-18, H-2K–H-2D* (Fig. 3.2). The greater the number of loci, the more important this factor must be. Also if histocompatibility loci sometimes occur in clusters because of duplication or other evolutionary factors, this would exaggerate this source of underenumeration.

### 3. *Loci That Do Not Segregate in a Given Cross*

The segregation method of histocompatibility gene counting obviously measures only those loci that segregate in the cross under study. If the two parent strains have the same allele at a locus, the locus goes undetected. The existence of multiple alleles at most loci favors detection, but does not ensure it. Data of Graff and Snell (1969) concerning the strain distribution of the known alleles of 8 loci permits a crude estimate of the importance of this factor. Strains B6 and DBA/2, the strains used by Brambilla *et al.*, had different alleles at 5 of the loci, the same allele at 2, and were indeterminate at another. This would suggest an underestimation of 25 to 37%. But this again may be a low figure, because laboratory strains of mice carry only a fraction of the polymorphism of wild populations and may never segregate at some loci.

### 4. *Loci Determining Alloantigens Not on Skin*

There is one final source of underenumeration whose importance can be scarcely guessed at, but which could be highly significant. Aside from the early estimates, which were based on tumor transplants, nearly all studies of *H* gene number have used skin grafts. If tissue-specific antigens are common, and we shall find some evidence that they are, studies with other tissues might tap an important source of unrevealed loci.

In conclusion, the figure of 44 histocompatibility loci derived from the study of Brambilla *et al.* must be a substantial underestimate. The true value, including weak loci, nests of closely linked loci, loci that do not segregate in a given cross, and loci whose end product is not represented on skin, probably is at least several times this figure.

### C. Studies with Species Other Than Mice

Studies with rats (Billingham *et al.*, 1962), chickens (Hala, 1969), and fish (Kallman, 1964) have all yielded estimates of *H* locus number similar to those derived from the earlier studies with mice. The Syrian hamster seems to present a special situation. One study (Billingham and Silvers, 1964) suggested the segregation of only 3 loci; a second study (Hildemann and Walford, 1960) indicated more loci, but exceptionally weak ones. There are reasons to believe that these results may convey a false picture, even for the hamster. All laboratory strains of the Syrian species come from only 1 male and 2 females captured in 1930. This would lead to a major underrepresentation of actual polymorphism. Also there are indications that the hamster immune system is unusual. In mice, the strong rejections due to *H-2* lead to the formation of antibody, and the same situation holds in most other species that have been studied. However, no antibody was found following comparably strong rejections in the hamster (Billingham and Silvers, 1964). Whatever the explanation of the unusual rejection behavior of the hamster, it is probably the exception and not the rule. The *H* gene number of the mouse is probably typical of most mammalian and perhaps most vertebrate species.

## IX. Mutations at Histocompatibility Loci

### A. Potential of *H* Genes for Mutation Studies

Histocompatibility genes offer a potential for mutation studies that is beginning to be both recognized and exploited. They afford several advantages. *H* genes typically behave as dominants; hence mutations can be detected in first generation offspring. Because of the rarity of genetic change, a model that, like *H* genes, permits a study of at least 40 loci at once has obvious attractions. While not as easy to spot individually as mutations with visible effects, *H* mutations are easy to detect as a group, since one graft tests for all loci. As we shall see, most *H* mutations involve the *gain* of antigenic activity. This may mean that they are more likely to be due to point mutation and less likely to be due to deletion than are the variants revealed by other widely used methods, especially as applied in the study of mutagens such as X rays. These are substantial recommendations.

The earliest evidence of *H* gene mutation came from the discovery of incompatibilities within inbred strains. Much more informative are the studies of Bailey and Kohn (1965), Egorov and Blandova (1972), and Kohn and Melvold (1974) specifically designed for the detection of mutation.

## B. Appearance of Histoincompatibilities in Inbred Lines

There have been a number of reports of the appearance of histoincompatibilities between related sublines. The data suggest that the likelihood of incompatibility and also its strength show a tendency to increase with the length of separation of the sublines, although with considerable variation according to the subline pair tested. This is what one would expect from the random nature of mutation. In one of the more thorough studies of this subject, Silvers and Gasser (1973) tested the survival of skin grafts exchanged between five pairs of mouse and one pair of rat sublines. Generations were estimated (perhaps generously) from the years since separation and were expressed as the sum of the separate generations accumulated by each subline. No incompatibilities were found between two subline pairs separated an estimated 29 and 42 generations, very weak incompatibilities between three subline pairs separated 123, 126, and 129 generations, and multiple (3 to 5) incompatibilities between one pair separated 119 generations.

## C. Design for a Mutation Study

The test system used by Bailey and Kohn (1965) in their *H* gene mutation study is shown in Figs. 3.4 and 3.5. The animals used were $F_1$ hybrids between strains C57BL/6 (B6) and BALB/c (C). Tail skin grafts were exchanged in a circle or ring between $F_1$ animals, each mouse donating a graft to and receiving a graft from each of its two neighbors. Using each mouse as both donor and recipient not only increased the chance of mutant detection, but also, as shown in the figures, made it possible to distinguish between gain, loss, and gain plus loss mutants. The use of $F_1$ hybrids was essential for the detection of loss

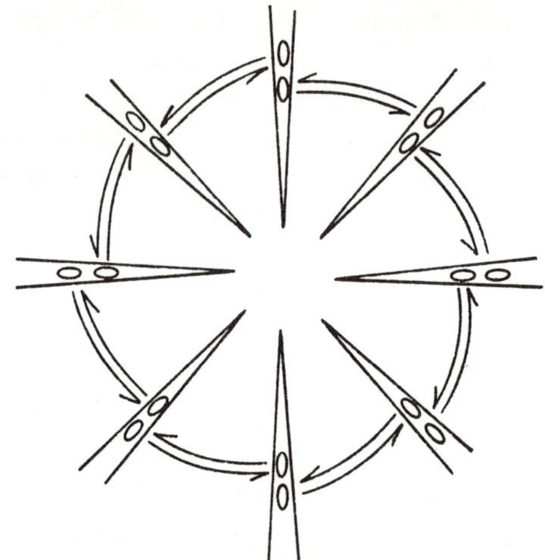

Fig. 3.4. Reciprocal circle system of tail skin grafting used by Bailey and Kohn (1965) in their study of histocompatibility gene mutation. Each mouse serves as both recipient and donor for each adjacent mouse in the circle. (From Bailey and Kohn, 1965. Reproduced from *Genetical Research* by permission of Cambridge University Press.)

mutations, or the loss component of gain plus loss mutations, since these would have a recessive expression; they would be covered up by the normal allele of homozygous animals. Presumed mutants were subjected

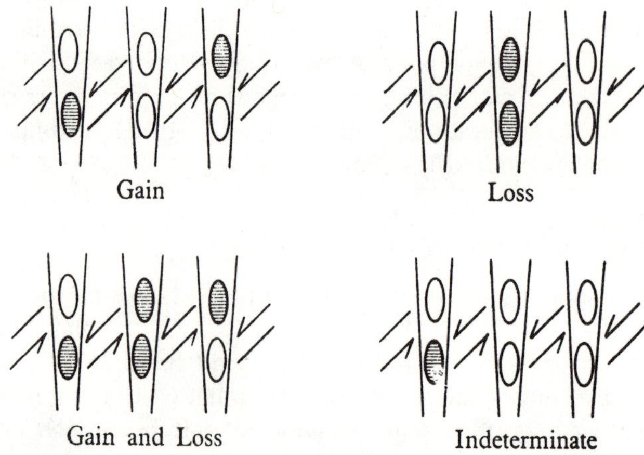


Fig. 3.5. Diagram showing how the reciprocal circle method of skin grafting can distinguish between gain, loss, and gain plus loss mutations. Shaded ovals represent rejected grafts, unshaded ovals accepted grafts. (From Bailey and Kohn, 1965. Reproduced from *Genetical Research* by permission of Cambridge University Press.)

to additional tests. The experiment was designed originally as a test for the induction of mutations by X rays, but since there was no difference between experimental and control groups, the data were pooled. This same system has been used by Bailey (1966) and by Kohn and Melvold (1974) in additional separate studies, and a similar but not identical system has been used by Egorov and Blandova (1972). The major difference in the study carried out by the Egorov and Blandova was in the inbred strains employed. The parents came from congenic strains differeing only at the *H-2* complex. Two congenic strain pairs were used, one on a strain A background, and the other on a B10 background. Since the $F_1$ mice tested by circle grafting were heterozygous only at *H-2*, loss mutations were detectable only at the *H* genes present in this complex.

## D. Spontaneous *H* Gene Mutation Rate

### 1. *Cumulative Rate at All H Loci*

Bailey and Kohn found 32 mutations in 2572 mice. Twenty-seven of these were subjected to a breeding test, and the incompatibility was found to be transmissible. A few of the rejections occurred in clusters, suggesting that the mutations causing them had originated prior to gametogenesis in the parent generation. This unfortunately makes an accurate estimate of mutation rate impossible. Uncorrected, the data show a mutation rate of 13.5 per $10^3$ zygotes or 6.75 per $10^3$ gametes.

In the subsequent study by Bailey (1966), 2055 $F_1$ mice were tested. Of these, 488 came, as in the earlier study, from untested parents and showed some clusters of histoincompatible animals, presumably due to the occurrence of *H* gene mutations prior to the parental generation. The apparent mutation rate was very high. The remaining 1967 $F_1$ mice were from parents that had been tested and proved to be histocompatible. Mutations must have occurred in the parents, although they could have occurred early in gametogenesis, in which case clustering would still be possible. The mutation rate was 5.4 per $10^3$ gametes. An X-rayed group showed essentially the same mutation rate. In the study by Kohn and Melvold (1974), 8200 $F_1$ mice from untreated parents yielded a rate of 1.28 per $10^3$ gametes, or 0.85 per $10^3$ gametes if clusters, presumably due to early mutation, are treated as single events. Five loss mutations are omitted in these calculations; three of these were believed to be due to loss of the X chromosome. In the study by Egorov and Blandova (1972) there was one mutation in 519 $F_1$ mice on the B10 background; a mutation rate of 0.96 per $10^3$ gametes. There were no mutations in the comparable group on a strain A background, but one mutation in an experimental group was shown to come from the untreated parent, and the authors estimate a spontaneous mutation rate in this group of 0.70 per $10^3$ gametes.

The mutation rates cited above are of course the rates for all *H* loci combined. The rate per locus can be estimated accurately only if we know the number of loci. If we assume 100 loci, the average rate should be of order of 8 per $10^6$ gametes per locus. Mutation rates probably vary tremendously from locus to locus (Schlager and Dickie, 1967; Cox, 1972; Searle, 1972), but this figure is certainly above the average. Rates determined for loci in mice producing visible effects range from 8.9 per $10^6$ gametes for forward mutations at five coat color loci to 0.5 per $10^6$ gametes for 14 loci with dominant expression. Half of the mutations included in this last figure were at one locus; a more typical rate for these loci would be 0.2 per $10^6$ gametes (Schlager and Dickie, 1967).

While circle skin grafts between $F_1$ animals give no clue as to the locus at which a histocompatibility mutation has occurred, it is possible, once a mutation is established, to test for the locus involved. The applicable tests are very similar to those used for the analysis of congenic resistant lines. Considerable progress has now been made in three different laboratories in analyses of this sort. The most detailed evidence so far available concerns the *H-2* complex.

### 2. *Mutations Involving the H-2 Complex*

In the studies of Bailey and Kohn, Bailey, and Egorov, 5 mutations involving some part of the *H-2* complex were found in 4827 mice (Egorov and Blandova, 1972). This gives the extraordinary mutation rate of 518 per $10^6$ gametes. Some of these mutants came from parents treated with mutagens. But Melvold and Kohn (1975) report eight independent *H-2* mutations in 26,316 mice. Because there were certain departures from the usual mating system, corrections have to be applied, but the authors calculate a mutation rate of 550 mutations per $10^6$ gametes, a figure very similar to that obtained by Egorov and Blandova. As an added curious feature, at least one of Bailey's mutants (Bailey, 1970), and all eight obtained by Melvold and Kohn, were shown to have occurred in the $H\text{-}2K^b$ allele derived from the B6 parent. This suggests the existence of a mutable gene at this locus.

### 3. *Mutations at Non-H-2 Loci*

By using, as tester stocks, the CR and RI strains developed by Bailey, non-*H-2* mutations can be divided into two groups: first, mutations at 28 loci by which B6 and BALB/c are known to differ; second, loci at which these strains probably do not differ. Melvold and Kohn (1975), in a large group of tested mice, found no mutations in the first category, 19 in the second. A precise mutation rate cannot be calculated from the latter figure. There were several clusters; there were some complications in the mating system; we do not know the number of loci involved. But the difference between the two groups is striking and suggests either that a mutable locus or mutable loci are at work or that there are a great many loci at which B6 and BALB/c have the same allele.

### 4. *Evidence from Mutation Studies Concerning the Number of H Loci*

Mutation studies, like studies using grafts made to segregating generation, emphasize the multiplicity of *H* loci. Specifically, they suggest that the number of loci at which two inbred strains, such as B6 and BALB/c, resemble each other may far exceed the 40 or so loci by which they are known or presumed to differ.

The evidence comes from two sources. Melvold and Kohn (1975), as we have noted, found a number of non-*H-2* mutations at loci at which B6 and BALB/c are presumed to have the same allele and none at 28 loci at which they are known to have different alleles. This suggests that the former category is more numerous than the later. Bailey (1968) has argued that the high frequency of mutations showing gains only, as contrasted with losses or gains plus losses, points in the same direction. Except for *H-2* mutations, where gains plus losses are the rule, the great majority of mutations in all studies have been manifest in the circle or ring test (Fig. 3.4) as gains only. Since a change in an antigen might be expected to cause a loss as well as a gain of antigen–antibody reactivity, this is a surprising result. But since the ring test does not reveal losses at those loci at which the $F_1$ test animals are homozygous, it may be that losses are occurring but simply not being revealed. The results again are explained by the postulate that homozygous *H* loci are much more numerous in the $F_1$ than heterozygous ones.

This interpretation requires one possible qualification. In studies of this sort, variants at a previously unmutated site of a known *H* locus might, under some circumstances, be indistinguishable from variants at a new locus. A change at a new site in a previously recognized antigen might, in some tests, look like a change in a previously unrecognized antigen. Where the RI strain distribution patterns of mutants have been determined, this possibility can be ruled out, since different patterns provide the ideal evidence that variants are at different loci. But data from this source are still lacking or incomplete. Hence Bailey (1968) qualifies a calculation from mutation data that there may be as many as 500 *H* loci by suggesting, as an alternative, that there may be fewer loci, but each with several mutable sites. Despite all qualifications, however, every new mutation study seems to bring forth new evidence emphasizing the extent and complexity of the *H* system.

### 5. *The Variability of the H Gene Mutation Rate*

In summarizing data on *H* gene spontaneous mutation rate (Section IX,A,1), we found that the cumulative rate in different studies varied from 5.4 per $10^3$ gametes to about 0.70 per $10^3$ gametes. Within the studies carried out by Bailey, moreover, there seemed to be variations when the data were broken down into five groups tested successively. Both Bailey (1966) and Kohn and Melvold (1974) believe that the variations are real. No firm explanation can be given. But Bailey (1966), noting an inverse relationship between the spontaneous *H* gene mutation rate and the degree of isolation and sanitation under which his colony was maintained, suggested that some mutations might be due to lysogeny, i.e., the incorporation of viral genomes into the parental chromosomes. Possibly there are other, unknown environmental factors influencing the *H* gene mutation rate. Kohn and Melvold (1974) believe their relatively low rate was obtained under conditions of sanitation and isolation equivalent to those prevailing in the test group that yielded Bailey's higher rate. Viral incidence, however, must be a very difficult parameter to estimate.

## X. Induced *H* Gene Mutations

The $F_1$ circle graft system has been used in three studies of the ability of known mutagenic agents to induce histocompatibility variants. The studies confirm the effectiveness of the system. Bailey and Kohn (1965) tested the mutagenic effect of X rays. The results were negative. Perhaps this is because a high proportion of presumed X-ray-induced mutations are actually small deletions, and the histocompatibility system is inappropriate for the detection of this kind of variant. Egorov and Blandova (1972) used diethyl sulfate as the mutagen. No mutations were found in the $F_1$ hybrids on a strain A background, but 14 appeared in 864 B6 $F_1$'s, for a rate of 5.8 per $10^3$ gametes. There was one mutation in the B6 $F_1$ controls. In a study by Kohn (1973), the mutagen selected was triethylenemelamine. No mutations were obtained when the treated parent was from B6, and 8 were obtained when the treated parent was from strain BALB/c.

While these should be regarded as pilot tests of the utility of *H* genes for mutation studies, they do indicate the potential value of the system.

The results were unexpected in a number of respects. X-rays proved ineffective; diethyl sulfate appeared to induce mutations in B6's but not A's, triethylenemelamine in BALB/c's but not B6's. This is not entirely surprising, since strain differences in mutation rate are well known in other species. In view of the very real threat imposed by possible mutagens in the environment, mutation studies in mammals are important, but they also are difficult. Because the *H* gene system tests for so many loci at once, it may very well become established as the system of choice.

## REFERENCES

Adams, R. A., D. I. Patt, and B. R. Lutz. 1956. Long term persistance of skin homografts in untreated hamsters. *Transplant Bull* **3**:41–42.

Bacon, L. D. 1970. Histoincompatibility associated with the Z-chromosome in chickens. *Transplantation* **10**:126–128.

Bailey, D. W. 1963. Histoincompatibility associated with the X chromosome in mice. *Transplantation* **1**:70–74.

Bailey, D. W. 1964. Genetically modified survival times of grafts from mice bearing X-linked histoincompatibility. *Transplantation* **2**:203–206.

Bailey, D. W. 1966. Heritable histocompatibility changes: Lysogeny in mice? *Transplantation* **4**:482–488.

Bailey, D. W. 1968. The vastness and organization of the murine histocompatibility gene system as inferred from mutation data. Pages 317–323 *in* J. Dausset, I. Hamburger, and G. Mathé, eds. Advances in transplantation. Munksgaard, Copenhagen.

Bailey, D. W. 1970. Analysis of a mutation at the histocompatibility-2 locus in mice. *Genetics* **64**:s3.

Bailey, D. W. 1971. Recombinant-inbred strains. An aid to finding identity, linkage, and function of histocompatibility and other genes. *Transplantation* **11**:325–327.

Bailey, D. W. 1975. Genetics of histocompatibility in mice. I. New loci and congenic lines. *Immunogenetics* **2**:249–256.

Bailey, D. W., and H. I. Kohn. 1965. Inherited histocompatibility changes in progeny of irradiated and unirradiated inbred mice. *Genet Res* **6**:330–340.

Bauer, J. A., Jr. 1960. Genetics of skin transplantation and an estimate of the number of histocompatibility genes in inbred guinea pigs. *Ann NY Acad Sci* **87**:78–92.

Bennett, D., and E. A. Boyse. 1973. Sex ratio in progeny of mice inseminated with sperm treated with H-Y antiserum. *Nature (Lond)* **246**:308–309.

Billingham, R. E., and W. K. Silvers. 1964. Syrian hamsters and transplantation immunity. *Plast Reconstr Surg* **34**:329–353.

Billingham, R. E., B. A. Hodge, and W. K. Silvers. 1962. An estimate of the number of histocompatibility loci in the rat. *Proc Natl Acad Sci USA* **48**:138–147.

Borland, R., Y. W. Loke, and P. J. Oldershaw. 1970. Sex differences in trophoblast behavior on transplantation. *Nature (Lond)* **228**:572.

Brambilla, G., M. Cavanna, S. Parodi, and L. Baldini. 1970. Time dependence of the number of histocompatibility loci in skin graft rejection of mice. *Experientia* **26**:1140–1141.

Celada, F., and W. J. Welshons. 1963. An immunogenetic analysis of the male antigen in mice utilizing animals with an exceptional chromosome constitution. *Genetics* 48:139–151.

Chai, C. K. 1973. The response of females to male grafts in inbred lines of rabbits. *J Hered* **64**:321–323.

Counce, S., P. Smith, R. Barth, and G. D. Snell. 1956. Strong and weak histocompatibility gene differences in mice and their role in the rejection of tumors and skin. *Ann Surg* **144**:198–204.

Cox, E. C. 1972. On the organization of higher chromosomes. *Nature (Lond), New Biol* **239**:133–134.

Egorov, I. K., and Z. K. Blandova. 1972. Histocompatibility mutations in mice: Chemical induction and linkage with the *H-2* locus. *Genet Res* **19**:133–143.

Eichwald, E. J., and C. R. Silmser. 1955. (Note without title.) *Transplant Bull* **2**:148–149.

Eichwald, E. J., C. R. Silmser, and N. Wheeler. 1957. The genetics of skin grafting. *Ann NY Acad Sci* **64**:737–740.

Eichwald, E. J., C. R. Silmser, and I. Weissman. 1958. Sex-linked rejection of normal and neoplastic tissue. I. Distribution and specificity. *J Natl Cancer Inst* **20**:563–575.

Feldman, M. 1958. The antigen determined by a Y-linked histocompatibility gene. *Transplant Bull* **5**:15–16.

Flaherty, L., and D. Bennett. 1973. Histoincompatibilities found between congenic strains which differ at loci determining differentiation antigens. *Transplantation* **16**:505–514.

Flaherty, L., and S. S. Wachtel. 1975. H(*Tla*) system: Identification of two new loci, *H-31* and *H-32*, and alleles. *Immunogenetics* **2**:81–85.

Fox, A. S., and S.-B. Yoon. 1958. Antigenic differences between males and females in *Drosophila* not attributable to the Y chromosome. *Transplant Bull* **5**:52–54.

Gillette, R. W., S. Cooper, and E. M. Lance. 1972. The reactivity of murine lymphocytes to epidermal cells. *Immunology* **23**:769–776.

Gilmore, D. G. 1967. Histocompatibility antigen in the heterogametic sex in the chicken. *Transplantation* **5**:699–706.

Gittes, R. F., and P. S. Russell. 1961. The male histocompatibility antigens in mouse endocrine tissues: Functional and histological evidence. *J Natl Cancer Inst* **26**:283–291.

Goldberg, E. H., E. A. Boyse, D. Bennett, M. Scheid, and E. A. Carswell. 1971. Serolological demonstration of H-Y (male) antigen on mouse sperm. *Nature (Lond)* **232**:478–480.

Goldberg, E. H., E. A. Boyse, M. Scheid, and D. Bennett. 1972. Production of H-Y antibody by female mice that fail to reject male skin. *Nature (Lond), New Biol* **238**:55–57.

Graff, R. J. 1971. The relationship between immunity and tolerance. II. *Curr Top Surg Res* 3:363–370.

Graff, R. J., and D. W. Bailey. 1973. The non-*H-2* histocompatibility loci and their antigens. *Transplant Rev* **15**:26–49.

Graff, R. J., and G. D. Snell. 1969. Histocompatibility genes of mice IX. The distribution of the alleles of the non-*H-2* histocompatibility loci. *Transplantation* **8**:861–876.

Graff, R. J., W. H. Hildemann, and G. D. Snell. 1966a. Histocompatibility genes of mice. VI. Allografts of mice congenic at various non-*H-2* histocompatibility loci. *Transplantation* **4**:425–437.

Graff, R. J., W. K. Silvers, R. E. Billingham, W. H. Hildemann, and G. D. Snell. 1966b. The cumulative effect of histocompatibility antigens. *Transplantation* **4**:605–617.

Hala, K. 1969. Syngeneic lines of chickens. III. The number of different histocompatibility loci between the lines. *Folia Biol (Praha)* **15**:136–140.

Hausman, S. J., and J. Palm. 1973. Serological detection of male-specific cell membrane antigen in the rat. *Transplant Proc* **5**:307–310.

Hildemann, W. H., and N. Cohen. 1967. Weak histoincompatibilities: Emerging immunogenetic rules and generalizations. Pages 13–20 *in* E. S. Curtoni, P. L. Mattiuz, and R. M. Tosi, eds. Histocompatibility testing 1967. Williams & Wilkins, Baltimore.

Hildemann, W. H., and R. L. Walford. 1960. Chronic skin homograft rejection in the Syrian hamster. *Ann NY Acad Sci* **87**:56–71.

Hildemann, W. H., Y. Mullen, and M. Inai. 1974. Anergy to dual H-X and H-Y antigens occurring in the same skin allografts between reciprocal $F_1$ hybrid mice. *Immunogenetics* **1**:297–303.

Hirsch, B. 1957. The influence of sex on transplantability of isologous thymic tissue in normal C57BL mice. *Transplant Bull* **4**:58.

Hoshino, K., and J. E. Moore. 1968. Sex-linked histoincompatibility of pituitary isografts in the C57BL strain of mice. *Int J Cancer* **3**:374–381.

Kallman, K. D. 1964. An estimate of the number of histocompatibility loci in the teleost *Xiphophorus maculatus*. *Genetics* **50**:583–595.

Kelly, W. D., J. M. Smith, C. Martinez, and R. A. Good. 1964. Induction of tolerance to skin grafts in mice with disrupted liver and kidney cells. *Proc Soc Exp Biol Med* **115**:8–10.

Klein, E., and O. Linder. 1961. Factorial analysis of the reactivity of C57BL females against isologous male skin grafts. *Transplant Bull* **27**:457–459.

Klein, J. 1973. List of congenic lines of mice. I. Lines with differences at alloantigen loci. *Transplantation* **15**:137–153.

Kohn, H. I. 1973. *H*-gene (histocompatibility) mutations induced by triethylenemelamine in the mouse. *Mutat Res* **20**:235–242.

Kohn, H. I., and R. W. Melvold. 1974. Spontaneous histocompatibility mutations detected by dermal grafts: Significant changes in rate over a 10-year period in the mouse *H*-system. *Mutat Res* **24**:163–169.

Koo, G. C., C. W. Stackpole, E. A. Boyse, U. Hammerling, and M. P. Lardis. 1973. Topographical location of the H-Y antigen on mouse spermatozoa by immunoelectron microscopy. *Proc Natl Acad Sci USA* **70**:1502–1505.

Lance, E. M., E. A. Boyse, S. Cooper, and E. A. Carswell. 1971. Rejection of skin allografts by irradiation chimeras: Evidence for skin-specific transplantation barrier. *Transplant Proc* **3**:864–868.

Lengerová, A. 1969. Immunogenetics of tissue transplantation. North-Holland, Amsterdam.

Melvold, R. W., and H. I. Kohn. 1975. Histocompatibility gene mutation rates: *H-2* and non-*H-2*. *Mutat Res* **27**:415–418.

Moretti, R. L., and P. B. Blair. 1966. The male histocompatibility antigen in mouse mammary tissue. I. Growth of male mammary gland in female mice. *Transplantation* **4**:596–604.

Mullen, Y., and W. H. Hildemann. 1972. X- and Y-linked transplantation antigens in rats. *Transplantation* **13**:521–529.

Scheid, M., E. A. Boyse, E. A. Carswell, and L. J. Old. 1972. Serologically demonstrable alloantigens of mouse epidermal cells. *J Exp Med* **135**:938–955.

Schlager, G., and M. M. Dickie. 1967. Spontaneous mutations and mutation rates in the house mouse. *Genetics* **57**:319–330.

Searle, A. G. 1972. Spontaneous frequencies of point mutations in mice. *Humangenetik* **16**:33–38.

Silvers, W. K., and R. E. Billingham. 1968. The *H-Y* transplantation antigen: A Y-linked or sex-influenced factor? *Nature* (*Lond*) **220**:401–403.

Silvers, W. K., and D. L. Gasser. 1973. The genetic divergence of sublines as assessed by histocompatibility testing. *Genetics* **75**:671–677.

Silvers, W. K., and S.-L. Yang. 1973. Male specific antigen: Homology in mice and rats. *Science* **181**:570–572.

Snell, G. D. 1958. Histocompatibility genes of the mouse. II. Production and analysis of isogenic resistant lines. *J Natl Cancer Inst* **21**:843–877.

Snell, G. D., and H. P. Bunker. 1965. Histocompatibility genes of mice. V. Five new histocompatibility loci identified by congenic resistant lines on a C57BL/10 background. *Transplantation* **3**:235–252.

Snell, G. D., and L. C. Stevens. 1961. Histocompatibility genes of mice. III. *H-1* and *H-4,* two histocompatibility loci in the first linkage group. *Immunology* **4**:366–379.

Snell, G. D., and J. H. Stimpfling. 1966. Genetics of tissue transplantation. Pages 457–491 *in* E. L. Green, ed. Biology of the laboratory mouse. McGraw-Hill, New York.

Snell, G. D., R. J. Graff, and M. Cherry. 1971. Histocompatibility genes of mice. XI. Evidence establishing a new histocompatibility locus, *H-12,* and a new *H-2* allele, $H\text{-}2^{bc}$. *Transplantation* **11**:525–530.

Staats, J. 1968. Standardized nomenclature for inbred strains of mice: Fourth listing. *Cancer Res* **28**:391–420.

Steinmuller, D., and J. S. Lofgreen. 1974. Differential survival of skin and heart allografts in radiation chimaeras provides further evidence for Sk histocompatibility antigen. *Nature* (*Lond*) **248**:796–797.

Vojtíšková, M., and M. Poláčková. 1966. An experimental model of the epigenetic mechanism of autotolerance using the H-Y antigen in mice. *Folia Biol* (*Praha*) **12**:137–140.

Vojtíšková, M., and M. Poláčková. 1973. Prolonged survival in syngeneic females of skin grafts from males pretreated with an antiandrogenic steroid. *Folia Biol* (*Praha*) **19**:381–384.

Wachtel, S. S., G. C. Koo, E. E. Zuckerman, U. Hammerling, M. P. Scheid, and E. A. Boyse. 1974. Serological crossreactivity between H-Y (male) antigens of mouse and man. *Proc Natl Acad Sci USA* **71**:1215–1218.

Wickstrand, C., and J. Haughton. 1974. The murine male antigen. I. Sensitive detection by the PEC transfer system. *Cell Immunol* **10**:226–237.

CHAPTER 4

# IMMUNOGENETIC METHODS



The purpose of this chapter is to provide the reader with a sufficient familiarity with serological and immunogenetic methods so that he can understand the data presented in subsequent chapters, particularly Chapters 5 and 6. Immunogenetic methods applicable to man will be described in Chapter 9. The methods summarized have been developed specifically for the mouse, or in a few cases the rat; some are not applicable to other species. The reader planning to use them should consult the original sources. We give only a limited bibliography. Some other papers on techniques will be found listed in Snell and Hummel (1966).

We shall deal exclusively with the production and testing of *alloantisera*, i.e., antisera produced by the allogeneic transfer of cells or tissues. The term *isoantisera* was formerly used in this sense, but has been dropped in transplantation studies because it implies transfer between isogeneic or genetically identical rather than transfer between allogenic or genetically disparate individuals of the same species.

## I. Titering Antisera

There are two basic methods of demonstrating alloantibodies in mice, the hemagglutination technique in which erythrocytes are the test cells and the cytotoxic test in which lymphocytes are typically the test cells. Other methods, for example, the coupling of antibody with fluorescent or electron-opaque compounds which permit their visualization under the light or electron microscopes, will be briefly mentioned in subsequent chapters.

### A. The Hemagglutination Technique

Mouse red cells do not agglutinate readily in alloantisera diluted in a saline medium unless developing agents, which augment the agglutination process, are added. The first successful hemagglutination technique for mice was developed by Gorer and Mikulska (1954). It employed dextran and human serum absorbed with mouse tissues to remove natural agglutinins. Such absorption is laborious. It is obviated in the PVP hemagglutination technique in which polyvinylpyrrolidone (PVP) in buffered saline is used as the diluent (Stimpfling, 1964). The test can be made slightly more sensitive by the addition of 0.1% bovine serum albumin (Snell *et al.*, 1971). A constant number of cells is used with serial dilutions of antiserum. Agglutination can be determined in various ways. A commonly used method is to centrifuge, and to estimate macroscopically the extent to which the sedimented pellet of red cells remains intact when subjected to gentle pipetting. The *titer* of an antiserum is the highest dilution at which unmistakable agglutination is still present. Reciprocal titers are frequently used, e.g., a titer of 1/128 is written 128.

Both the dextran and the PVP methods give good results with the rat (Palm, 1962).

### B. Cytotoxic Techniques

#### 1. Complement

Cytotoxic techniques require the use of a foreign serum as a source of complement, in addition to cells and antiserum. Rabbit and guinea pig sera are both used; rabbit serum generally yields the higher titers and is preferred (Haughton and McGehee, 1969). There are great differences in the complement from individual rabbits, and indeed from the same rabbit at different times. Often natural cytotoxins are present which have to be absorbed with mouse cells (Snell *et al.*, 1971), but sera can be found where this is not necessary. If absorption is used, the presence of EDTA helps to reduce the loss of complement activity (Boyse *et al.*, 1970).

### 2. *The Dye Exclusion Test*

The cytotoxic test, as originally developed by Gorer and O'Gorman (1956), used as the test of cell death the ability of living but not dead cells to exclude dyes. The test in essentially the original form is still widely employed (Boyse *et al.*, 1964). Lymphocytes are obtained from either lymph nodes or thymus. Because of the absence or near absence of B cells (Chapter 5, Section I,A) in the thymus, lymphocytes from the two sources may give quite different results. The proportion of dead (stained) cells is determined under the microscope. An economical microcytotoxic assay has been described (Pincus and Gordon, 1971).

### 3. *The Radioactive Chromium Release Assay*

The widely used and quantitatively precise Sanderson–Wigzell assay employs, as the measure of cytotoxicity, the absorption by living cells, and subsequent release following cell death, of $^{51}$Cr (Snell *et al.*, 1971). After incubation and centrifugation, the activity is read as the percentage of radioactivity found in the supernatant. The titer of the antiserum is usually taken as the dilution giving 50% of the release above the background value.

Several useful variants of the test have been described. Treatment of spleen cell suspensions with Tris-buffered isotonic ammonium chloride has been used to selectively lyse the red cells that otherwise interfere with the use of spleen lymphocytes in cytotoxic tests (Boyle, 1968). One advantage of using spleen is that it can be removed by a simple operation, thus keeping the donor alive. An even simpler method, effective at least for H-2 antisera, is to absorb the antiserum with washed peripheral blood cells and measure the residual activity by chromium release (David and Shreffler, 1972). A method for the preparation of dermal cell suspensions by the trypsinization of tail skin permits the extension of the chromium release assay to an entirely different category of cells (Cooper and Lance, 1971).

## II. The Production of Antisera

### A. Immunization and Bleeding

There are so many possible variations in immunization schedules that it is impossible, practically speaking, to scientifically select the ideal schedule. A great variety of schedules give adequate results. Quite probably the efficacy of a schedule depends on the antigen employed and the test used to demonstrate antibody. A method found satisfactory at The Jackson Laboratory for the production of alloantisera in mice uses injections of thymus cells (one 4-week-old donor per 25 recipients) on days 0 and 40, and injections of thymus, spleen, and submaxillary gland (one donor per 10 recipients) on days 47 and 54. Cell suspensions are prepared in the cytosieve (see Chapter 2, Section IV). Injections are intraperitoneal. Mice are bled on days 61 and 64, then given booster injections and bled twice on alternate weeks (Snell *et al.*, 1973). The long interval between first and second injections was chosen because of evidence that the priming influence of an initial injection continues to rise for about 6 weeks before leveling off (e.g., Fecsik *et al.*, 1964). The submaxillary gland was included because it is a good source of H-2 antigen. Subsequent studies suggest that it may contribute a plasma cell stimulating factor (Naughton *et al.*, 1969), but the actual utility of this, if any, has not been determined.

Barth *et al.* (1965) analyzed the antibody classes produced as a result of various immunization schedules and found substantial differences. A long interval between first and second injections was favorable to the production of IgG1 ($7S\gamma_1$). There are also strain differences. Strain C57BL/6 is particularly prone to the formation of IgM.

Bleeding is usually accomplished either from the lateral tail veins (Stimpfling *et al.*, 1964) or from the orbital sinus (Stone, 1954). Ascitic fluid, which can be obtained from mice in large quantities, contains antibody (Lieberman *et al.*, 1962), but we have found it to be, in several respects, a less satisfactory source than serum.

### B. Definitions

We shall use the term *antigen* to mean the whole antigen molecule. To function as an *alloantigen*, an antigen must exist in at least two alternative or allelic forms. It is only because of the existence of multiple forms that it is possible to expose individuals of the donor's own species to the substance in a foreign and hence antigenic form. To have alternative forms, an antigen must have a *variable region* or regions. It is this variable region which is directly involved in the antigen–antibody reaction, and which we may therefore call the *antigenic site.*

One of the basic units in immunogenetic thinking is the concept of *specificity*. Specificities, like the species of the systematist, are so variable as to lack sharp boundaries. This makes definition difficult. They are also of two complementary kinds. We may say, as an approximation, that an *antigen specificity* means any allelic form of a reactive site with which a given antibody combines. An *antibody specificity* means the antibody combining region reactive with a given antigen specificity. These are definitions of specificity in terms of physical entities. There is also, as we shall see later, an operational definition of specificity. We do not know to what extent the two meanings are really the same.

Antigens are designated by the same symbols as the loci, genes, or alleles that determine them, except that they are set in Roman type rather than italics. Genetic combinations used in producing antisera are also set in Roman type, e.g., H-$2^{a}$ anti-H-$2^{b}$. Specificities are designated by numbers. When appropriate, these may be appended to a gene symbol (e.g., 8 or H-2.8).

## C. Methods of Approximating Monospecificity

### 1. *Complexity of Antisera*

One of the important requirements in immunogenetic analysis is the achievement of something approximating monospecificity in test antisera, or at least of a test situation where only one specificity is revealed. A good deal of effort in immunogenetic studies is devoted to this goal. Let us consider the problems involved.

If individual, A, is immunized with tissues from unrelated individual, B, the resulting A anti-B serum will contain a diversity of antibodies. As immunization is continued, the spectrum of antibodies will change. Some of the early antibodies will fade out, others will appear. Four sources of diversity can be distinguished: (1) There are many alloantigens and, potentially, a corresponding number of antibodies. If donor and host differ at *H-2*, anti-H-2 is sure to be present, but other disparities can lead to other antibodies, although these are usually slower in appearing and harder to demonstrate. Since the demonstration of diverse alloantigens is where all immunogenetics begins, the first job of the immunogeneticist is to analyze antibody diversity arising from this source. (2) Some alloantigens probably have more than one variable region, and hence more than one potentially reactive site. Of course, every reactive site can engender its own antibodies. This source of atibody multiplicity is harder to pin down than source (1), but it is theoretically important and is receiving increasing attention. (3) There can be multiple antibodies reactive with a single specificity, distinguishable on the basis of the affinity with which they combine. Antibodies with high affinity tend to appear late in the immunization procedure and to show more cross-reaction than antibodies with low affinity (Gershon and Kondo, 1972; Underdown and Eisen, 1971). The immunogeneticist is not often concerned with this source of antibody diversity unless he is dealing with a situation where cross-reactions occur not only within specificities but between specificities or between antigens. Such situations are untidy and there is a tendency to sweep them under the carpet, but they are probably quite common, and for any real understanding of alloimmune reactions they have to be understood. (4) Antibodies belonging to any one of the different antibody classes (IgM, IgG, etc.) may form against a single antigenic site. Usually several such classes are present in any one antiserum. This, for the immunogeneticist, is the least important source of antibody diversity. However, if he is using a test involving complement, his results can be distorted by a high proportion of noncomplement-binding antibody (Miller and DeWitt, 1972).

To deal with source (1) of antibody variability, the desideratum is an antiserum reactive with a single antigen. To deal with source (2), the desideratum is an antiserum reactive with a single specificity. Several measures may be used to reach or approximate these desired states.

### 2. *Use of Inbred Strains*

Where inbred strains are available, it is possible to draw on reservoirs of genetically uniform individuals that, at least in the case of mice, have been extensively typed for alloantigen-determining genes. This makes it possible to select recipient–donor combinations with an advanced knowledge, not available in species where inbred lines are lacking, of the antibodies that will be formed. Even with inbred strains, however, there is an element of unpredictability, since there is a surprising degree of nongenetic individual variation in the immune response. One might expect that if pools of antiserum from a number of individuals are used, these individual variations would average out. This is not always the case, however. Of course different bleedings can be quite different. But also different pools produced under presumably identical conditions can have differences in titer and occasionally differences in the specificities present (G. D. Snell and M. Cherry, unpublished observations). The reasons for this are not fully understood; however, some of the variation in antibody response may be due to the generation of a part of the diversity of each individual's armament of antibody-producing cell clones through a random mutational process and some to seemingly minor environmental factors, such as order of injection, to which mice are surprisingly susceptible (McArthur *et al.,* 1971).

### 3. *Use of Congenic Strains*

The most important single agent in the approximation of monospecificity in alloantisera in mice is the congenic strain (see Chapter 2, Section II). If donor and recipient have been so contrived as to differ at a single alloantigen-determining locus, the resulting antiserum of necessity can react only with the end product of that one locus. This property of congenic strains was promptly exploited in the serological analysis of *H-2* (Hoecker *et al.,* 1954).

Congenic strains are now available which differ at many alloantigen-determining loci, and they are being put to work in the production of simplified antisera. There is one limitation in their use. Evidence is accumulating that when donor–recipient combinations approach a state of unitary alloantigenic disparity, they become poor antibody procedures. Immune response genes (Chapter 7) enter into this situation, but even in the presence of favorable alleles at immune response loci, antibody may be difficult to obtain. Even in the case of the notably "strong" *H-2K* locus, congenic lines derived by mutation may not yield antibody. This difficulty in getting antibody in truly monospecific combinations may be attributable to the need for cell collaboration in the immune response and hence for the presence of more than one "handle" that the cells can get hold of. The two reactive sites can be on the same molecule or apparently in some cases on different molecules on the same cell (Schierman and McBride, 1972; Stimpfling and McBroom, 1971).

### 4. *Use of Hybrid Recipients*

While the use of congenic strains as donor–recipient pairs in the production of antisera accomplishes a marked and predictable simplification in the resulting antibody, it still often falls far short of achieving monospecificity. This is particularly true in the case of *H-2* and even of the subunits of *H-2* (*H-2K* and *H-2D*) when studied separately. This is partly due to the presence of multiple reactive sites and partly due to differences in the cross-reactivity of antibodies generated against the same site [factors (2) and (3), Section II,C,1].

This problem can be solved in considerable part by the use of $F_1$ hybrids as recipients. When properly selected, each parent will possess, and therefore block the formation of antibodies against, certain specificities lacking in the other parent but present in the donor. Thus a monospecific (or approximately monospecific) anti-H-2.9 can be produced

TABLE 4.1
THE USE OF A HYBRID RECIPIENT TO YIELD A MONOSPECIFIC ANTI-H-2.9

| | *H-2* type | Specificities present | | | | | | | | | | | |
|---|---|---|---|---|---|---|---|---|---|---|---|---|---|
| Recipient parent 1 | *H-2*$^d$ | 3 | 4 | | | 8 | | 13 | | 27 | 28 | 29 | 31 |
| Recipient parent 2 | *H-2*$^s$ | 3 | | 5 | 7 | | | | 19 | | 28 | | |
| $F_1$ | | 3 | 4 | 5 | 7 | 8 | | 13 | 19 | 27 | 28 | 29 | 31 |
| Donor | *H-2*$^f$ | | | | 7 | 8 | 9 | | | 27 | | | |
| Resulting antibody | | | | | | | 9 | | | | | | |

by making a B10.D2 (*H-2*$^d$) $\times$ A.SW (*H-2*$^s$) anti-B10.M (*H-2*$^f$) as shown in Table 4.1.

The use of hybrid recipients offers additional advantages. The antibody response is often better (Stimpfling and Pandis, 1969), and the yield of serum is higher.

### 5. *Absorption*

Another method used in the simplification of complex antisera is *absorption.* This can be accomplished by mixing tissues of the absorbing strain with the antiserum to be absorbed, incubating, and removing the absorbing cells and bound antibody by centrifugation. Often more than one absorption is necessary for complete removal of the unwanted antibody. Tissues commonly used for absorption in mice are the lymphoid organs and the liver. An alternative method, very effective in mice, is *in vivo* absorption (Amos, 1955). The antiserum is injected intraperitoneally, about 0.3 ml per mouse, and the mouse bled 2 to 24 hours later. Absorption of antibodies reactive with recipient antigens is usually complete. Unabsorbed antibodies are diluted about 1 in 10 or 1 in 12, but this is a perfectly acceptable dilution for high titered antisera. For quantitating antigens, serial dilutions of absorbing cells or other absorbing material can be used (Snell *et al.*, 1971).

Absorbing an A anti-B with strain C has exactly the same effect on the end product as making an (A $\times$ C) anti-B. In either case, antibodies reactive with the antigens of both A and C are excluded. The use of the hybrid is the simpler procedure. However, when the use of a hybrid recipient still yields a polyspecific antiserum, absorption is the only alternative for simplification.

### 6. *The Use of Diverse Test Strains*

Even when an antiserum is not monospecific, a test system can often be set up which, in effect, reveals only antibodies of one specificity.

This is accomplished by taking test cells from strains not used as recipient, donor, or absorber. Thus if an (A × B) anti-C contains two antibodies, an anti-x and an anti-y, a test against cells of strain D that is x+, y−, is a test for anti-x only, and a test against C following absorption with D is a test for anti-y only. A test against the donor, C, without absorption would not resolve the two antibodies. Tests of this sort can be used to compare different antisera or the consequences of absorbing one antiserum with different strains.

## III. Genetic Tests

### A. Determination of Locus

For the immunogeneticist, one of the major objectives in the study of alloantisera is the identification of alloantigen-determining loci. Three basic methods are available.

#### 1. *Use of Congenic Lines*

If the antiserum under study is made with a congenic pair whose defining alloantigen-determining locus is already known, the question as to the locus responsible for the alloantigenic activity is already answered. An unanalyzed congenic pair is no better in this respect than any noncongenic recipient–donor combination. Occasionally an antibody of unknown genetic determination can be run down by testing against congenic pairs of known alloantigenic disparity. If one member of the pair reacts and the other does not, the antibody must be a product of the defining alloantigen. This sort of test is especially indicated where strains A.B(1), A.B(2), A.B(3), etc., are available for testing an A anti-B or a B anti-A. This test can, of course, be complicated by the presence in a congenic strain of a passenger alloantigenic disparity.

#### 2. *Use of Recombinant Inbred Strains*

The utility of recombinant inbred (RI) strains as a tool for the identification of histocompatibility loci has already been discussed (Chapter 2, Section III,D). RI strains are quite as effective in the identification of serologically studied loci, and for exactly the same reasons. The only requirement for their use with a particular antiserum is that, of the two strains from which the RI lines are derived, one should be positive with the antiserum, and the other should be negative. Some of the details of the methods employed, and the limitations of these methods, will become apparent when we discuss actual cases in Chapter 5.

### 3. *Use of Segregating Generations*

If appropriate RI strains are not available, or if they fail to give the critical information, recourse must be had to serotyping of $F_2$ or backcross generations. If the unknown antibody gives a reaction pattern different than that of a known antibody, it must be determined by a different locus.

## B. Determination of Specificity

In Section II,B we gave definitions of specificity in terms of antigen and antibody structure. These definitions point to characteristics of antigen and antibody of basic importance for an understanding of the immunogenetics of alloantigens. They indicate what we would like to know, but at present can only conceptualize inferentially. The firm knowledge that we have from alloimmune tests is that certain antisera react with certain strains and not with others. This is the basis for the *operational definition of specificity.*

If possible, we start with an *operationally monospecific antiserum,* i.e., an antiserum that cannot be further split by absorption. It reacts with certain strains, and absorption with any one of these strains clears it for all the others. A particular specificity is thereby identified. Strains that react possess the specificity, strains that do not lack it. In more general terms, a specificity, operationally defined, is a property common to those strains that react positively with a presumed monospecific antiserum. If the specificity is x, the antiserum is an anti-x. And any other antiserum that gives the same strain distribution pattern of positive reactions we assume to be also an anti-x.

An example of specificities thus defined is given in Table 4.2, which summarizes the information about H-2 specificities available in 1954. Each vertical column represents results with a different antibody. Since the strain distribution of positive reactions is different for each antibody, each antibody defines a different specificity. Specificity 2 is present only in strain B6 (of the strains included in the table), 3 in all strains but B6, 4 in strains A and DBA/2, etc.

In practice, it is often impossible to obtain even an operationally monospecific antiserum. Thus, as can be seen from Table 4.2, if anti-3 and anti-4 are both present in the same antiserum, the 4 cannot be removed without removing the 3. To accomplish this would require a strain which is 4-positive and 3-negative, and no such strain is known. Such situations are common. To deal with them, we must resort to the device outlined in Section II,C,6. Thus, to type for 3 with an anti-3,4 we resort to a test based on absorption. If, after absorption with the

TABLE 4.2
*H-2* CHART[a]

| Strain | Specificities 2 | 3 | 4 | 5 | 11 | 16 | 17 | 19 |
|---|---|---|---|---|---|---|---|---|
| A | — | 3 | 4 | 5 | 11 | — | — | — |
| B6 | 2 | — | — | 5 | — | — | — | — |
| DBA/2 | — | 3 | 4 | — | — | — | — | — |
| C3H | — | 3 | — | 5 | 11 | — | — | — |
| P | — | 3 | — | 5 | — | 16 | — | — |
| DBA/1 | — | 3 | — | 5 | — | — | 17 | — |
| A.SW | — | 3 | — | 5 | — | — | — | 19 |

[a] Data of Hoecker *et al.* (1954).

strain to be typed, the antiserum no longer reacts with a 3-positive 4-negative test strain, e.g., A.SW, we type it as possessing 3.

One other complication frequently encountered in both *H-2* and HLA serology requires mention. Strains sometimes absorb an antibody, and hence must be regarded as positive, even though they do not react with the antibody by direct hemagglutination or direct cytotoxicity. In HLA serology, this situation is referred to as CYNAP (cytotoxic negative, absorption positive). This is an added reason why, in serotyping, a test by absorption is often mandatory.

## REFERENCES

Amos, D. B. 1955. The persistance of mouse iso-antibodies *in vivo*. *Br J Cancer* **9**:216–221.

Barth, W. F., C. L. McLaughlin, and J. L. Fahey. 1965. The immunoglobulins of mice. VI. Response to immunization. *J Immunol* **95**:781–790.

Boyle, W. 1968. An extension of the $^{51}$Cr-release assay for the estimation of mouse cytotoxins. *Transplantation* **6**:761–764.

Boyse, E. A., L. J. Old, and I. Chouroulinkov. 1964. Cytotoxic test for the demonstration of mouse antibody. *Methods Med Res* **10**:39–47.

Boyse, E. A., L. Hubbard, H. E. Stockert, and M. E. Lamm. 1970. Improved complementation in the cytotoxic test. *Transplantation* **10**:446–449.

Cooper, S., and E. M. Lance. 1971. A serological method for detecting the surface antigens of epidermal cells. *Transplantation* **11**:108–110.

David, C. S., and D. C. Shreffler. 1972. Adaptation of the $^{51}$Cr cytotoxic assay for rapid *H-2* classifications on peripheral blood cells. *Transplantation* **13**:414–420.

Fecsik, A. I., W. T. Butler, and A. H. Coons. 1964. Studies on antibody production. XI. Variation in the secondary response as a function of the length of the interval between two antigenic stimuli. *J Exp Med* **120**:1040–1049.

Gershon, R. K., and K. Kondo. 1972. Degeneracy of the immune response to sheep red cells. *Immunology* **23**:321–334.

Gorer, P. A., and Z. B. Mikulska. 1954. The antibody response to tumor inoculation. Improved methods of antibody detection. *Cancer Res* **14**:651–655.

Gorer, P. A., and P. O'Gorman. 1956. The cytotoxic activity of isoantibodies in mice. *Transplant Bull* **3**:142–143.

Haughton, G., and M. P. McGehee. 1969. Cytolysis of mouse lymph node cells by alloantibody: A comparison of guinea pig and rabbit complements. *Immunology* **16**:447–461.

Hoecker, G., S. Counce, and P. Smith. 1954. The antigens determined by the *H-2* locus: A Rhesus-like system in the mouse. *Proc Natl Acad Sci USA* **40**:1040–1051.

Lieberman, R., N. Mantel, W. Humphrey, Jr., and J. G. Blakely. 1962. Studies of antibodies in ascitic fluid of individual mice. *Proc Soc Exp Biol Med* **110**:897–903.

McArthur, J. N., P. D. Dawkins, and M. J. H. Smith. 1971. Of mice and means. *Nature* (*London*) **229**:66.

Miller, C., and C. DeWitt. 1972. Rat alloantibody responses against strong and weak histocompatibility antigens. *J Immunol* **109**:919–926.

Naughton, M. A., J. Koch, H. Hoffman, V. Bender, H. Hagopian, and E. Hamilton. 1969. Isolation and activity of a thymocyte-transforming factor from the mouse submaxillary gland. *Exp Cell Res* **57**:95–103.

Palm, J. 1962. Current status of blood groups in rats. *Ann NY Acad Sci* **97**:57–68.

Pincus, J. H., and R. O. Gordon. 1971. A microsasay for the detection of murine H-2 antigens. *Transplantation* **12**:509–513.

Schierman, L. W., and R. A. McBride. 1972. Immune response to minor histocompatibility antigens. Augmentation by major histocompatibility antigens. *Transplantation* **13**:97–100.

Snell, G. D., and K. P. Hummel. 1966. Bibliography of techniques. Pages 655–661 *in* E. L. Green, ed. Biology of the laboratory mouse. McGraw-Hill, New York.

Snell, G. D., P. Démant, and M. Cherry. 1971. Hemagglutination and cytotoxic studies of *H-2*. I. H-2.1 and related specificities in the EK crossover regions. *Transplantation* **11**:210–237.

Snell, G. D., M. Cherry, I. F. C. McKenzie, and D. W. Bailey. 1973. *Ly-4,* a new locus determining a lymphocyte cell-surface alloantigen in mice. *Proc Natl Acad Sci USA* **70**:1108–1111.

Stimpfling, J. H. 1964. Methods for the detection of hemagglutinins in mouse isoantisera. *Methods Med Res* **10**:22–26.

Stimpfling, J. H., and C. R. McBroom. 1971. The effect of *H-2* on the humoral antibody response to a non-H-2 blood group antigen. *Transplantation* **11**:87–89.

Stimpfling J. H., and D. E. Pandis. 1969. The effect of heterozygosity on the humoral antibody response in mice. *Folia Biol* (*Praha*) **15**:233–238.

Stimpfling, J. H., E. A. Boyse, and R. Mishell. 1964. The preparation of isoantisera in laboratory mice. *Methods Med Res* **10**:18–21.

Stone, S. H. 1954. Method for obtaining venous blood from the orbital sinus of the rat or mouse. *Science* **119**:100.

Underdown, B. J., and H. N. Eisen. 1971. Cross-reactions between 2,4-dinitrophenyl and 5-acetouracil groups. *J Immunol* **106**:1431–1140.

CHAPTER 5

# SEROLOGICALLY DEMONSTRATED MEMBRANE ALLOANTIGENS OF MICE



The number of membrane alloantigens of mice detected by serological techniques is still small compared to the number of known histocompatibility (H) alloantigens, but this group is rapidly expanding. It includes erythrocyte (blood group) alloantigens demonstrated by hemagglutination, lymphocyte alloantigens demonstrated by lymphocytotoxicity, and a small but potentially important group found on a diversity of other cells by cytotoxic techniques. Since the common property of all these alloantigens, including, in all probability, the histocompatibility alloantigens, is their presence in or on the cell membrane where they are vulnerable to antibodies and/or immune effector cells, we may refer to them as *cell membrane alloantigens,* and the loci which determine them as *cell membrane alloantigen determining* or *CMAD loci.* In this chapter we shall deal with the serologically demonstrated CMAD loci of mice, but not, except for purposes of comparison, with *H* loci or the CMAD loci in the *H-2* complex. These are covered in Chapters 3 and 6. Similar loci in rats will be noted where comparisons are of interest. Information on *Ir* loci, which influence the immune response to cell membrane alloantigens, will be found in Chapter 7.

Rules for the designation of CMAD loci are discussed in Snell (1971). This paper also lists revised symbols and the symbols they replace. In general, loci are designated by symbols in the form *Ea-1, Ea-2* (erythrocyte alloantigen loci) or *Ly-1, Ly-2* (lymphocyte alloantigen loci). Alleles are designated by the addition of superscript letters, e.g., $Ea\text{-}1^a$, $Ea\text{-}1^b$, and specificities by appending numbers, e.g., Ly-1.1, Ly-1.2. The usual convention is to associate specificity 1 with allele *a,* specificity 2 with allele *b.* Absence of reactivity with any known antibody may be indicated by a minus (—). Symbols used to represent genes are distinguished from the same symbols used to represent antigens or specificities by being set in italics.

## I. Erythrocyte and Lymphocyte Alloantigens of Mice

The known blood group loci and a partial strain distribution of alleles of these loci are shown in Table 5.1. For the data in this and other tables in this chapter we are indebted to sources too numerous to list. Linkages, where known, are indicated in Fig. 3.2. Further details will be found in Snell (1971), Snell and Cherry (1972), and Staats (1972).

One locus listed in Table 5.1, because of its unique properties, deserves special mention. Rubinstein *et al.* (1974) have described a locus, *Eam,* in mice which determines electrophoretic mobility and agglutinability of erythrocytes. There appear to be only two alleles, $Eam^h$ (high) and $Eam^l$ (low). This interesting finding confirms and explains strain differences in the hemagglutination reaction which have been suspected for a long time.

Because lymphocytes can be obtained in substantial numbers as single-cell suspensions, they are a favorable material for the study of cell surface alloantigens. Excluding the *H-2* complex alloantigens, nine such alloantigens are now known on the lymphocytes of mice, and the number is certain to expand.

TABLE 5.1
STRAIN DISTRIBUTION OF KNOWN SPECIFICITIES OF MURINE ERYTHROCYTE ALLOANTIGENS AND OF THE Eam POLYMORPHISM[a]

| | Locus | | | | | | | |
|---|---|---|---|---|---|---|---|---|
| Strain | *Ea-1* | *Ea-2* | *Ea-3* | *Ea-4* | *Ea-5* | *Ea-6* | *Ea-7* | *Eam* |
| C57BL/10 | —[b] | 2 | —[c] | 2 | —[c] | 1 | 2 | *l* |
| C57L | | 2 | 1 | 1 | | | 2 | *l* |
| A | | 2 | — | 1 | 1 | 1 | 2 | *h* |
| BALB/c | | 2 | — | 1 | | 2 | 2 | *l* |
| SJL | | 2 | | 1 | | | 2 | *h* |
| 129 | | 2 | | 1 | 1 | 1 | — | *h* |
| DBA/2 | — | 2 | | 1 | — | 2 | 2 | *h* |
| C3H/He | — | 2 | — | 1 | — | 1 | — | *h* |
| AKR/J | | 2 | | 1 | | 1 | 2 | *h* |
| RF/J | | 1 | | 1 | — | 2 | 2 | *l* |

[a] The data in Table 5.1 are taken in part from uncited sources as well as from sources cited in the text.

[b] All laboratory stocks tested for *Ea-1* have null allele *Ea-1*$^0$. Alleles *Ea-1*$^a$ and *Ea-1*$^b$ are found only in wild populations.

[c] Antisera identifying *Ea-3* and *Ea-5* have each been reported from only one laboratory.

Because one of the important properties of the lymphocyte alloantigens is their unequal representation on the different classes of lymphocytes, we need, before discussing them, to describe these classes. We give here only a bare outline, without documentation. Further details will be found in Chapter 13.

### A. CLASSES OF LYMPHOCYTES

The two major classes of lymphocytes are bone marrow-derived or *B lymphocytes* and thymus-derived or *T lymphocytes.* T lymphocytes originate in the bone marrow, but reach functional maturity only after residence in the thymus. The standard marker for B cells is easily demonstrable immunoglobulin bound to the cell surface. Plasma cells, which produce and shed antibody, are derived from B cells.

T cells can be divided into two functional classes. *T helper* cells make up much of the circulating pool of lymphocytes. They are called helper cells because they collaborate with B cells in the secondary antibody response to many antigens. *T effector cells* can cause specific cytotoxic destruction of allogeneic target cells. They play a major role in graft rejection.

We now turn to a description of the individual lymphocyte alloantigens. We shall consider first three antigens, Thy-1, Tla, and $G_{IX}$, which are characteristic of T lymphocytes.

## B. Thy-1 or $\theta$

### 1. *Genetics*

The Thy-1 or $\theta$ alloantigen of mice, now recognized as the standard marker for T cells, was discovered by Reif and Allen (1964). Reciprocal antisera prepared in strains AKR and C3H by the injection of thymocytes had high cytotoxic titers for thymocytes of the donor strain. Since AKR and C3H are both $H\text{-}2^k$, an H-2 antibody was ruled out. When tested against a panel of inbred strains, only AKR and RF were positive with the C3H anti-AKR; all other strains were negative with this antiserum but positive with the AKR anti-C3H.

In subsequent studies this antigen was shown to be determined by a single locus, *Thy-1*. This locus symbol replaces $\theta$, the symbol originally used by Reif and Allen. Strain AKR is assigned the $Thy\text{-}1^a$ allele and the Thy-1.1 specificity, strain C3H the $Thy\text{-}1^b$ allele and the Thy-1.2 specificity (Table 5.2) (Snell and Cherry, 1972). *Thy-1* has been located in chromosome 9 (Itakura *et al.*, 1972) (Fig. 3.2).

### 2. *Tissue Distribution*

Reif and Allen (1964) made their anti-Thy-1 antisera by the injection of thymus cell suspensions, and found that the antisera reacted with and were absorbed by thymus lymphocytes to a much greater degree than by node or spleen lymphocytes. They concluded that the Thy-1 antigen is specific for lymphocytes of thymic origin. This has been confirmed in numerous studies. Thus Raff and Wortis (1970) found a near absence of Thy-1-bearing lymphocytes in *nude* mice which have congenital absence of the thymus. Thy-1 can be induced in a fraction of presumably predetermined bone marrow cells by minute quantities of a thymic hormone, *thymin* (Basch and Goldstein, 1974). Some nonspecific agents, e.g., poly(AU), can cause the same transformation (Scheid *et al.*, 1972). Thymus derived lymphocytes cultured *in vitro* progressively lose their Thy-1, but retain helper cell activity (Pierce, 1973).

Reif and Allen (1964) tested the ability of various tissues other than the lymphoid tissues to bind anti-Thy-1 and found a high absorptive capacity in brain. Almost no Thy-1 antigen was present in the brain of newborn mice, but the level rose rapidly during the first two postnatal weeks and reached adult level at about 40 days (Reif and Allen, 1966). The antigen occurs in both white and gray matter, but is most easily

TABLE 5.2
STRAIN DISTRIBUTION OF KNOWN SPECIFICITIES OF CELL SURFACE ALLOANTIGENS OF MURINE LYMPHOCYTES AND LYMPHOID-DERIVED CELLS[a]

| Strain | Locus | | | | | | | | | | |
|---|---|---|---|---|---|---|---|---|---|---|---|
| | *Thy-1* | *Tla* | *Ly-1* | *Ly-2,3* | *Ly-4* | *Ly-5* | *Ly-6* | *Ly-7* | *Pca-1* | *Mph-1* | *Mls* |
| C57BL/10 | 2 | — | 2 | 2,2 | 2 | 1 | + | − | − | + | *b* |
| C57L | 2 | — | 2 | 2,2 | 2 | 1 | + | + | | | *b* |
| A | 2 | 1,2,3 | 2 | 2,2 | 1 | 1 | − | + | + | + | *c* |
| BALB/c | 2 | 2 | 2 | 2,2 | 1 | 1 | − | + | + | + | *b* |
| SJL | 2 | 1,2,3 | 2 | 2,2 | ? | 2 | + | + | + | | |
| 129 | 2 | 2 | 2 | 2,2 | 1 | 1 | + | + | − | + | |
| DBA/2 | 2 | 2 | 1 | 1,2 | 1 | 1 | +? | + | − | + | *a* |
| C3H/He | 2 | — | 1 | 1,2 | 1 | 1 | − | ? | + | + | *c* |
| I/St | 2 | — | 2 | 1,2 | | 1 | | | − | − | |
| AKR/J | 1 | — | 2 | 1,1 | ? | 1 | + | + | + | + | *a* |
| RF/J | 1 | — | 2 | 1,1 | 1 | 1 | + | + | + | + | |

[a] The data in Table 5.2 are taken in part from uncited sources as well as from sources cited in the text.

detected in myelinated areas (Moore *et al.*, 1971). This antigen has also been found in epidermal cells, mammary glands, and tumors of mammary gland origin (John *et al.*, 1972; Scheid *et al.*, 1972; Hilgers *et al.*, 1975). Despite its presence on epidermal cells, skin grafts with a Thy-1 disparity are rejected very weakly if at all.

### 3. *Anti-Thy-1 Antisera*

While strains AKR and C3*H*, originally used by Reif and Allen (1964) in the production of anti-Thy-1, are both *H-2*$^{k}$, they are not congenic. Hence antisera made in these strains may be expected to have multiple non-H-2 antibodies. And indeed, contaminants are present (see, e.g., Baird *et al.*, 1971). Since strains congenic for *Thy-1* are now available (Klein, 1973), their use for antiserum production is recommended. Titers are increased by the use of an appropriate hybrid for the recipient.

### 4. *The Rat Homolog of Thy-1*

Micheel *et al.* (1973) and Douglas (1972) have shown that brain and thymocytes of rats possess an antigen which reacts with anti-Thy-1.1. The reciprocal antigen was not found. However, Lubaroff (1973) was able to prepare a thymus-specific alloantibody in rats of the black-hooded (BH) strain. Only further tests can show whether this corresponds to the mouse anti-Thy-1.

## C. The Thymus-Leukemia Alloantigen (TL or Tla)

*Tla* is a locus, closely linked to *H-2* (Fig. 3.2), which determines an alloantigen of thymus lymphocytes and of thymus-derived leukemias. It has the unusual property that the antigen may be expressed on leukemias of normally negative strains. Also, as expressed on leukemias, it is sometimes serologically distinct from the antigen on normal thymocytes. It is because of these properties that it was called the thymus-leukemia antigen (Old *et al.*, 1963; Boyse *et al.*, 1969). The antigen is usually designated by the symbol TL, but we shall use Tla, in conformity with the rule that gene and antigen have the same symbol, except that the antigen symbol is not italicized.

There are four alleles and four specificities. Table 5.3 gives the expression of the various specificities in the different alleles, with separate listings for normal thymocytes and thymus-derived leukemias, since the expression is different on the two cells types. The *Tla*$^{b}$ allele is serologically unexpressed on normal thymocytes, but is manifest on some leukemias, the specificities which are then present being 1, 2, and 4. Although specificities 1 and 2 are associated only with the *Tla*$^{a}$ allele on normal cells, they occur on all Tla-positive leukemias. Specificity 4 occurs only

TABLE 5.3
ALLELES AND SPECIFICITIES OF THE *Tla* LOCUS[a]

| Allele | Type strain | Serologically demonstrable specificities: Of normal thymocytes | Of positive leukemias |
|---|---|---|---|
| *Tla*[a] | A | 1 2 3 | 1 2 3 |
| *Tla*[b] | C57BL/6 | — | 1 2 4 |
| *Tla*[c] | DBA/2 | 2 | 1 2 4 |
| *Tla*[d] | BALB/c | 2 | 1 2 |

[a] From Boyse *et al.* (1969).

on leukemias. A partial strain distribution of the different serotypes is given in Table 5.2.

Presumably the leukemogenic virus responsible for the transformation of lymphocytes to the leukemic form has something to do with the accompanying changes in the antigen structure, but the mechanisms involved have not been elucidated (Boyse *et al.*, 1969).

The Tla antigen, unlike the Thy-1 antigen, does not persist on thymic lymphocytes after they leave the thymus. Probably it disappears before emigration. Thymic cell preparations introduced into the bloodstream lose demonstrable Tla within 24 hours (Lance *et al.*, 1971). Also unlike Thy-1, Tla is not known to occur on any cell types other than thymocytes. The *Tla* locus is associated with a histocompatibility effect, but this is probably due to linked *H* loci (Chapter 3).

The original anti-Tla antisera were produced by the inoculation of leukemias, but thymus injections are also effective. However, Tla.4, since it is limited to leukemic cells, can be produced only against these cells. Tla.2 tends to be weak. Contrary to what might be expected, injection of lymphoid cells other than thymocytes, although they are Tla-negative, will induce anti-Tla. This, however, is contingent on the presence of an intact thymus. Presumbaly the thymus acts by release of a Tla-inducer (Boyse *et al.*, 1969; Old *et al.*, 1968; Komuro *et al.*, 1973).

The Tla antigen shows some interesting relationships to H-2, and particularly to H-2D. The *H-2K*, *H-2D*, and *Tla* loci are in one small chromosome region, arranged in the order named. Chemically, the H-2 and the Tla antigens are similar (Chapter 11). Tests of the blocking action of different antibodies sequentially absorbed, indicate that Tla and H-2D are close together on the cell surface (Boyse *et al.*, 1968b). The amount of demonstrable H-2D is substantially greater in the presence of the null *Tla*$^b$ allele than in the presence of *Tla*$^a$. There are also interactions of *Tla* alleles with each other not seen with most loci. Thus the heterozygote *Tla*$^a$/*Tla*$^c$, though it carries only one allele (*Tla*$^a$) specifying Tla.1 and Tla.3, has as much 1 and 3 demonstrable on the cell surface as the *Tla*$^a$/*Tla*$^a$ homozygote (Boyse *et al.*, 1968c). These phenomena suggest interesting interactions of chemically, sterically and perhaps phylogenetically related membrane components, but the mechanisms involved remain obscure.

## D. The $G_{IX}$ Antigen

A cell surface antigen, $G_{IX}$, of mouse thymocytes and leukemias has, seemingly, the unusual property of being not only a product of a locus or loci within the mouse genome, but of being identical with, or with part of, an envelope glycoprotein, gp69/71, of a murine RNA leukemia virus. Genetic studies of $G_{IX}$ reveal a number of complexities not easily interpreted.

$G_{IX}$ is identified by an antiserum prepared in rats against a rat leukemia induced by MuLV, a mouse leukemia virus. Different mouse strains react at different levels with this antiserum. A cross between high-reacting strain 129 and low-reacting strain B indicated a two-gene determination. The postulated loci were designated *Gv-1* and *Gv-2*. Linkage studies placed *Gv-1* in chromosome 17 at a distance from *H-2D* of 36 crossover units. However, when different stocks were used, *Gv-1* appeared to be at the distal end of chromosome 4. *Gv-2* was located at the distal end of chromosome 7 (Fig. 3.2).

One explanation that has been proposed for these odd results is that the *Gv-1* locus is an example of a viral gene that is reverse-transcribed into the mouse genome. The seemingly different locations of *Gv-1* in different stocks would then be explained as the result of incorporation of the same viral gene in chromosome 4 in one stock and chromosome 17 in another. Two "mutations" that have converted the $G_{IX}$-negative stocks C57BL/6 and C57BR/cd to a $G_{IX}$-positive genotype are perhaps examples of the postulated incorporation of the viral genome. (Stockert *et al.*, 1971, 1975; Strand *et al.*, 1974; Obata *et al.*, 1975; F. Lilly, personal communication.)

## E. Some Additional Alloantigens of T Cells

Besides the anti-Thy-1 and anti-Tla antibodies, several other alloantibodies are known which react specifically with thymus-derived lymphocytes (T cells). Like anti-Thy-1 but unlike anti-Tla, they react with thymocytes that have left the thymus, and hence with a proportion of node and spleen cells. As would be expected with antigens confined to T cells, reactivity is lacking in neonatally thymectomized mice. However, as is also true of both Thy-1 and Tla, reactivity can be specifically induced in some non-thymus-processed cells by a thymic hormone and nonspecifically induced by some other substances. (Boyse *et al.*, 1968a; Boyse *et al.*, 1971; Boyse and Bennett, 1974; Cherry and Snell, 1969; Itakura *et al.*, 1972; Komuro and Boyse, 1973; Komuro *et al.*, 1974; Schlesinger and Yron, 1970.)

The alloantigens with which these antibodies react are determined by three or possibly four loci. Locus *Ly-1* (formerly *Ly-A* or $\mu$) is identified by two reciprocal antisera. It is in chromosome 19 (Fig. 3.2). Another locus, or possibly a pair of linked loci, is identified by four antibodies forming reciprocal pairs. Originally, the symbols *Ly-B* and *Ly-C* were assigned, but since no recombinants were found in 370 backcross mice, and absorption of antibody against one of the postulated antigens was found to block absorption of antibody against the other, a single locus interpretation seems preferable. The provisional designation is *Ly-2,3*. The locus is in chromosome 6 (Fig. 3.2), close to the $\kappa$ light chain immunoglobulin locus (Gottlieb, 1974). No recombinants have been found. The last locus in this group, *Ly-5*, linkage undetermined, is also identified by reciprocal antisera (Komuro *et al.*, 1974). A partial strain distribution of the known specificities determined by these loci is given in Table 5.2.

An antigen with the properties of the Ly antigens of mice has been reported in rats (Fabre and Morris, 1974).

None of the antigens specified by these loci has been found on any cell except the T lymphocyte. In this respect they differ from Thy-1 which occurs also on brain and epidermal cells. It is possible that differences in distribution on T cells will be discovered, thereby identifying sub-populations of these cells (Boyse and Bennett, 1974). The Ly antibodies give a proportionately slightly stronger reaction with nodes and spleen as compared with thymus than does anti-Thy-1. The two types of antibody also have slightly different effects on the homing tendencies of thymic lymphocytes (Schlesinger *et al.*, 1973). Some further details are given in Chapter 13, Sections II,A and II,B.

### F. Some Alloantigens of B Cells

Three murine alloantigens have been reported which are the inverse of Ly-1, 2, 3, and 5 in that they are demonstrable not on T but on B lymphocytes (Snell *et al.*, 1973; Cherry *et al.*, 1976). Alloantigen Ly-4 was originally identifiable by only one antibody, but the reciprocal antibody has now been found. Reciprocal antisera are not yet known for Ly-6 and Ly-7. Test cells are prepared from lymph nodes. Infrequent reactions seen with thymus cells are probably due to contaminant antibodies. The usual titers found with node cells in the chromium lable cytotoxic test are of the order of 1/40, substantially lower than those often seen with some of the T-cell-reactive antibodies. The maximum lysis tends to be low, presumably because only lymphocytes of marrow origin (B cells) are reacting. A partial strain distribution of the specificities that characterize the three alloantigens is given in Table 5.2. In the case of Ly-6 and Ly-7, positive reactions with the single antiserum known for each antigen are indicated by a +; specificity numbers have not been assigned.

The strain distribution pattern in recombinant inbred strains, and tests in appropriate backcross generations and with congenic strains, show the loci determining Ly-4, Ly-6, and Ly-7 to be independent of each other and of known loci determining serologically demonstrated cell membrane alloantigens. *Ly-6* and *Ly-7* are also independent of known *H* loci. Unexpectedly, in view of the low probability of identical CXB recombinant inbred strain patterns occurring by chance, *Ly-4, H-2, Ea-4,* and *H-3* all have the same pattern. Other evidence shows the *Ly-4* is distinct from *H-2* and *Ea-4;* the identity of the CXB patterns is fortuitous. *Ly-4* and *H-3*, however, also show similar patterns in the AKXL recombinant inbred lines, and tests with appropriate congenic pairs prove that these loci are either identical or closely linked. This places the *Ly-4* gene in chromosome 2.

Studies of the distribution of the Ly-4 antigen on different classes of lymphocytes have shown that it is, with certain possible qualifications, specific for B cells. It is thus antithetical to Thy-1 (Aoki *et al.*, 1974; McKenzie and Snell, 1975; McKenzie, 1975). The number of cells reacting in the different lymphoid organs by cytotoxicity and as determined by immunoelectron microscopy was roughly the reciprocal of the number of cells reacting with anti-Thy-1. In tests in which the two antibodies were applied sequentially, anti-Ly-4 killed many cells not killed by anti-Thy-1, and *vice versa.* In athymic mice, the proportion of lymphocytes killed by anti-Ly-4 was greatly increased. No Ly-4 was demonstrable on kidney, liver, brain, or red cells. In tests of cells defined by function, it was shown that Ly-4 is present on antigen reactive cells, memory cells, antibody-forming cells, and antibody-forming cell precursors. In the electron microscope study, anti-Ly-4 appeared to react with a few macrophages in the thymus, lymph nodes, and spleen. In an *in vivo* test, the antiserum was shown to suppress antibody formation.

These results indicate that Ly-4 is typical of bone marrow-derived (B) lymphocytes. It is present also, however, on some lymphocytes still within the marrow, some B cell derivatives, and about 5% of thymus lymphocytes. Its presence on this last category of cells may account for the successful production of anti-Ly-4 by an immunization schedule in which the first two injections include thymus cells only (Chapter 4). It is of course also possible that Ly-4 is present on thymus or other cell types in a masked form not demonstrable by the usual tests.

Sachs *et al.* (1973) have published a preliminary report of a BALB/c anti-DBA/2 lymphocytotoxic antibody which seems to identify a new antigen. Legrand and Dausset (1975) have reported a B cell alloantigen in humans. The Ia antigens of mouse B cells will be examined in Chapter 6. A cell surface polymorphism of B cells controlled by the *Mls* locus (Table 5.2) is described in Chapter 8.

## II. Miscellaneous Cell Surface Alloantigens

There probably are many cell surface alloantigens present on and perhaps specifically characteristic of cell types other than erythrocytes and lymphocytes, but detection has been slow because of the difficulty of preparing single cell suspensions suitable for study. Several such alloantigens, however, are now known, and the number is likely to grow rapidly. Two, Sk and H-Y, which are also histocompatibility antigens, are described in Chapter 3. Three others are described here.

### A. A Plasma Cell Alloantigen, Pca-1

Takahashi *et al.* (1970a,b) by immunizing DBA/2 mice with a BALB/c plasma cell tumor, obtained a cytotoxic antiserum of distinctive properties. Reactivity segregated independently from that of other known membrane alloantigens. A new locus was indicated, and the symbol *Pca-1* was assigned. The strain distribution of activity is shown in Table 5.2. No reciprocal antibody has been reported, but the search for such an antibody is limited by the scarcity of plasma cell tumors.

Cytotoxicity and absorption tests showed the reactive antigen to be present on myelomas, hemolytic plaque-forming cells of the spleen, and cells from liver, kidney, brain, spleen, and to a limited degree lymph nodes. No antigen was demonstrable on thymocytes, peritoneal cells, blood lymphocytes, bone marrow cells, erythrocytes, or an ascites sarcoma. In a cell transfer study, although treatment of donor spleen cells with anti-Thy-1 abolished ability to transfer the antibody response to sheep erythrocytes, presumably due to the elimination of T helper cells, anti-Pca-1 had no effect. This indicates that Pca-1 is not present on those B cells that are destined to become antibody producers. It appears not to be present on T cells. Whether it is absent from all lymphocytes is not entirely clear.

## B. Mph-1, An Alloantigen of Murine Peritoneal Exudate Cells

Archer and Davies (1974) have demonstrated an alloantigen of peritoneal exudate cells obtained by the intraperitoneal injection of starch or acetone-dried *Shigella shigae*. The antiserum was produced by immunization of I/St mice with B10.M exudate cells. An anti-H-2 was present, but after this was removed by absorption with B10.M lymph nodes, activity against peritoneal cells remained. All strains except the recipient, I/St, reacted (Table 5.2). Attempts to produce a similar antibody using other more readily available tissues were unsuccessful.

Genetic studies indicate control by a locus closely linked to *p* in chromosome 7 (Fig. 3.2). *H-4* is also very close to *p*. Since the induced peritoneal exudate cells carrying the antigen were presumably macrophages, the symbol *Mph-1* (macrophage-1) was assigned. The authors suggest that Mph-1 may be characteristic of one class of macrophages rather than of macrophages in general.

## C. Sperm Alloantigens Determined by the *T* Locus

The murine *T* locus is a CMAD locus of unusual properties. The *T* allele, discovered by Dobrovolskaïa-Zavadskaïa (1927), is a lethal causing a shortened tail in heterozygotes. In subsequent years, additional mutant alleles were discovered which produce a variety of morphological, physiological, and genetic effects. It was not until 1972 that Bennett *et al.* showed that *T* determines an alloantigen expressed on sperm. It is linked to *H-2* on chromosome 17 (Fig. 3.2) and may be, in certain evolutionary respects, a part of the *H-2* supergene (Snell, 1968). Before discussing the serological studies, a brief outline of the genetics of the locus is necessary. The literature is extensive; some representative recent papers on which we have drawn are Bennett and Dunn (1967), Boyse and Bennett (1974), Dunn and Bennett (1971), Geyer-Duszynska (1964), and Lyon and Meredith (1964).

Beside the wild type (+) allele and the original *T* mutant allele, the locus determines an extensive series of alleles or pseudoalleles designated $t^1$, $t^2$, etc., or $t^{w1}$, $t^{w2}$, etc., if they have been found in wild mice. These may produce any of the following effects, singly or in a variety of combinations.

1. Combined with *T* they may change the short tail of the *T*/+ mouse to a tailless condition. It is because of this effect that most of them have been discovered.

2. They may be lethal, causing death at any stage from 4 days of embryo age to birth, or they may be semilethal. Mice heterozygous for different *t* lethal mutants may be viable. Complementation groups can thus be distinguished.

3. If not lethal, they may cause, when homozygous or when in combination with other alleles, varying degrees of sterility.

4. They usually restrict crossing over in the *T–H-2* region.

5. They often produce distorted segregation ratios, the *t* gene being transmitted by +/*t* or *T*/*t* heterozygous males to more than, and sometimes many more than, 50% of zygotes. This is probably due to different activity levels of the two classes of sperm. A consequence of the distorted ratios is to preserve *t* alleles in wild populations, despite their lethality.

These manifold effects may be due to a series of closely linked loci rather than to a single locus. Some of the manifestations of the postulated chromosome region, e.g., the reduction of crossing over, may be due to the association of *t* effects with deletions.

The alloantigenic expression of the *T* complex was discovered with antisera produced by injecting mutant sperm into normal males. The antisera were absorbed with normal sperm to remove the sperm autoantibody which is present in all anti-sperm antisera. The antisera thus produced were shown, by the dye exclusion method, to be cytotoxic for donor sperm. The *T*-locus antigen thus demonstrated was not found on other adult cells (Bennett *et al.*, 1972).

Studies with antisera produced against sperm of different *t* genotypes showed that distinct *t* alleles determine distinct alloantigens. It was further demonstrated that, in heterozygotes, one-half or less of the sperm reacted with antibody directed against one of the two t antigens carried by the heterozygote. The number of sperm reacting with a double antiserum made against both the represented alloantigens was double that observed when one alloantigen alone was reacting (Yanagisawa *et al.*, 1974a,b). This indicates that sperm of *t* heterozygotes are of two antigenic classes, and hence that haploid spermatocytes are capable of generating the *t* gene end product. Whether this is a rare or a common situation is not yet known, but haploid expression may also occur with the H-Y antigen of mice and the AB and HLA antigens of man (Chapter 3; Boyse and Bennett, 1974; Shahani and Southam, 1962; Beatty, 1970; Fellous and Dausset, 1970; Halim *et al.*, 1974).

The existence in +/*t* and *T*/*t* males of two antigenically distinct classes of sperm may well account for the distorted segregation ratios produced by such males. Seemingly one class of sperm must suppress the motility of the other, although the mechanism by which such suppression might occur is unknown.

Besides being present on sperm, a *T*-determined antigen is present on undifferentiated teratomas and, as might be expected from the morphological nature of teratomas, probably also on cleaving embryos (Vitetta *et al.*, 1975). A teratoma of a strain 129 male developed by Stevens (1967) was split into undifferentiated and differentiated cell lines maintained in culture. Injection of cells of one of the undifferentiated lines into male 129 mice yielded an antiserum that reacted with all the undifferentiated cell lines, with male germ cells, and with morulae of all strains tested but not with the differentiated cell lines. Absorption of this antiserum, and of an anti-sperm serum, with spermatozoa carrying different *T* alleles, yielded evidence that the teratoma antigen was, in fact, specified by the *T* locus. That the *T* locus is normally functional in early development, and hence that the T antigen should be present then, is indicated by the early lethality caused by some *t* alleles. The H-2 antigen was absent from the primitive teratoma used to produce the antibody with anti-T-like properties, just as it is absent from early embryos.

## III. Distribution of Alloantigens in Different Tissues

While our knowledge of the tissue distribution of cell membrane alloantigens is still in a very primitive state, it is worth summarizing for two reasons. It is a major source of information of the extent of overlap between the groups of CMAD loci demonstrated by different techniques. It provides at least a little insight into possible functions of membrane alloantigens.

Edidin (1972) has reviewed evidence concerning the tissue distribution and cellular location of transplantation antigens, particularly H-2 and HLA.

For our purposes, a comparison of a representative group of CMAD loci is important. As illustrative of erythrocyte alloantigens, we draw to a limited extent on studies of human blood groups. As many of the assembled data as possible are presented in Table 5.4. The table is limited to those alloantigens and those tissues for which substantial data are available. In the next to the last column, the histocompatibility effect of each alloantigen is given, if known.

Most data on tissue distribution of alloantigens have been obtained by absorption. An antiserum is incubated with a homogenate of the tissue to be typed, and the resulting absorbed serum tested against

TABLE 5.4
THE TISSUE DISTRIBUTION AND HISTOCOMPATIBILITY EFFECT OR NONEFFECT OF SOME CELL MEMBRANE ALLOANTIGENS OF MICE AND HUMANS

| Antigen | Presence in[a] | | | | | | | | | | | | | Fraction with antigen[b] |
|---|---|---|---|---|---|---|---|---|---|---|---|---|---|---|
| | Red cells | Thymus | T lymphocytes | Spleen, lymph nodes | B lymphocytes | Plasma cells | Brain | Kidney | Liver | Lung | Testis, spermatozoa | Skin, epidermal cells | Skin $H$ effect | |
| ABO | + | + | | + | | | + | + | + | + | + | + | + | 9/9 |
| Ea-2 | 4+ | 3+ | | 4+ | | | 4+ | 3+ | 4+ | 4+ | 4+ | − | − ± | 8/9 |
| Ea-4 | 4+ | 1+? | | − 3+ | | | − | 2+ | − | 2+ | − | | − | 5/8 |
| Ea-5 | 4+ | | | 1+ | | | 1+ | 4+ | − 2+ | 2+ | 3+ | | | 7/7 |
| Ea-6 | 4+ | | | 1 3+ | | | 3+ | 1+ | 2+ | 2+ | 3+ | | − | 7/7 |
| H-2 | 1+ | 2+ | | 4+ | | + | 1+ | 1 2+ | 3+ | 2+ | + | 2+ | + | 10/10 |
| HLA | + | | | 4+ | | | 1+ | 2+ | 3+ | 3+ | + | + | + | 8/8 |
| H-Y | | + | | + | | | + | + | + | + | + | + | + | 8/8 |
| Pca-1 | − | − | | + | − | + | + | + | + | | − | − | | 4/9 |
| Sk | − | − | | − | | − | + | | | | − | + | + | 2/7 |
| Thy-1 | − | + | + | + | − | − | + | − | − | − | − | + | weak? | 3/10 |
| Ly-1 | − | + | + | + | − | − | − | − | − | − | − | − | −? | 1/10 |
| Ly-2,3 | − | + | + | + | − | − | − | − | − | − | − | − | −? | 1/10 |
| Ly-5 | − | + | + | + | − | | − | − | − | | − | − | | 1/8 |
| Tla | − | + | − | − | − | − | − | − | − | − | − | − | −? | 1/10 |
| Ly-4 | − | −? | −? | + | + | | − | − | − | | | | | 1/6 |

[a] + indicates presence of antigen; − indicates its absence. Where quantitative absorption data are available, the relative quantity of antigen in different tissues is indicated by numerals placed before the + (4+ = maximum amount, 1+ = minimum amount). In a few cases where there are conflicting reports, two different values are given. The data in the table come from numerous uncited sources as well as from sources cited in the text.

[b] In calculating the fraction of typed tissues in which the indicated antigen is present, thymus and T (thymus-derived) lymphocytes are treated as a single tissue, and spleen, lymph nodes, and B (bone marrow-derived) lymphocytes as a single tissue. Where thymus and T lymphocytes are discordant, the pair is scored according to the behavior of the thymus. Where spleen and/or lymph nodes and B lymphocytes are discordant, the pair is scored according to the behavior of the B lymphocytes.

appropriate cells for residual activity. If serial dilutions of the absorbing tissue are employed, this method of typing can give roughly quantitative data on the amount of antigen present. Where quantitative estimates are available, they are indicated in the table by the use of numerals. The given values should be regarded as only an approximate indication of relative antigen concentrations. Typing has also been done by the use of fluorescent labeled antibody [e.g., the typing of ABO, Szulman (1960)] and by direct cytotoxicity [e.g., the typing of epidermal cells, Scheid *et al.* (1972)].

The data are subject to several limitations. There are a number of cases in which tissues were typed as negative, then later retyped by a more sensitive method and found to be positive. Thus the H-2 antigen was originally thought to be absent from brain and spermatozoa, but has since been shown to be present. Some of the negatives in the table may be similarly in error. Typing by absorption with a tissue homogenate of an organ such as kidney gives no information concerning the differences in antigen concentration on the radically different cell types of which such an organ may be composed. Immunofluorescent microscopy overcomes this limitation, and in a few cases has added important details which would otherwise be missed. Thus, although the ABO human blood group antigen is, as shown by numerous studies, widely distributed, its distribution between different cell types within the various organs is extremely unequal. It is, in fact, largely or entirely confined to the endothelium of blood vessels, the stratified epithelia, and (in secretors and to a much more limited extent nonsecretors) various secretions (Szulman, 1960). And finally, the data are based on a very incomplete and possibly biased sample of all tissues and antigens.

Table 5.4 shows that if both tissue distribution and the degree of representation on different tissues is taken into account, there is great individuality in the different alloantigens. The probably homologous antigens H-2 and HLA are the one, not unexpected, exception. These show a striking similarity. There is one minor quantitative difference: H-2 can easily be demonstrated on red cells by agglutination; HLA can be demonstrated on red cells only by very refined techniques. Except for this pair of presumed homologues, the pattern for each antigen is as unique as a fingerprint.

Another aspect of tissue distribution revealed by Table 5.4 is a tendency for the alloantigens to occur on all tissues or on only one. The relevant information is given in the last column and footnote *b*. If we treat H-2 and HLA as a single entity, there are 15 alloantigens listed. Five of these occur in all tested tissues, 5 in only one. This is not a normal distribution. The Mph-1 antigen, since the injection of cell types other than peritoneal macrophages failed to induce antibody, may also belong in the group with single-tissue representation, but we have not included it in the table because of the absence of data from absorption. The T antigen is on two cell types, spermatozoa and cells of the early embryo.

The antigens with restricted distribution have been referred to as *differentiation antigens,* implying that they appear at specific stages in differentiation and play a role in determining the properties of individual cell types (Boyse and Old, 1969).

Table 5.4 is a condensation of a large volume of data and of necessity omits some valuable material. A few items that are not covered deserve mention. We have already noted that the ABO blood group antigen, although present in all organs, appears to show a restricted distribution within organs (Szulman, 1960). H-2 and HLA are present in all adult tissues tested and perhaps are present on all nucleated cells of the adult. HLA in soluble form has been found in normal human serum and in seminal plasma (Billing *et al.,* 1973; Singal and Berry, 1972). H-2 is not present in the cleaving embryo prior to implantation (Edidin, 1972).

The presence of the H-2 antigen on all cells except those of the earliest developmental stages and the presence of the T antigen only on the cells of the early developmental stages (with the one exception of sperm) establish a reciprocal relationship between the two antigens. The linkage of *T* and *H-2* and the chemical similarity of their end products (Vitetta *et al.,* 1975) adds interest to this evidence for sequential expression.

The non-H-2 histocompatibility antigens constitute a major void in our knowledge concerning the tissue distribution of cell membrane alloantigens. If an antigen is demonstrable serologically, its tissue distribution can be studied by the methods of antibody absorption or immunofluorescence. Since workable antisera against H antigens other than H-2 are seemingly very difficult to produce, these methods are not applicable, at least at present, to most *H* loci. We do have limited information about H-3 and H-13. These (or possibly one of these without the other) have been demonstrated on peritoneal macrophages, cleaving ova, and spermatozoa (DeAngelis and Haughton, 1971; Palm *et al.,* 1971; Vojtíšková *et al.,* 1968).

One source of information concerning tissue distribution that does apply to *H* loci is experiments in which immunity or tolerance have been induced to skin grafts by prior injection of lymphoid tissues. With the use of congenic lines, it has been shown that there is cross-immunity between thymus and skin for 10 *H* loci (Graff *et al.,* 1966; see also Chapter 3). Where congenic lines are not used, so that donor and recipient have multiple *H* differences, immunization experiments are subject to a major limitation as a source of evidence concerning tissue distribution. Accelerated rejection of the test graft does not mean that all the alloantigenic disparities of donor and host are shared by the graft and the immunizing cells. The sharing of a single disparity is enough to cause acceleration. If the strains used differ at *H-2*, the overriding action of the H-2 antigen (already known to be widely distributed) will obscure any possible non-H-2 activity. The induction of tolerance is more informative because the full acceptance of the test graft requires that tolerance be induced to each and every one of the antigenic disparities. There have been many tolerance studies, employing both mice and rats, in which tolerance to a test skin graft has been induced across multiple histocompatibility barriers. With respect to the wide sharing of H antigens by lymphoid cells and skin, most of these add little to the original tolerance experiments of Billingham *et al.* (1956). Other studies have shown that, in rats, tolerance can be induced to kidneys and hearts, and that, in poultry, tolerance to skin can be induced by erythrocytes (Barker *et al.*, 1971; Feldman *et al.*, 1968; Kinsky and Mitchison, 1963). Poultry are a somewhat special case, since the red cells of birds are nucleated, but these studies do point to a wide distribution of H antigens.

While the authors of these and other similar experiments have all reported a substantial induction of tolerance, there have been signs of residual incompatibility. Late rejection of skin grafts can be accounted for by the Sk antigen, which is confined to murine skin and brain (Table 5.4), and to the probable existence of a homologous antigen in other species. The study by Barker *et al.* (1971) also points to some disparities in the antigens on cells from the different lymphoid organs that were used to induce tolerance and on hearts and skin that were used as targets. Studies of this sort provide only indirect evidence as to the tissue distribution of H antigens, but they do suggest that while many H antigens are widely shared, there are also cases of restricted distribution.

## IV. The Problem of Overlap between Alloantigens Demonstrated by Different Techniques

CMAD loci have been demonstrated by three basic techniques: histogenetic techniques, using skin or tumor transplants, which are the source of information concerning *H* loci; agglutination of red cells (*Ea* loci); and cytotoxicity of lymphocytes or other nucleated cells (*Ly* loci, *Thy-1*, *Sk*, etc.). A basic question in immunogenetics is the extent to which loci demonstrated by these different methods overlap. What proportion of the loci defined by any one method can also be recognized by one or both of the others? We believe we can now say, with caution, that the degree of duplication is surprisingly small.

It will be well to consider first some of the problems in gathering and interpreting relevant data.

Determination of the histocompatibility effect, if any, of a locus originally demonstrated serologically is a time-consuming and uncertain process. Except for a locus imposing a very strong barrier to transplants, which, in the mouse, means essentially only *H-2,* the histocompatibility effect of any one locus can be determined only through the production and testing of a congenic line. This takes several years. And even after 10 or 12 generations of backcrossing, the marker locus will still carry with it many adjacent genes, and one of these and not the marker itself may be the source of any histocompatibility effect. The study of Flaherty and Bennett (1973) (reviewed in Chapter 3) shows that this is a very real problem. These factors are the source of several blanks or uncertainties in the column on skin *H* effect in Table 5.4.

The problem of measuring overlap would be simplified if we could say with confidence that the demonstration of an alloantigen on epidermal cells was proof that it has a histocompatibility effect, or that its presence on red cells or lymphocytes was a guarantee of its demonstrability by hemagglutination or lymphocytotoxicity. Presence and demonstrability by the usual tests probably go hand in hand in most cases, but there seem to be exceptions or partial exceptions. Thus Thy-1, although easily demonstrable on epidermal cells, is at most a weak histocompatibility antigen, causing or being associated with only infrequent rejection of skin grafts in a congenic strain pair (Scheid *et al.,* 1972; John *et al.,* 1972). The Ea antigens listed in Table 5.4 may represent another category of exceptions. All four have been demonstrated in the lymphoid organs and, therefore, are presumably on lymphocytes, but only Ea-2 seems to be demonstrable by lymphocytotoxicity (Popp, 1969; M. Cherry, unpublished data).

With these reservations in mind, let us consider the evidence for the presence or absence of overlap. We are considering only overlap between categories of loci defined by the three standard methods that we have been discussing.

*H-2* is the classic case of complete overlap. It is demonstrable by skin grafting, by hemagglutination, and by lymphocytotoxicity. The human ABO is a histocompatibility as well as a blood group locus, and may also be demonstrable by lymphocytotoxicity (Möller and Eklund, 1965). *Ea-2* of mice is demonstrable by both hemagglutination and lymphocytotoxicity. The murine *Thy-1,* a very strong locus by lymphocytotoxicity, may have a very weak histocompatibility expression. Of the 16 antigens listed in Table 5.4, these are the only proved cases of overlap. The clearest cases of lack of overlap are provided by the antigens of restricted distribution, called differentiation antigens. Five antigens in the table seem to occur only on lymphocytes and are correspondingly demonstrable only by lymphocytotoxicity. If differentiation antigens turn out to be very common, overlap will be correspondingly infrequent. One of the obscure areas is the extent to which *H* loci will turn out to be demonstrable serologically. If *H-3* and *Ly-4* are one and the same, a possibility in view of their close linkage, this will emphasize the possibility of *H* loci also being *Ly* or *Ea* loci.

Despite the uncertainties, the data seem to reinforce the view that there is both a great diversity and a surprising number of CMAD loci.

## REFERENCES

Aoki, T., I. F. C. McKenzie, M. M. Sturm, and M. Liu. 1974. Distribution of the alloantigen Ly-4.2 on murine B-cells. *Immunogenetics* **1**:291–296.

Archer, J. R., and D. L. A. Davies. 1974. Demonstration of an alloantigen on the peritoneal exudate cells of inbred strains of mice and its association with chromosome 7 (linkage group I). *J Immunogen* **1**:113–123.

Baird, S., J. Santa, and I. Weissman. 1971. Anti-theta antisera may contain anti-allotype contamination. *Nature (Lond), New Biol* **232**:56.

Barker, C. F., D. M. Lubaroff, and W. K. Silvers. 1971. Lymph node cells: Their differential capacity to induce tolerance of heart and skin homografts in rats. *Science* **172**:1050–1052.

Basch, R. S., and G. Goldstein. 1974. Induction of T-cell differentiation *in vitro* by thymin, a purified polypeptide hormone of the thymus. *Proc Natl Acad Sci USA* **71**:1474–1478.

Beatty, R. A. 1970. The genetics of the mammalian gamete. *Biol Rev* **45**:73–119.

Bennett, D., and L. C. Dunn. 1967. Studies of effects of *t*-alleles in the house mouse on spermatozoa. I. Male sterility effects. *J Reprod Fertil* **13**:421–428.

Bennett, D., E. Goldberg, L. C. Dunn, and E. A. Boyse. 1972. Serological detection of a cell-surface antigen specified by the *T* (brachyury) mutant gene in the house mouse. *Proc Natl Acad Sci USA* **69**:2076–2080.

Billing, R. J., K. K. Mittal, and P. I. Terasaki. 1973. Isolation of soluble HL-A antigens from normal human sera by ion exchange chromatography. *Tissue Antigens* **3**:251–256.

Billingham, R. E., L. Brent, and P. B. Medawar. 1956. Quantitative studies on tissue transplantation immunity. III. Actively acquired tolerance. *Phil Trans R Soc Lond* [Biol Sci] **239**:357–414.

Boyse, E. A., and D. Bennett. 1974. Differentiation and the cell surface; Illustrations from work with T cells and sperm. Pages 155–176 *in* G. M. Edelman, ed. Cellular selection and regulation in the immune response. Raven, New York.

Boyse, E. A., and L. J. Old. 1969. Some aspects of normal and abnormal cell surface genetics. *Annu Rev Genet* **3**:269–290.

Boyse, E. A., M. Miyazawa, T. Aoki, and L. J. Old. 1968a. Ly-A and Ly-B: Two systems of lymphocyte isoantigens in the mouse. *Proc R Soc Lond (Biol)* **170**:175–193.

Boyse, E. A., L. J. Old, and E. Stockert. 1968b. An approach to the mapping of antigens on cell surface. *Proc Natl Acad Sci USA* **60**:886–893.

Boyse, E. A., E. Stockert, and L. J. Old. 1968c. Isoantigens of the *H-2* and *Tla* loci of the mouse. Interactions affecting their representation on thymocytes. *J Exp Med* **128**:85–95.

Boyse, E. A., E. Stockert, and L. J. Old. 1969. Properties of four antigens specified by the *Tla* locus. Similarities and differences. Pages 353–357 *in* N. R. Rose and F. Milgrom, eds. International convocation on immunology. Karger, Basel.

Boyse, E. A., I. Katsuaki, E. Stockert, C. A. Iritani, and M. Miura. 1971. *Ly-C*, a third locus specifying alloantigens expressed only on thymocytes and lymphocytes. *Transplantation* **11**:351–352.

Cherry, M., and G. D. Snell. 1969. A description of mu: A non-*H-2* alloantigen in C3H/Sn mice. *Transplantation* **8**:319–327.

Cherry, M., G. D. Snell, I. F. C. McKenzie, B. A. Taylor, and D. W. Bailey. 1976. Loci determining murine lymphocyte alloantigens. I. *Ly-6* and *Ly-7*. *Immunogenetics,* in press.

DeAngelis, W. J., and G. Haughton, 1971. Detection of weak histocompatibility antigens on mouse peritoneal macrophages. *Transplant Proc* **3**:202–206.

Dobrovolskaïa-Zavadskaïa, N. 1927. Sur la mortification spontanée de la queue chez la souris nouveau-née et sur l'existence d'une caractère héréditaire (facteur) "non-viable." *C R Soc Biol (Paris)* **97**:114–116.

Douglas, T. C. 1972. Occurrence of a theta-like antigen in rats. *J Exp Med* **136**:1054–1062.

Dunn, L. C., and D. Bennett. 1971. Further studies of a mutation (low) which distorts transmission ratios in the house mouse. *Genetics* **67**:543–558.

Edidin, M. 1972. The tissue distribution and cellular location of transplantation antigens. Pages 125–140 *in* B. D. Kahan and R. A. Reisfeld, eds. Transplantation antigens: Markers of biological individuality. Academic Press, New York.

Fabre, J. W., and P. J. Morris. 1974. The definition of a lymphocyte-specific alloantigen system in the rat (*Ly-1*). *Tissue Antigens* **4**:238–246.

Feldman, J. D., E. Pick, S. Lee, W. K. Silvers, and D. B. Wilson. 1968. Renal homotransplantation in rats. II. Tolerant recipients. *Am J Pathol* **52**:687–700.

Fellous, M., and J. Dausset. 1970. Probable haploid expression of HL-A antigens on human spermatozoon. *Nature (Lond)* **225**:191–193.

Flaherty, L., and D. Bennett. 1973. Histoincompatibilities found between congenic strains which differ at loci determining differentiation antigens. *Transplantation* **16**:505–514.

Geyer-Duszynska, I. 1964. Cytological investigations on the *T*-locus in *Mus musculus L. Chromosoma* **15**:478–502.

Gottleib, P. D. 1974. Genetic correlation of a mouse light chain variable region marker with a thymocyte surface antigen. *J Exp Med* **140**:1432–1437.

Graff, R. J., W. H. Hildeman, and G. D. Snell. 1966. Histocompatibility genes of mice. VI. Allografts in mice congenic at various non-*H-2* histocompatibility loci. *Transplantation* **4**:425–437.

Halim, A., K. Abbasi, and H. Festenstein. 1974. The expression of the HL-A antigens on human spermatozoa. *Tissue Antigens* **4**:1–6.

Hilgers, J., J. Haverman, R. Nusse, W. van Blitterswijk, F. Cleton, P. Hageman, R. van Nie, and J. Calafat. 1975. Immunological, virological and genetical aspects of mammary tumor virus (TMV) induced cell surface antigens; The presence of these antigens as well as the Thy-1.2 antigen on murine mammary gland and tumor cells. *J Natl Cancer Inst* **54**:1335–1342.

Itakura, K., J. Hutton, E. Boyse, and L. J. Old. 1972. Genetic linkage relationships of loci specifying differentiation alloantigens in the mouse. *Transplantation* 13:239–243.

John, M., E. Carswell, E. A. Boyse, and G. Alexander. 1972. Production of $\theta$ antibody by mice that fail to reject $\theta$ incompatible skin grafts. *Nature (Lond)*, New Biol **238**:57–58.

Kinsky, R., and N. A. Mitchison. 1963. Tolerance of skin induced by erythrocytes in poultry. *Transplantation* **1**:224–231.

Klein, J. 1973. List of congenic lines of mice. I. Lines with differences at alloantigen loci. *Transplantation* **15**:137–153.

Komuro, K., and E. A. Boyse. 1973. *In vitro* demonstration of thymic hormone in the mouse by conversion of precursor cells into lymphocytes. *Lancet* **1**:740–743.

Komuro, K., E. A. Boyse, and L. J. Old. 1973. Production of TL antibody by mice immunized with TL— cell populations. A possible assay for thymic hormone. *J Exp Med* 137:533–536.

Komuro, K., K. Itakura, E. A. Boyse, and M. John. 1974. Ly-5; a new T-lymphocyte antigen system. *Immunogenetics* **1**:452–456.

Lance, E. M., S. Cooper, and E. A. Boyse. 1971. Antigenic change and cell maturation in murine thymocytes. *Cell Immunol* **1**:536–547.

Legrand, L., and J. Dausset. 1975. Immunogenetics of a new lymphocyte system. *Transplant Proc* **7**:5–8.

Lubaroff, D. M. 1973. An alloantigenic marker on rat thymus and thymus derived cells. *Transplant Proc* **5**:115–118.

Lyon, M. F., and R. Meredith. 1964. Investigation of the nature of *t*-alleles in the mouse. II. Genetic analysis of an unusual mutant allele and its derivatives. *Heredity* **19**:313–325.

McKenzie, I. F. C., and G. D. Snell. 1975. Ly-4.2: A cell membrane alloantigen of murine B lymphocytes. II. Functional studies. *J Immunol* **114**:856–862.

McKenzie, I. F. C., and G. D. Snell. 1975. Ly-4.2: A cell membrane alloantigen of murine B lymphocytes. I. Population studies. *J Immunol* **114**:848–855.

Micheel, B., G. Pasternak, and J. Steuden. 1973. Demonstration of $\theta$-AKR differentiation antigen in rat tissue by mouse alloantiserum. *Nature (Lond), New Biol* **241**:221–222.

Möller, E., and A. E. Eklund. 1965. Cytotoxic effect of iso-antibodies directed against ABO and Rh antigens on human lymph node cells. *Nature (Lond)* **206**:731–732.

Moore, M. J., P. Dikkes, A. E. Reif, F. C. A. Romanul, and R. L. Sidman. 1971. Localization of theta alloantigens in mouse brain by immunofluorescence and cytotoxic inhibition. *Brain Res* **28**:283–293.

Obata, Y., H. Ikeda, E. Stockert, and E. A. Boyse. 1975. Relation of $G_{IX}$ antigen of thymocytes to envelope glycoprotein of murine leukemia virus. *J Exp Med* **141**:188–197.

Old, L. J., E. A. Boyse, and E. Stockert. 1963. Antigenic properties of experimental leukemias. I. Serological studies *in vitro* with spontaneous and radiation-induced leukemia. *J Natl Cancer Inst* **31**:977–986.

Old, L. J., E. Stockert, E. A. Boyse, and J. H. Kim. 1968. Antigenic modulation. Loss of TL antigen from cells exposed to TL antibody. Study of the phenomenon *in vitro*. *J Exp Med* **127**:523–539.

Palm, J., S. Heyner, and R. L. Brinster. 1971. Differential immunofluorescence of fertilized mouse eggs with *H-2* and non-*H-2* antibody. *J Exp Med* **133**:1282–1293.

Pierce, C. W. 1973. Immune responses *in vitro*. VII. Loss of susceptibilty of functional θ-bearing cells to cytotoxic action of anti-θ serum and complement *in vitro*. *Cell Immunol* **9**:465–473.

Popp, D. M. 1969. Histocompatibility-14: Correlation of the isoantigen rho and *R-Z* locus. *Transplantation* **7**:233–241.

Raff, M. C., and H. H. Wortis. 1970. Thymus dependence of θ-bearing cells in the peripheral lymphoid tissues of mice. *Immunology* **18**:931–942.

Reif, A. E., and J. M. V. Allen. 1964. The AKR thymic antigen and its distribution in leukemias and nervous tissues. *J Exp Med* **120**:413–433.

Reif, A. E., and J. M. V. Allen. 1966. Mouse nervous tissue iso-antigens. *Nature* (*Lond*) **209**:523.

Rubinstein, P., N. Liu, E. W. Streun, and F. Decary. 1974. Electrophoretic mobility and agglutinability of red blood cells: A "new" polymorphism in mice. *J Exp Med* **139**:313–322.

Sachs, J. A., B. Huber, J. Penã-Martinez, and H. Festenstein. 1973. Genetic studies and effect on skin allograft survival of DBA/2DAG, *Ly*, and *M*-locus antigens. *Transplant Proc* **5**:1385–1387.

Scheid, M. P., E. A. Boyse, E. A. Carswell, and L. J. Old. 1972. Serologically demonstrable alloantigens of mouse epidermal cells. *J Exp Med* **135**:938–955.

Schlesinger, M., and I. Yron. 1970. Serological demonstration of a thymus-dependent population of lymph-node cells. *J Immunol* **104**:798–804.

Schlesinger, M., Z. Shlomai-Korzash, and E. Israel. 1973. Antigenic differences between spleen-seeking and lymph node-seeking thymus cells. *Eur J Immunol* **3**:335–339.

Shahani, S., and A. L. Southam. 1962. Immunofluorescent study of the ABO blood group antigens in human spermatozoa. *Am J Obstet Gynecol* **84**:660–666.

Singal, D. P., and R. Berry. 1972. Soluble HL-A antigens. Localization in the human seminal plasma fraction. *Transplantation* **13**:441–442.

Snell, G. D. 1968. The *H-2* locus of the mouse: Observations and speculations concerning its comparative genetics and its polymorphism. *Folia Biol* (*Praha*) **14**:335–358.

Snell, G. D. 1971. The histocompatibility systems. *Transplant Proc* **3**:1133–1138.

Snell, G. D., and M. Cherry. 1972. Loci determining cell surface alloantigens. Pages 221–228 *in* P. Emmelot and P. Bentvelzen, eds. Viruses and host genome in oncogenesis. North-Holland Publ., Amsterdam.

Snell, G. D., M. Cherry, I. F. C. McKenzie, and D. W. Bailey. 1973. *Ly-4*, a new locus determining a cell-surface alloantigen in mice. *Proc Natl Acad Sci USA* **70**:1108–1111.

Staats, J. 1972. Standardized nomenclature for inbred strains of mice: Fifth listing. *Cancer Res.* **32**:1609–1646.

Stevens, L. C. 1967. The biology of teratomas. *Adv Morphol* **6**:1–28.

Stockert, E., L. J. Old, and E. A. Boyse. 1971. The $G_{IX}$ system. A cell surface alloantigen associated with murine leukemia virus: Implications regarding chromosomal integration of the viral genome. *J Exp Med* **133**:1334–1355.

Stockert, E., E. A. Boyse, T. Obata, H. Ikeda, N. H. Sarkar, and H. A. Hoffman. 1975. New mutant and congenic mouse stocks expressing the murine leukemic virus-associated thymocyte surface antigen $G_{IX}$. *J Exp Med* **142**:512–517.

Strand, M., F, Lilly, and J. T. August. 1974. Host control of endogenous murine leukemia virus gene expression: Concentrations of viral proteins in high and low leukemia mouse strains. *Proc Natl Acad Sci USA* **71**:3682–3686.

Szulman, A. E. 1960. The histological distribution of blood group substances A and B in man. *J Exp Med* **111**:785–800.

Takahashi, T., L. J. Old, and E. A. Boyse. 1970a. Surface alloantigens of plasma cells. *J Exp Med* **131**:1325–1341.

Takahashi, T., E. A. Carswell, and G. J. Thorbecke. 1970b. Surface antigens of immunocompetent cells. I. Effect of $\theta$ and PC.1 alloantisera on the ability of spleen cells to transfer immune responses. *J Exp Med* **132**:1181–1190.

Vitetta, E., K. Artzt, D. Bennett, E. A. Boyse, and F. Jacob. 1975. Structural similarities between a product of the *T/t*-locus isolated from sperm and teratoma cells and H-2 antigens isolated from splenocytes. *Proc Nat Acad Sci USA* **72**:3215–3219.

Vojtíšková, M., M. Poláčková, and Z. Pokorná. 1968. Histocompatibility antigens on mouse spermatozoa. *Folia Biol* (*Praha*) **15**:322–331.

Yanagisawa, K., D. Bennett, E. A. Boyse, L. C. Dunn, and A. Dimeo. 1974a. Serological identification of sperm antigens specified by lethal *t*-alleles in the mouse. *Immunogenetics* **1**:57–67.

Yanagisawa, K., D. R. Pollard, D. Bennett, L. C. Dunn, and E. A. Boyse. 1974b. Transmission ratio distortion at the *t*-locus: Serological identification of two sperm populations in *t*-heterozygotes. *Immunogenetics* **1**:91–96.

CHAPTER 6

# SEROLOGICALLY AND HISTOGENETICALLY DEMONSTRATED LOCI OF THE *H-2* COMPLEX

## I. Introduction

### A. The Complexity of *H-2*

The term *histocompatibility-2* (*H-2*), originally used as the designation of what was supposed to be a single locus, now embraces a complex of linked loci of diverse but often seemingly related manifestations and functions. *H-2* was first defined through the demonstration by Gorer (1936, 1942) of the association of a major histoincompatibility and an erythrocyte antigen. Control of both manifestations by a single locus was postulated. Linkage between the postulated locus and the genes *Fu* and *T* in chromosome 17, linkage group IX, was later demonstrated (Gorer *et al.*, 1948; Allen, 1955). Subsequent studies showed that *H-2* consists of at least two loci separable by crossing over, and that in the same, small chromosome region are other loci determining a bewildering variety of phenomena, but phenomena often tied to a membrane alloantigen or some form of immune responsiveness. Functional and perhaps phylogenetic interrelationships seem to be implied.

### B. Definitions and Symbols

Since *H-2* is divisible by crossing over, it is properly referred to as the *H-2 loci* or the *H-2 system.* To distinguish individual *H-2* loci one from another, capital letters are appended, e.g., *H-2K* and *H-2D*. Linked alleles of the *H-2* system which, because of the closeness of the linkage, tend to be inherited as a unit, are called *haplotypes.* Individual haplotypes, like individual alleles, are distinguished by superscript small letters, e.g., $H\text{-}2^a$, $H\text{-}2^b$. Since the number of halotypes now exceeds 26, double letter superscripts have become necessary. The convention has been adopted (Snell *et al.*, 1964) of adding letters from the first half of the alphabet to designate minor variants, e.g., $H\text{-}2^{ba}$, from the second half to designate major variants, e.g., $H\text{-}2^{qp}$. The chromosome region embraced by *H-2* is referred to as the *H-2 complex* (Klein *et al.*, 1974a). Shreffler (1974) includes as part of complex the additional short chromosome segment from *H-2* to and including *Tla* (Fig. 3.2).

Because of gaps in our knowledge and the intergradation of phenotypes, there is some ambiguity as to just what loci within the *H-2* complex are part of the *H-2* system. We shall see that there are two loci which, because of similarity of phenotype and of the chemistry of the end product, clearly belong within this system, and others for which *H-2* properties have been suggested.

Reviews of *H-2* complex research will be found in Démant (1973),

Iványi and Forejt (1974), Klein (1975a), and Shreffler and David (1975).

## C. Comparative Genetics

A major histocompatibility system similar to and presumably homologous with the *H-2* system of the mouse has been demonstrated in all mammals for which adequate data are available, and may occur in species as remote as the chicken. Evidence for a major system sufficient to assign a symbol implying homology to *H-2* has been found for man (HLA, Chapter 9), chimpanzees [ChL-A, Balner *et al.* (1971)], Rhesus monkeys [RhL-A, Balner *et al.* (1971)], dog [DL-A, Dausset *et al.* (1971)], swine [SL-A, Vaiman *et al.* (1973)], rabbits [rabbit *H-1* Démant (1966) or *Hg*, Colberg *et al.* (1969)—there is some lack of agreement with regard to this species], and rats [Rt *H-1* or *Ag-B*, Stark and Kren (1969), Palm and Wilson (1973)]. Evidence in regard to a major *H* system in cattle is still ambiguous, but some cattle lymphocytotoxic antisera appear to cross-react with the human HLA antigen. Absorption with cattle red cells does not remove the cross-reacting antibody, so the determining locus presumably is not the complex B blood group locus (Iha *et al.*, 1973). Antisera reactive with certain specificities of the murine *H-2* system cross-react with some specificities of the human HLA system (Ivašková and Iványi, 1974). The *B* locus in chicken is both a blood group and a histocompatibility locus, and may, like *H-2*, be divisible by crossing over (Pazderka *et al.*, 1975; Hála *et al.*, 1976). In a phylogenetically more remote vertebrate, the newt, skin graft experiments have not revealed a major *H* system (Cohen and Hildemann, 1968). Evidence in regard to major histocompatibility systems has been reviewed by Iványi (1970).

Where a clear homology exists, the functionally interrelated systems of linked loci marked by *H-2* and its homologues in other species are referred to as the *major histocompatibility complex* or MHC.

## D. Early Studies

Gorer's original discovery of *H-2* was based on the use of tumor transplants and red cell typing (Gorer, 1936, 1942). Gorer and O'Gorman (1956) later showed that H-2 can be demonstrated on lymphocytes by the dye exclusion cytotoxic test. The *H-2* system was thus amenable to study by all three of the basic techniques of mammalian cell membrane immunogenetics, an advantage not enjoyed by any other system or locus. Histogenetic methods were used successfully in early studies to demonstrate many of the known *H-2* haplotypes, and in development of congenic resistant (CR) lines, which played and continue to play an important role in *H-2* work (Snell *et al.*, 1953; Snell, 1958). At the same time, Gorer and his students were using serological methods to identify a steadily growing number of H-2 specificities. Histogenetic methods are still the basic tool in mutation studies, and the $F_1$ test remains a valuable adjunct to serological techniques in the identification of new haplotypes and new alleles. However, by far the larger part of *H-2* investigations now are based on serological methods. Therefore, in the following sections we shall pass over the earlier histogenetic studies and describe *H-2* largely in terms of serological findings. Reviews of *H-2* studies will be found in Démant (1973), Klein and Shreffler (1971), Shreffler and David (1975), Snell *et al.* (1973), and Snell and Stimpfling (1966).

## II. Recombination Studies

### A. H-2 Specificites as Markers

Hemagglutination studies of *H-2* carried out by Gorer and his former students soon revealed a high degree of complexity. More and more specificities were identified, each defined by a characteristic strain distribution pattern, and each proved by linkage tests or the use of congenic stocks to be determined either by one locus or by a small chromosome region. Multiple "alleles"—we would now say multiple haplotypes—were also identified. To make this accumulated information usable, it was presentd in *H-2* papers in the form of a chart.

An *H-2* chart published in 1959, with modifications to make it conform to current terminology, is shown in Table 6.1. Seven haplotypes and 12 specificities are included. A type strain for each haplotype is also shown. Some haplotypes were found in more than one strain. Thus $H\text{-}2^d$ occurred in DBA/2, BALB/c, and the congenic resistant strain B10.D2.

### B. Crossover Studies

The existence of multiple H-2 specificities suggested the hypothesis that different specificities are determined by different, but closely linked loci. This could be tested by serotyping a backcross and looking for new combinations of specificities. It will be seen from Table 6.1 that there are several strain combinations that would provide multiple serological markers. Thus haplotypes $H\text{-}2^a$ and $H\text{-}2^b$ differed at the then known speci-

TABLE 6.1
AN *H-2* CHART OF 1959, SHOWING SEVEN HAPLOTYPES, THE SPECIFICITIES BY WHICH EACH WAS DEFINED, AND THE TYPE STRAIN[a,b]

| *H-2* haplo-type | Specificity | | | | | | | | | | | | Type strain |
|---|---|---|---|---|---|---|---|---|---|---|---|---|---|
| *a* | — | 3 | 4 | 5 | 6 | — | 8 | — | 11 | — | — | — | A |
| *b* | 2 | — | — | 5 | 6 | — | — | — | — | — | — | 33[c] | C57BL/10 |
| *d* | — | 3 | 4 | — | 6 | — | 8 | — | — | — | 31 | — | DBA/2 |
| *f* | — | — | — | — | 6 | 7 | 8 | 9 | — | — | — | — | A.CA |
| *k* | — | 3 | — | 5 | — | —[d] | 8 | — | 11 | — | — | — | C3H |
| *r* | — | 3 | — | 5 | ? | — | 8 | — | 11 | — | — | — | RIII |
| *s* | — | 3 | — | 5 | 6 | 7 | — | — | — | 19 | — | — | A.SW |

[a] Adapted from Hoecker *et al.*, 1959.
[b] *H-2* specificities were originally designated by letters, but this was later changed to a numerical system (Snell *et al.*, 1964). This table is modified accordingly.
[c] Specificity 33, not shown in the table of Hoecker *et al.* (1959) is added from the work of Gorer and Mikulska (1959).
[d] $H\text{-}2^k$ is now known to have a weak variant of specificity 7.

ficities 2, 3, 4, 8, 11, and 33, and haplotypes $H\text{-}2^d$ and $H\text{-}2^b$ by 2, 3, 4, 5, 8, 31, and 33. Using these haplotypes, Gorer and Mikulska (1959) set up $H\text{-}2^d/H\text{-}2^b \times H\text{-}2^b/H\text{-}2^b$ and $H\text{-}2^a/H\text{-}2^b \times H\text{-}2^b/H\text{-}2^b$ backcrosses and, out of slightly fewer than 300 backcross mice, obtained the three recombinants shown in Table 6.2. The serotypes of the recombinant chromosomes, as confirmed by progeny testing, were 31,2; 11,2; and 33,3,4. The last two of these were reciprocals obtained from the same $F_1$. The three were assigned, in terminology as now revised (Snell *et al.*, 1964), the haplotype symbols $H\text{-}2^g$, $H\text{-}2^h$, and $H\text{-}2^i$. The recombinant frequency for the total experiment was 1.02%.

The demonstration that crossing-over could occur within *H-2* compelled a reinterpretation of its structure. It appeared that there were at least two closely linked loci rather than one. The postulated loci were assigned the symbols *K* and *D*, from the letter symbols then used for specificities 11 and 4. These were later changed to *H-2K* and *H-2D*, although *K* and *D* are still used as abbreviations. *H-2K* was shown to be at the centromeric end of *H-2* (Lyon *et al.*, 1968). Hence, following the convention that in chromosome maps the centromere is placed either at the left or at the top, the two loci are placed in the order *H-2K–H-2D*.

Since the original experiments of Gorer and co-workers, other crossover studies have been carried out (e.g., Stimpfling and Richardson, 1965; David and Shreffler, 1972), and many recombinants found. At least 33 are

TABLE 6.2
*H-2* RECOMBINANTS OBTAINED BY BACKCROSSING $H\text{-}2^d/H\text{-}2^b$ AND $H\text{-}2^a/H\text{-}2^b$ $F_1$ MICE TO $H\text{-}2^b/H\text{-}2^b$ [a]

| Heterozygous parent | | Recombinant chromosome | |
|---|---|---|---|
| Haplotype | Serotype[b] | Haplotype | Serotype |
| $H\text{-}2^d$ / $H\text{-}2^b$ | 31 3 4 / 33 2 | $H\text{-}2^g$ | 31 2 |
| $H\text{-}2^a$ / $H\text{-}2^b$ | 11 3 4 / 33 2 | $H\text{-}2^h$ | 11 2 |
| $H\text{-}2^a$ / $H\text{-}2^b$ | 11 3 4 / 33 2 | $H\text{-}2^i$ | 33 3 4 |

[a] From Gorer and Mikulska (1959).
[b] Vertical lines show the location and direction of the recombination.

still in existence (Klein, 1975a). In addition to the recombinants found in crossover studies, there are six haplotypes that because of the specificities they determine and in some cases also because of the known history of the type strains, presumably arose as accidental crossovers in outcrossed stocks. Thus, as first pointed out by Gorer, and as can be seen from Table 6.1, $H\text{-}2^a$ does not have any specificities that are not found in $H\text{-}2^d$ and $H\text{-}2^k$, and hence $H\text{-}2^a$ might have arisen from these two haplotypes by recombination.

The combined *H-2* crossover studies indicate a recombination frequency between *H-2K* and *H-2D* of about 0.5% (Shreffler, 1974). Crossing over between *H-2D* and *Tla* is about 1%. This degree of crossing over leaves room for a number of unidentified loci in the *H-2* complex—but a number that is impossible to estimate with any precision at the present time because of uncertainty concerning the number of functional genes in mammals. Two of the necessary statistics are known with at least some degree of precision. The haploid number of nucleotides in the mouse genome is placed at $6.5 \times 10^9$ (Sparrow *et al.*, 1972). With respect to the number of crossover units or cM, both chiasmata counts (Slinzynsky, 1955) and the linkage map (M. Green, personal communication) lead to an estimate of about 2000. The number of amino acids for which the average gene codes is poorly known. The fraction of the total DNA that, because it consists of repeated sequences (Kolata, 1973) or of "fossil" genes or "junk" (Ohno, 1972), does not code for functional genes is currently subject to the most varied estimates. O'Brien

(1973) presents rather persuasive evidence that most of the DNA codes for functional genes, although many of these may be regulatory rather than structural. If we assume that the average protein molecule consists of 400 amino acids and that 3/5 of the genome is repeat sequences, we arrive at a figure of about 1000 genes per cM (compare Shreffler, 1974). But if we accept the estimate of mammalian gene number proposed by some geneticists on the basis presumed mutation rate and the tolerable load of mutant genes (review in Ohno, 1972), the figure becomes about 15 genes per cM. The second estimate, which would allow for only 7 or 8 genes between *H-2K* and *H-2D,* is almost certainly too low, but the first estimate may be too high, at least with respect to structural genes.

The availability of many *H-2* recombinants has been the key to the genetic analysis of the *H-2* complex.

## III. The *H-2*-Linked *Ss* Serum Protein Locus

*Ss* is a locus in the middle of the *H-2* complex, discovered and analyzed by Shreffler and co-workers, which determines the amount and structure of a serum β-globulin (review in Shreffler and David, 1975). The protein either is, or is associated with, a component of complement (Čapková and Démant, 1974). This ties it to immune processes. There is also a similarity in the subunit structure of the Ss protein and the *H-2* gene product (Klein, 1975b). Analysis of crossovers has shown *Ss* to be essentially in the middle of the *H-2* region. Seventeen of the known cases of recombination can be placed to the left of *Ss,* i.e., between *H-2K* and *Ss,* and 19 to the right.

*Ss* is now recognized as being a locus (or possibly loci) of considerable complexity, with numerous alleles. It controls quantitative differences in the level of the Ss serum protein, which can be demonstrated with rabbit antisera, and structural differences, which are recognized through the use of alloantisera. There is one allele determining the structural variant which is sex limited; the variant protein, when this allele is present, occurs only in males. We need not go into further details. The important point in this context is that there are many alleles. This increases the value of *Ss* as a marker, since it segregates in virtually every cross. The current convention is to designate each allele with the haplotype symbol of its associated nonrecombinant *H-2* haplotype. Thus the *Ss* allele of $H\text{-}2^b$ is $Ss^b$, that of $H\text{-}2^d$ is $Ss^d$, and that of $H\text{-}2^d/H\text{-}2^b$ recombinant $H\text{-}2^g$ is $Ss^d$, since it was derived from $H\text{-}2^d$.

A locus has been identified in the human HLA complex which determines a component of complement and may well be a homologue of the murine *Ss* locus (Teisberg *et al.*, 1975; Wolski *et al.*, 1975).

To cope with this added complexity of the *H-2* chromosome region, we need additional terminology. The *genotype* of any particular haplotype is the sequence of alleles at known or relevant loci included in this haplotype. Thus the genotype of $H\text{-}2^b$ is $H\text{-}2K^b\ Ss^b\ H\text{-}2D^b$. This, where appropriate, may be abbreviated $K^b\ Ss^b\ D^b$. The *serotype* of a particular haplotype is the list of known or relevant specificities determinated by that haplotype.

## IV. The Occurrence of the Same Specificity at Both Ends of *H-2*

One of the surprising findings in regard to *H-2* is that there are several specificities that occur at both the *K* and *D* ends of the system. The failure to realize this in some of the early studies led to an interpretation of *H-2* structure which is now rejected, and ultimately led to considerable confusion before the problem was resolved. There is now extensive evidence for the repetition of specificities. In order to understand this evidence, we have to introduce some more of the many complexities that characterize *H-2*.

In *H-2* recombination studies, there have been frequent instances of serologically identical crossovers occurring more than once. Despite the serological identity, it was not to be expected that the actual point of exchange would be identical. And indeed, when *Ss* was added to the map, it turned out that the exchange points in serologically similar recombinants were often on opposite sides of *Ss*.

This created a nomenclature problem; haplotype symbols were necessary that would distinguish all recombinants, including those that at first appeared similar. The convention adopted was the addition of a number to the haplotype symbol as defined by serotype alone. Thus $H\text{-}2^{h2}$ and $H\text{-}2^{h3}$ are two successive recombinants from the same type of cross and of the same serotype. A more complex symbol, conforming to the accepted rule for variants that are members of a series (Staats, 1968), was originally used.

Table 6.3 shows seven recombinants from two different crosses and of four different serotypes. Two of the recombinants are the same as $H\text{-}2^h$ and $H\text{-}2^i$ of Table 6.2, but additional specificities and information concerning *Ss* are included in Table 6.3. The seven recombinants provide evidence that three *H-2* specificities, 1, 3, and 35, are each determined by two genes, one on each side of *Ss*, and presumably corresponding to *H-2K* and *H-2D*.

TABLE 6.3

EVIDENCE FOR THE OCCURRENCE OF H-2 SPECIFICITIES 1, 3, AND 35 IN BOTH *H-2K* AND *H-2D* [a]

| Heterozygous parent | | Recombinant chromosome | |
|---|---|---|---|
| Haplotype | Serotype | Haplotype | Serotype |
| *H-2*$^a$ / *H-2*$^b$ | 11 1 3 $Ss^d$ 3 35 4<br>33 35 $Ss^b$ 2 | *H-2*$^{h2}$ | 11 1 3 $Ss^d$ 2 |
| | 11 1 3 $Ss^d$ 3 35 4<br>33 35 $Ss^b$ 2 | *H-2*$^{h4}$ | 11 1 3 $Ss^b$ 2 |
| | 11 1 3 $Ss^d$ 3 35 4<br>33 35 $Ss^b$ 2 | *H-2*$^i$ | 33 35 $Ss^b$ 3 35 4 |
| | 11 1 3 $Ss^d$ 3 35 4<br>33 35 $Ss^b$ 2 | *H-2*$^{i5}$ | 33 35 $Ss^d$ 3 35 4 |
| *H-2*$^d$ / *H-2*$^k$ | 31 3 $Ss^d$ 3 35 4<br>11 1 3 $Ss^k$ 1 32 | *H-2*$^{a1}$ | 11 1 3 $Ss^k$ 3 35 4 |
| | 31 3 $Ss^d$ 3 35 4<br>11 1 3 $Ss^k$ 1 32 | *H-2*$^{o1}$ | 31 3 $Ss^k$ 1 32 |
| | 31 3 $Ss^d$ 3 35 4<br>11 1 3 $Ss^k$ 1 32 | *H-2*$^{o2}$ | 31 3 $Ss^d$ 1 32 |

[a] Data used in this table came from the following sources: Démant *et al.*, 1971; Klein and Shreffler, 1971; Shreffler *et al.*, 1966; Shreffler and David, 1975; Snell and Cherry, 1974; Snell *et al.*, 1971b; Stimpfling and Richardson, 1965.

Let us consider first the case of H-2.1. This segregated in both crosses, being present in the *H-2*$^a$ parent of the first cross and the *H-2*$^k$ parent of the second. H-2.1, in the first cross, segregated with H-2.11. All four recombinants from this cross listed in the table place it to the left of *Ss*. But in the second cross, 1 segregated with 32 in a coupling relationship and with 4 in a repulsion relationship. H-2.4 we have already placed in *H-2D* (Table 6.2), and since the three recombinants of this cross show 32 to be separable from 11 and 31, it also is placed in *H-2D*. Recombinants *H-2*$^{a1}$ and *H-2*$^{o2}$ not only place 1 at the right end of *H-2*, but also to the right of *Ss*. The simplest interpretation of these data is that there are loci both at the left and right of *Ss* which determine specificity 1. *H-2*$^k$ has alleles determining 1 at both these loci, *H-2*$^a$ at only one, and *H-2*$^b$ and *H-2*$^d$ at neither. The loci need not be the same as the loci determining 11 and 31, on the one hand, and 4 and 32, on the other, but there is no evidence that requires the postulation of additional loci.

The evidence for a locus determining 3 on both sides of *Ss* is essentially similar to that for H-2.1, and need not be examined in detail. The evidence for H-2.35 is somewhat different. In the first cross in Table 6.3, both parents have 35. But one of the recombinant serotypes, *H-2*$^{h}$, lacks 35. This probably could be explained in terms of some sort of gene interaction, but the simplest explanation is that in the *H-2*$^{a}$ parent the 35 determinant is in *H-2D*, and in the *H-2*$^{b}$ parent the 35 determinant is in *H-2K*. Recombinants occurring in one direction get both 35's, recombinants occurring in the other direction get neither.

Other specificities for which similar evidence of dual sites exist are 5, 28, and 36. H-2.6 is placed by serological studies in *H-2D* but by a molecular study in *H-2K* (Hauptfeld and Klein, 1975). Perhaps this means it also is determined by dual sites. Additional examples are likely to turn up. There is other convincing evidence for dual sites besides that given in Table 6.3 (see, e.g., Shreffler *et al.*, 1966; Murphy and Shreffler, 1975a; Hauptfeld and Klein, 1975), but it would be redundant to cite it. Dual sites probably also occur in the two loci of HLA, the human homologue of *H-2* (Chapter 9).

By immunizing with one skin graft and testing with another, from appropriately selected haplotypes, it has been shown that there are cross-reactions in the histocompatibility effects of *H-2K* and *H-2D*. The data suggest that the demonstrated cross-reactions correspond to the cross-ractions of specificities 3 and 36 (Murphy and Shreffler, 1975b).

The recombination anomalies created by the existence of dual sites were originally explained by postulating the existence of additional *H-2* loci besides *H-2K* and *H-2D*. As many as six loci were at one time suggested. This was an entirely logical interpretation of the data then extant, but was rendered untenable when multiple recombinants typed for *Ss* became available. It was then inescapable that the same determinant could exist on both sides of the *Ss* marker.

In designating divisible H-2 specificities, the specificity number may be preceded by a K or a D to indicate which locus determines it, e.g., H-2K.3 or K3.

## V. Classification of H-2 Specificities

### A. Private Specificities

It will be seen from the *H-2* chart in Table 6.1 that five of the twelve listed specificities, 2, 9, 19, 31, and 33, occur in single haplotypes, whereas four others, 3, 5, 6, and 8, occur in five or six out of seven listed haplotypes. This is an asymmetrical distribution. The chart in Table 6.1 includes far fewer specificities and haplotypes than are found in more recent charts, but this tendency to high or low representation in the known haplotypes remains unchanged. The unevenness of the distribution is made more striking if we examine, in more detail, some of the specificities which, like H-2.4, occur in only two or three haplotypes. H-2.4 is found in $H\text{-}2^d$, $H\text{-}2^a$, and $H\text{-}2^i$. Two of these, $H\text{-}2^a$ and $H\text{-}2^i$, are recombinants of which $H\text{-}2^d$ was one of the parental haplotypes. The corresponding genotypes are $H\text{-}2^d$: $H\text{-}2K^d$ $H\text{-}2D^d$; $H\text{-}2^a$: $H\text{-}2K^k$ $H\text{-}2D^d$; $H\text{-}2^i$: $H\text{-}2K^b$ $H\text{-}2D^d$. Specificity 4 is located at the right end of *H-2* (Table 6.2) which places it in *H-2D*. The only *H-2* allele, therefore, in which it occurs, is $H\text{-}2D^d$. Thus although it occurs in three haplotypes, it occurs in only one allele. In this sense its distribution is as restricted as 2, 9, etc.

We shall call the H-2 specificities which recur in a single allele *private specificities*, adopting a term originally used by Amos (1962), and the more widely distributed specificities, *public specificities*. We shall find that private and public specificities are distinguished by other characteristics in addition to their frequency of occurrence.

The most important property of the private specificities is that they can be arranged in two allelic or mutually exclusive series, one series determined by *H-2K* and the other by *H-2D* (Snell *et al.*, 1971a). Thus the recombination data in Table 6.3 show that 31 and 33 can be placed in *H-2K* and 2, 4, and 32 can be placed in *H-2D*. There is one exception. Private specificities occurring in haplotypes that have not been involved in a recombination, or whose recombinants have not been fully analyzed, cannot yet be assigned to one or the other end of *H-2*. Thus H-2.18, the private specificity of $H\text{-}2^r$, is unassignable. But H-2.19, a private specificity of $H\text{-}2^s$, originally unassignable, was shown by the $H\text{-}2^{qp}$ recombinant derived from an $H\text{-}2^q/H\text{-}2^s$ heterozygote, to be divisible into H-2.19, assignable to *H-2K*, and H-2.12, assignable to *H-2D*. H-2.9 has likewise been moved from the unassignable to the assignable category (Klein *et al.*, 1975c). We may safely assume that all private specificities will, in due course, be assignable to either the *H-2K* or the *H-2D* allelic series.

The private specificities generally give rise to particularly strong antisera, with H-2K antisera on the average being stronger than H-2D (Snell *et al.*, 1971a; McKenzie and Snell, 1973). The different specificities differ in the relative ease with which they are demonstrable by hemagglutination as compared with lymphocytotoxicity. H-2.33 is demonstrable only by cytotoxicity, except when tested in the autoanalyzer, which reveals a hemagglutinating component. H-2.32 gives at best weak hemagglutination reactions; H-2.4 gives strong and dependable hemagglutination reactions but it also generates good cytotoxic antibodies (Gorer and

Mikulska, 1959; Douglas and Nieman, 1973; M. Cherry and G. D. Snell, unpublished date).

## B. Public Specificities

### 1. *Confusion with Ia Specificities*

Some specificities associated with the *K* end of the *H-2* complex and originally assigned to H-2 public group, now turn out to be determined by the *Ia* loci (Section VIII,B). This has been shown for 34 and 46 (Staines *et al.*, 1974). It is probably true of 53, a cytotoxic specificity showing the low maximum lysis characteristic of Ia specificities. Some other public specificities may turn out to be similarly misclassified. But specificities manifesting hemagglutinating as well as lymphocytotoxic activity in all probability are *H-2* determined.

### 2. *Diversity of Public Specificities*

Public specificities may occur in anywhere from two known alleles, e.g., H-2.25, to the great majority of alleles at one locus, e.g., H-2.6. There appears to be some tendency toward either narrow or wide distribution (Snell *et al.*, 1973). Thus, after correcting for specificities now reclassified as part of the *Ia* system, we find 17 specificities that occur in two or three alleles, 4 associated with four to eight alleles, and 5 with nine to eleven alleles.

Besides the differences in distribution, there are other indications of diversity among the public specificities. Some tend to induce weak antibodies, others give antibodies of good titer. Some give rise to predominantly hemagglutinating antibodies (e.g., 3, 41, 42), some to good cytotoxic as well as hemagglutinating antibodies (1, 11, 28), and a few to exclusively cytotoxic antibodies (35, 36). As we have already pointed out (Section IV), some are represented in both *H-2K* and *H-2D*. Most of these specificities which are determined by both loci are widely distributed (e.g., 1, 3, 5, 28). Specificities 35 and 36 appear to be, but are not necessarily, an exception. At least some of the widely distributed specificities have two other properties that set them apart: because of lack of uniformity from allele to allele they have to be defined in terms of families of similar but nonidentical antibodies; they may fall into alleic series. These points require additional discussion.

### 3. *Specificities Defined by Antibody Families*

Specificity H-2.1 will serve to illustrate the widely distributed, nonuniform specificities defined by antibody families. Table 6.4 shows the haplotype distribution of reactivity of five anti-1 sera, of an anti-45 that

TABLE 6.4
HAPLOTYPE DISTRIBUTION OF H-2 SPECIFICITY 1, AS DEFINED BY FIVE DIFFERENT ANTISERA, AND OF THE RELATED SPECIFICITIES 45 AND 5[a]

| | Grade of reaction of indicated antiserum[b] | | | | | | |
|---|---|---|---|---|---|---|---|
| Haplotype | *i* × *f* *pa* | *b* × *d* *v* | *b* × *f* *o* | *s* × *f* *p* | *d* × *p* *s* | *b* *ja* | *d* × *f* *i* |
| *a* | 4 | 4? | 4 | 4? | 4 | 4 | 4 |
| *h* | 4 | 4 | 4 | 4 | 4 | 4 | 4 |
| *k* | 4 | 4 | 4 | 4? | 4 | 4 | 4 |
| *m* | 4 | 4 | 4 | 4 | 4 | 4 | 4 |
| *r* | 3 | 3 | 3 | 3 | 3 | 3 | 2 |
| *q* | 2 | 3 | 3 | 3 | 2 | 3 | 2 |
| *v* | 3 | 3 | 2 | 2? | 2 | 3 | 2 |
| *o* | 2 | 3 | 3 | 2 | 2? | 1 | 2 |
| *s* | 3 | 3 | 2 | 0 | 3 | 3 | 2 |
| *p* and *pa* | 3 | 3? | 2 | 3 | 0 | 1 | 2 |
| *j* and *ja* | 1 | 0 | 0 | 0 | 0 | 3 | 1–2 |
| *u* | 1 | 0 | 0 | 1 | 0? | 1 | 2 |
| *b* | 0 | 0 | 0 | 0 | 0 | 0 | 3 |
| *i* | 0 | 0 | 0 | 0 | 0 | 0 | 3 |
| *d* | 0 | 0 | 0 | 0 | 0 | 0 | 0 |
| *f* | 0 | 0 | 0 | 0 | 0 | 0 | 0 |
| *g* | 1? | 0 | 0 | 1? | 0 | 0 | 0 |
| Possible antibodies | 1,16, 38 | 1, 21 | 1, 3, 31, 32 | 1, 16, non-H-2? | 1, 19, non-H-2? | 15, 45, non-H-2? | 5, 33 |

[a] Data on which grades of reaction of anti-1 and anti-5 sera are based were taken from Snell *et al.* (1971b). Data for anti-45 came from Čapková and Démant (1972) and from G. D. Snell and M. Cherry (unpublished).

[b] The headings to the columns show the haplotypes of the recipient–donor pairs used in the production of the antisera. Except for the anti-15, 45, the recipients were all $F_1$ hybrids. The grades of reaction are derived from a combination of data from hemagglutination and cytotoxic reactions, and from both direct reactions and absorption studies. 4 indicates maximum activity, 0, no activity. The individual grades should be regarded as indications of trends or tendencies, not as precise values.

is clearly a member of the 1 family, and of an anti-5 that defines a closely related specificity. With respect to the anti-1 sera and the anti-45, the haplotypes fall into three groups. The first four haplotypes in the table, all of which carry allele $H\text{-}2K^k$ and private specificity 23, originally derived from haplotype $H\text{-}2^k$, are strong and consistent reactors. Quantitative absorption studies show that these four possess substantially more 1 activity than the other haplotypes. Indeed, they absorb more anti-1 than the donors used in producing the antisera (Snell *et al.*, 1971b). The next eight haplotypes in the table grade from moderately strong to weak and uncertain reactors. Each of the last four failed to react with at least one of the antisera. Two of them, *s* and *p*, were in fact represented in the recipients of two of the antisera. If H-2.1 were a uniform entity, no anti-1 could have been present in these instances. The last haplotype in group two, $H\text{-}2^u$, is such a weak reactor that it could equally well have been placed in the last group. This group, containing five haplotypes, is nonreactive except for two very weak and questionable reactions shown by $H\text{-}2^g$.

Specificity H-2.5 shows a haplotype distribution identical to H-2.1 except that it is present also in $H\text{-}2^b$ and the derivative haplotype $H\text{-}2^i$. The reactions also show the same gradations in strength as H-2.1.

Widely distributed specificities H-2.3 and H-2.28 show similar gradations in their haplotype distribution (Snell and Cherry, 1974; Snell *et al.*, 1974). H-2.28 can be, and originally was, divided into three separate specificities, 27, 28, and 29, with similar but nonidentical haplotype distributions (Stimpfling and Pizarro, 1961). We would interpret a recent study of Murphy and Shreffler (1975a) as indicating that specificities 13, 35, and 36 constitute a family. Like the 1 and 28 families, specificities of the 36 family occur in both *H-2K* and *H-2D*. Other widely distributed public specificities have not been subjected to the sort of study with multiple antisera necessary to determine if they also show graded levels of activity and uncertain limits.

### 4. *Allelism of Widely Distributed Specificities*

Allelism of widely distributed public specificities at present can be said with any assurance to exist only for 1 and 28. These do seem to show a mutually exclusive relationship in both *H-2K* and *H-2D* (Snell *et al.*, 1973, 1974). Thus $H\text{-}2^k$ has K1 and D1 and lacks 28, $H\text{-}2^o$ has K28 and D1, $H\text{-}2^a$ has K1 and D28, and $H\text{-}2^b$ has K28 and D28 and lacks 1. There are, however, some haplotypes, particularly those for which well-analyzed recombinants are not available, for which the data are very inconclusive. There are also great differences in the strength of the reactions. H-2.5, which seems to belong in this family of specificities, closely paralleling H-2.1 in its haplotype distribution, overlaps 28. This, however, all fits in the picture of the variability of this category of specificities in different haplotypes.

Anti-1, anti-5, and anti-28 sera show good titers by both hemagglutination and cytotoxicity. This further emphasized their similarity.

There are many parallels between 1 and 28 and the HLA specificities 4a and 4b (Chapter 9).

### 5. *Interpretation*

The source of the diverse reactions with alloantigens that, on genetic grounds, can be interpreted as a single molecule is one of the oldest puzzles of immunogenetics. Is it cross-reactions with a single site? Is it multiple sites on a single molecule? Or is it, perhaps, the unsuspected existence of multiple antigens determined by closely linked genes? There is a growing suspicion in the case of *H-2* that it may be all three.

Certainly some of the narrowly distributed public specificities are easily interpreted as the product of cross-reactions between the same sites that determine their private specificities. However, a good case can also be made for multiple sites (Snell *et al.*, 1973), and Hess and Davies (1974a) have postulated that the private and public specificities are not merely determined by different sites, but by different loci. The end result, according to this concept, is a hybrid molecule containing a private and any one of a number of alternative public specificities.

Perhaps the test case will ultimately be provided by specificities 1 and 28. If there are any specificities with serological properties that set them apart from the others it is these two, and indeed there is now evidence that they may be determined by a locus distinct from but very closely linked to the locus that determines the private specificities (Démant *et al.*, 1976; Lemonnier *et al.*, 1975).

Irrespective of where it is located, the 1–28 site, on serological grounds, must be interpreted as highly variable. Although all known allelic forms of the H-2 antigens, with possible minor exceptions, express either one or the other of these specificities, the specificities appear to be not quite the same in any two alleles for which there is adequate evidence. Of course there must be two major forms of the site, one associated with specificity 1, the other with 28, but the 1's and the 28's themselves seem also to vary. The range of antigenic variation is obviously much less than that manifested by the private specificities, but the total polymorphism may be much the same.

One possible structural interpretation of the serological data is that the two major forms of the 1–28 site are determined by differences in amino acids with high antigenic potency, e.g., tyrosine and lysine, the minor forms by differences in amino acids low in the antigenic hierarchy (Gill 1973).

## VI. *H-2* Polymorphism

The *H-2* system, and in fact the whole *H-2* chromosome region to and including the *T* locus, shows an extraordinary polymorphism. With the possible exception of a few genes between *H-2* and *T*, all loci in this region seem to exist in numerous allelic forms. We are concerned here with the polymorphism of *H-2*. Part of the diversity of *H-2* is due to the existence of two or possibly more than two *H-2* loci whose alleles can be combined and recombined in a variety of relatively stable haplotypes. However, even if we consider the different loci separately we find much variation.

A recent *H-2* chart shows 12 *H-2K* alleles and 10 *H-2D* alleles (Snell *et al.*, 1973). This does not include mutants and minor variants. These alleles have been detected exclusively in inbred strains of mice available in and usually originating in the United States. It is known that these strains had a restricted origin (Staats, 1966). The ancestral mice were derived from a limited number of imports from European biologists or fanciers with perhaps a small admixture of Japanese waltzing strains, and the stocks of European fanciers themselves, which are probably ancestral to nearly all laboratory mice, were doubtless a miniscule sample of wild mice in general. Yet all *H-2* haplotypes in European inbred strains are turning out to be new ones (Anna Dux, personal communication). We may thus infer that the polymorphism of wild mice should substantially exceed that of their domestic relatives.

There is now evidence confirming this inference. Klein (1974) has analyzed the *H-2* haplotypes of wild mice trapped on farms in the Ann Arbor area. To avoid the confusion that would result from trying to type *H-2* heterozygotes, the separate *H-2* chromosomes of the wild mice were isolated by backcrossing, with appropriate serotyping, to inbred backgrounds. In the course of backcrossing, alloantisera were produced in inbred recipients against the wild haplotypes. Thirty chromosomes from mice trapped in different locations have now been isolated and typed. Every one of them has a different *H-2* haplotype.

The serological results with the wild mice confirmed the validity of the distinction between public and private specificities. When typed with standard antisera, mice from 75 to 95% of the localities where mice were caught reacted with the different public antibodies, mice from 0 to 10% of the localities reacted with the different private antibodies. Of seven known private specificities tested, only four were found in any of the wild mice. Antisera made against wild chromosomes identified 12 new private specificities, each of which presumably is separable into *K* and *D* components.

Iványi and Micková (1972), in a similar study of wild mice in Czechoslovakia, found reactions with five private antibodies, but added the observation that, when tested by absorption, the wild mice did not remove all activity.

The conclusion to which both studies point is that the *H-2* haplotypes of wild mouse isolates are usually different, not only from the haplotypes of laboratory mice, but from each other. That the wild antigens do react with some private antibodies points to a likeness between some wild and domestic alleles. One absorption test suggests that the likeness, sometimes at least, does not extend to identity.

The data do not permit any quantitative estimate of the number of *H-2* alleles, but it clearly is enormous. Combining analyses of American and European inbred strains and of wild mice, we can say that about 40 alleles at each locus are now known, although some are still poorly characterized. Seemingly hundreds of others must exist in mice throughout the world.

Another contribution of these studies of wild mice was their confirmation of the already suspected deme structure of wild populations. Mice trapped in the same location tended to have the same *H-2* alleles; mice trapped in other locations, even on the same farm, usually had different alleles. A result of this sort of deme structure should be considerable inbreeding. It is not surprising, therefore, that in a skin graft study Micková and Iványi (1972) found evidence for heterozygosity in wild mice at only 3 to 6 histocompatibility loci. Since all of these were often weak, homozygosity at *H-2* may have been common.

## VII. The *H-2* Chart

Since data on H-2 specificities first began to accumulate, it has been customary to summarize the information in *H-2* charts. The charts have grown more and more complex and are now organized in several different ways. Table 6.5 is a chart from which many specificities and recombinant haplotypes and some nonrecombinant haplotypes are omitted. It does, however, give the more widely used haplotypes and specificities and should be adequate for many uses. The footnotes give some details not amenable to presentation in the table. Sources of additional information are listed in Table 6.6.

## VIII. Other CMAD Loci in the *H-2* Complex

Besides *H-2K* and *H-2D* there are several other serologically or histogenetically defined cell membrane alloantigen determining (CMAD) loci in the *H-2* complex. We consider these loci in this section. These may

TABLE 6.5
CONDENSED *H-2* CHART[a]

| Haplotype | Recombinant origin | Specificities: *H-2K* Private | *H-2K* Public 1,[b] 28 | 3 | 5 | 8 | 11 | 25 | 36[c] | 38 | *H-2G* 7 | *H-2D* Private | *H-2D* Public 1,[b] 28 | 3 | 5 | 6[f] | 13 | 36[c] | 41 | 42 | 43 | 55 |
|---|---|---|---|---|---|---|---|---|---|---|---|---|---|---|---|---|---|---|---|---|---|---|
| Nonrecombinant | | | | | | | | | | | | | | | | | | | | | | |
| *b* | | 33[d] | 28 | | 5 | | | | 36 | | | 2 | 28 | | | 6 | | | | | | |
| *d* | | 31 | 28 | 3 | | 8 | | | | | | 4 | 28 | 3 | | 6 | 13 | 36 | 41 | 42 | 43 | |
| *f* | | 26 | 28? | | | 8 | | | | | 7 | 9 | 28 | | | 6 | | | | | | |
| *k* | | 23 | 1 | 3 | 5 | 8 | 11 | 25 | | | 7w | 32[d] | 1 | 3 | 5 | | | | | | | |
| *p, pa* [g] | | K16[e] | 1 | | 5 | 8 | | | | 38 | 7 | D16[e] | 1 | 3 | 5? | 6 | | 36 | 41 | | | |
| *q* | | 17 | 1 | 3 | 5 | | 11 | | | | | 30 | 28 | 3? | | 6 | 13 | 36 | | | | 55 |
| *r* | | K18[e] | 1 | 3 | 5 | 8 | 11 | 25 | | | | D18[e] | 28 | | | 6 | | | | | | |
| *s* | | 19 | 1 | | 5 | | | | | | 7 | 12 | 28 | 3 | | 6 | | 36 | | 42 | | |
| *v* | | K21[e] | 1 | | 5 | | | | | | | D21[e] | 28 | 3 | | ? | | 36 | | | 43 | 55 |
| Recombinant[h] | | | | | | | | | | | | | | | | | | | | | | |
| *a* | *k/d* [i] | 23 | 1 | 3 | 5 | 8 | 11 | 25 | | | | 4 | 28 | 3 | | 6 | 13 | 36 | 41 | 42 | 43 | |
| *h2* | *a/b* | 23 | 1 | 3 | 5 | 8 | 11 | 25 | | | | 2 | 28 | | | 6 | | | | | | |
| *i5* | *b/a* | 33 | 28 | | 5 | | | | 36 | | | 4 | 28 | 3 | | 6 | 13 | 36 | 41 | 42 | 43 | |
| *j ja* [i] | *?/b* | 15 | 45 | | | | | | | 38 | 7 | 2 | 28 | | | 6 | | | | | | |
| *m* | *k/q* | 23 | 1 | 3 | 5 | 8 | 11 | 25 | | | 7w | 30 | 28 | 3? | | 6 | 13 | 36 | | | | 55 |
| *o1* | *d/k* | 31 | 28 | 3 | | 8 | | | | | 7w | 32 | 1 | 3 | 5 | | | | | | | |
| *qp* | *q/s* | 17 | 1 | 3? | 5 | | 11 | | | | | 12 | 28 | 3 | | 6 | | 36 | | 42 | | |
| *u* | *?/d* | 20 | ? | 3? | 5 | | | | | | | 4 | 28 | 3 | | 6 | 13 | 36 | 41 | 42 | 43 | |

[a] Based on the following sources: G. D. Cherry and M. Snell (unpublished); David *et al.*, 1975a; Démant, 1973; Klein *et al.*, 1975b,c; Klein and Shreffler, 1971; Murphy and Shreffler, 1975a; Shreffler and David, 1975; Snell *et al.*, 1973.

[b] Specificities 1, 28, and 45 are placed in the same column to indicate their probable allelism (Section V,B,4). Because of their variability from allele to allele, 1 and 28 can only be defined in terms of families of antibodies. Specificity 45 is a member of the 1 family. Anti-45 is the only anti-1 that reacts at more than a weak level with haplotypes *j* and *ja*. H-2.28 can be split into three specificities, 27, 28, and 29, with a similar strain distribution. The three usually occur together, but $H\text{-}2^f$ has 27 only, $H\text{-}2^s$ 28 only, and $H\text{-}2^o$ 29 only. $H\text{-}2^i$ has been typed as lacking 27 (Démant, 1973).

[c] H-2.36 resembles H-2.1 and 28 in that it is defined by a family of similar but not identical antibodies. It includes specificity 13 (shown separately in the chart) and 35 (not shown). We identify *v* as possessing 36 because of reactions reported by Murphy and Shreffler (1975a). H-2.36 is a cytotoxic specificity. Specificities 41, 42, and 43 comprise a family closely resembling 36, but absent from $H\text{-}2^b$ and defined by hemagglutination.

[d] H-2.33 is a strong cytotoxic specificity but is not demonstrable by the usual humagglutination techniques. It is demonstrable on bromelin-treated red cells used in the autoanalyzer (Douglas and Nieman, 1973). Some other specificities, e.g., H-2.32, are difficult to demonstrate by hemagglutination.

[e] Because of the lack of well analyzed recombinants derived from haplotypes, *p*, *pa*, *r*, and *v*, the private antisera associated with these haplotypes are not separable into *K* and *D* end specificities. Presumably they will be separable when recombinants are available. We have entered the same specificity number for both *H-2K* and *H-2D*, preceded by a K or D.

[f] Specificity 6 has been placed by serological and crossover studies in *H-2D*, but a molecular study places it in *H-2K* (Hauptfeld and Klein, 1975). Possibly this means that it is determined by sites in both *H-2K* and *H-2D*.

[g] Haplotypes *p* and *pa* are serologically similar and perhaps indistinguishable but with different *Ss* alleles.

[h] The list of recombinants in Table 6.5 is very incomplete. In particular, repeat recombinants of the same serotype are not shown. The serotype of any recombinant not listed can be figured out, using information as to the *H-2K* and *H-2D* alleles of the recombinant (Fig. 6.3 or Shreffler and David, 1975), and information from the table under nonrecombinants as to the specificities determined by these alleles. Thus recombinant $H\text{-}2^g$ ($K^d$ $D^b$) has the combined specificities of the *K* end of *d* and the *D* end of *b*. Six haplotypes, *a*, *i*, *ja*, *m*, *qp*, and *u*, listed under recombinants are presumed to be recombinants because their *H-2K* and/or *H-2D* serotype duplicates that of a known nonrecombinant. They were not detected in a cross designed to produce recombinants.

[i] This column gives the haplotypes of the parental strains from which each recombinant arose. The haplotype listed first is the one which gave rise to the *K* end of the recombinant, that listed second is the one which gave rise to the *D* end. In the case of the six recombinants not detected in a planned cross (footnote *g*), there is an element of uncertainty in these listings. Thus since haplotype *a* is $Tla^a$ whereas *d* is $Tla^c$, the ancestral *D* end of $H\text{-}2^a$, from which its *Tla* allele would have been derived, was probably present in a haplotype similar to rather than identical with the existing $H\text{-}2^d$.

[j] Haplotypes *j* and *ja* are almost or quite identical serologically and in terms of graft compatibility, but have different *Ss* alleles.

TABLE 6.6
SOURCES OF INFORMATION ON THE *H-2* COMPLEX

| Reference | Type of information |
|---|---|
| Démant (1973) | *H-2* chart with complete list of *H-2* specificities, but includes some specificities now classified as part of the *Ia* system |
| Démant (semiannual) | New *H-2* haplotypes and specificities are recorded semiannually by Peter Démant in Mouse Membrane Alloantigen News, which is issued by M.R.C. Laboratory Animals Centre, Woodmanstern Road, Carshalton, Surrey, England, as part of Mouse News Letter; results of *H-2* typing of previously untyped inbred strains are also given |
| Klein (1975a) | Book reviewing all aspects of the *H-2* complex |
| Klein (1973) | List of congenic strains of mice |
| Klein *et al.* (1974a) | Genetic nomenclature for the *H-2* complex |
| Shreffler and David (1975) | List of *H-2* recombinants and their genotypes (Table 2), also a list of parental haplotypes of various recombinants (Table 12) |
| Snell and Cherry (1972); Frelinger *et al.* (1974a) | *Tla* specificities of different inbred congenic, and recombinant strains |
| Snell *et al.* (1973) | An *H-2* chart arranged to show probable structural and phylogenetic relationship |
| Staats (1968) | An alphabetical list of inbred strains, with information on various characteristics, including *H-2* and *Tla* type |
| Staats (1972) | An alphabetical list of various mouse polymorphic loci, including *H-2*, together with the inbred strains which carry each allele |

be identical with loci defined by other methodologies, e.g., the mixed lymphocyte reaction (Chapter 8), but this has not been proved.

## A. REGIONS OF THE *H-2* COMPLEX

For purposes of describing the *H-2* complex, it has proved convenient to divide the chromosome segment bounded on the left by *H-2K* and on right by *H-2D* into four regions (Klein *et al.*, 1974a). The regions, from left to right, are designated *K, I, S,* and *D*. Regions *K, S,* and *D* are marked, respectively, by the *H-2K, Ss,* and *H-2D* loci. The *I* region is defined by loci that we shall examine in Section VIII,B and in Chapter 7. As we shall see in Section VIII,D, a *G* region has recently been added. The precise boundaries of the regions are at present indeterminate. Ultimately they will probably be defined in terms of specific recombinants. The *I* region is divided into subregions.

## B. The *Ia* Loci

### 1. *Production and Testing of Antisera*

*Ia* is the generalized symbol for a serologically defined CMAD group of loci in the *I* region (*Ia* = *I* region associated). Work on the loci is reviewed in Shreffler and David (1975). Van Leeuwen *et al.* (1973) have presented evidence for what appears to be a human homologue.

The antisera that led to the discovery of *Ia* were produced in recombinant recipient–donor pairs matched at *H-2K* and *H-2D* but differing at *Ss*. The strain pairs were congenic, so that all background genes were shared. The formation of anti-H-2 antibodies, or of non-H-2 antibodies determined by loci unlinked to the *H-2* complex, was thus excluded. David *et al.* (1973) made reciprocal antisera using the two recombinant haplotypes $H\text{-}2^{t1}$ and $H\text{-}2^{t2}$. The first of these has the genotype $K^s$ $Ss^k$ $D^d$, the second has the genotype $K^s$ $Ss^s$ $D^d$. Antisera made with these haplotypes in donor and recipient could not be directed against antigens determined by the terminal portions of the *H-2* complex; they had to be directed against a product of the central region. Similar antisera were made by Hauptfeld *et al.* (1973) using the haplotype pair $H\text{-}2^{y1}$ (genotype $K^q$ $Ss^d$ $D^d$) and $H\text{-}2^{y2}$ (genotype $K^q$ $Ss^q$ $D^d$). Recipient mice were immunized by multiple injections of lymphoid cells.

Reciprocal antisera made in both haplotype pairs contained antibodies demonstrable by lymphocytotoxicity. Tested by either the chromium release or the dye exclusion methods against lymph node lymphocytes, the antisera showed excellent titers but reacted against only a fraction of the cells. The maximum release of radioactivity in the chromium tests was sometimes only 15% above control levels.

That lymphocytotoxic antibodies directed against a non-*H-2* component of the *H-2* complex may coexist with H-2 antibodies has been shown by Sachs and Cone (1973). A B10.A (genotype $K^k$ $Ss^d$ $D^d$) anti-B10.D2 (genotype $K^d$ $Ss^d$ $D^d$) reacted with C57BL/10 (genotype $K^b$ $Ss^b$ $D^b$) node or spleen lymphocytes by cytotoxicity, giving a moderate titer but conspicuously low lysis (Fig. 6.1). A determinant gene to the left of *Ss* was indicated. Thymus lymphocytes were essentially non-reactive, though, as expected, they reacted in the same test with an anti-H-2. The only predicted antibody in the antiserum was an anti-H-2K.31. Specificity 31 is lacking in C57BL/10. The absence of a known H-2 specificity to account for the reaction with B10, and the unusual serological properties of the antibody, pointed to a non-H-2 antigen determined by the K end of *H-2*.

Archer *et al.* (1974) showed that a B10.D2 ($H\text{-}2^d$) anti-B10.M ($H\text{-}2^f$), after exhaustive absorption with erythrocytes which should remove H-2

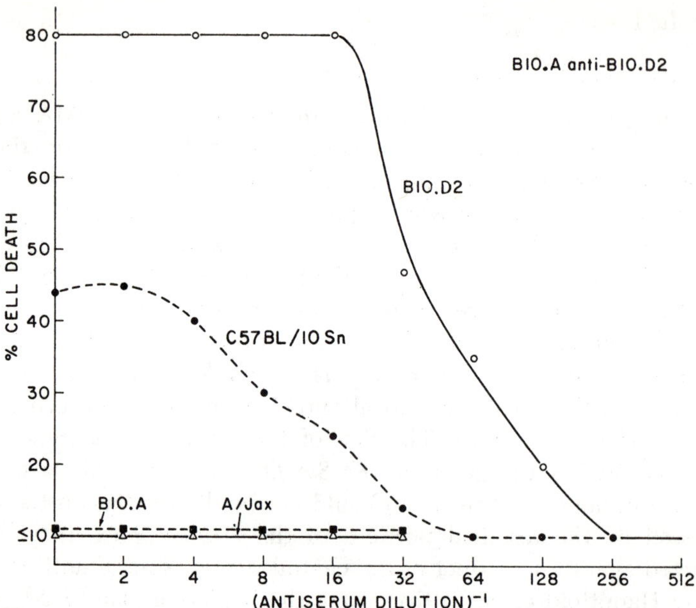


FIG. 6.1. Cytotoxic reactions, as measured by the dye exclusion method, of a B10.A anti-B10.D2 tested against lymph node cells from strains B10.D2 and C57BL/10Sn. The reaction with B10.D2 was due to anti-H.2.31, the reaction with C57BL/10Sn to an anti-Ia antibody probably directed against specificity Ia.8. Note the low maximum cell killing given by the anti-Ia, presumably caused by the nonreactivity of the antibody with the thymus-derived lymphocytes that make up about half the cell population of lymph nodes (Sachs and Cone, 1973).

antibodies, was still reactive against lymph node cells. The reaction showed the low maximum lysis characteristic of anti-Ia antibodies. Although the antibodies remaining after absorption were primarily reactive with B cells, thymocytes could absorb them. The authors add the interesting observation that the erythrocyte-absorbed antiserum was quite as effective in enhancing the survival of B10.M → B10.D2 skin grafts as was the unabsorbed antiserum.

Using the same method of red cell absorption, Davies and Alkins (1974) produced a rat analogue of the mouse anti-Ia. After three absorptions with red cells, a lymphocytotoxic antibody showing low maximum lysis remained and was not further reduced by additional absorptions. This was tested for enhancing capacity against abdominal heart transplants. In the strain combination used, anti-donor alloantibody increased the survival of most such grafts from 8–10 days, the value seen in controls, to 100 + days. The red cell absorption did not diminish the enhancing capacity. The authors speculate that anti-Ia operates via donor lymphocytes carried over in the graft.

## 2. *The Genetics of Ia*

The recipient–donor combinations, in which the anti-Ia antisera so far described were made, served to localize the determinant locus or loci between *H-2K* and *H-2D* or, in the case of the B10.A anti-B10.D2, in the left end of *H-2*. More precise localization has been achieved by the production of additional antisera, and by the *Ia* typing of appropriate panels of recombinant haplotypes. This work was facilitated by genetic studies previously carried out on *I*-region loci concerned in the immune response which we shall review in Chapter 7. It is now established as the result of these tests that *Ia* maps between *H-2K* and *Ss*, and that it consists of multiple loci. Three loci appear to have been identified which may tentatively be called *Ia-1*, *Ia-2*, and *Ia-3*. The total evidence for these loci is complex. We shall merely describe one example of the sort of data by which they are established.

Figure 6.2 shows some of the results obtained with two anti-Ia antisera and indicates how these lead to the postulate of two *Ia* loci, *Ia-1* and *Ia-3*, at the K end of *H-2*. Line 1 of the figure shows the genotypes of recipient and donor of an H-2$^{a}$ anti-H-2$^{d}$. This is the Sachs and Cone antiserum already mentioned. Because haplotypes *a* and *d* share *Ss*$^{d}$ and *H-2D*$^{d}$, the antibody must be formed against the product of a gene to the left of *Ss*. Line 2 shows the genotypes of recipient and donor of

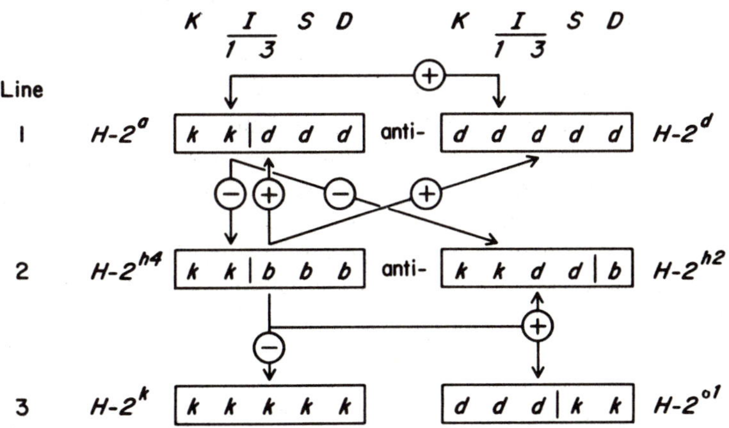


FIG. 6.2. Diagram showing and analyzing the reactions of a B10.A (*H-2*$^{a}$) anti-B10.D2 (*H-2*$^{d}$) studied by Sachs and Cone (1973) and of a 4R (*H-2*$^{h4}$) anti-2R (*H-2*$^{h2}$) studied by David *et al.* (1974). See text for details. Plus (+) indicates reaction; minus (—) indicates absence of reaction.

an H-$2^{h4}$ anti-H-$2^{h2}$, studied by David *et al.* (1974). Because haplotypes *h4* and *h2* share *H-2*$K^k$ and *H-2*$D^b$, the antibody cannot be directed against the *H-2K* or the *H-2D* gene products. It also cannot be directed against the *Ss* gene product even though donor and recipient differ at *Ss*. This follows from the negative reaction of the antibody with *H-2*$^k$, yet its positive reaction with *H-2*$^{o1}$ despite the presence of the same *Ss* allele, *Ss*$^k$, in both haplotypes (Fig. 6.2, line 3). If the antibody were directed against *Ss* we would expect the same reaction in both cases. We conclude that the reactive product must be determined by a locus or loci between *H-2K* and *Ss*.

Referring again to the H-$2^{h4}$ anti-H-$2^{h2}$ of line 2, we see that the donor allele at the postulated locus must be of *d* origin, the recipient allele of *b* origin. We are dealing with a b anti-d. Thus the antisera of both lines 1 and 2 are directed against *d* gene products. We would then predict that the antibody of line 2 would react with donor of line 1, as indeed it does.

While the antibody of line 2 is negative with H-$2^k$, it is positive with H-$2^a$, the *recipient* of line 1. Since the *H-2*$^a$ haplotype has a left end from *H-2*$^k$, a right end from *H-2*$^d$, the reaction must be determined by the right or *H-2*$^d$ end. A reaction with the *H-2K* gene product is ruled out. However, and this is the key point, the locus determining the line 2 antibody must be not only to the right of *H-2K* but also to the right of the locus determining the line 1 antibody. Line 1 recipient *H-2*$^a$ has to be of *k*-type at the first or left-hand locus, of *d*-type at the second or right-hand locus. The presence of two loci determining Ia-type antisera is thereby established.

Similar evidence from these and other antisera splits the *Ia* region into at least three loci, *Ia-1, Ia-2,* and *Ia-3.* The analysis was greatly aided by the prior demonstration of three immune response loci in the same chromosome region, a subject we do not treat until Chapter 7. We shall pass over details of the evidence, but we give in Fig. 6.3 the haplotype, genotype, and exchange points of some of the recombinants that have proved to be critical in analyzing the fine genetic structure of the *H-2* complex. A more complete listing will be found in Shreffler and David (1975).

### 3. *Ia Specificities*

Analysis of the various Ia antisera has shown them to be serologically complex. The application of the same methods by which multiple H-2 specificities have been demonstrated has led to the detection of 17 Ia specificities (Shreffler and David, 1975; C. S. David, personal communication). A partial strain distribution of the specificities is given in Table 6.7, and, at the bottom of the table, the as yet imperfect information

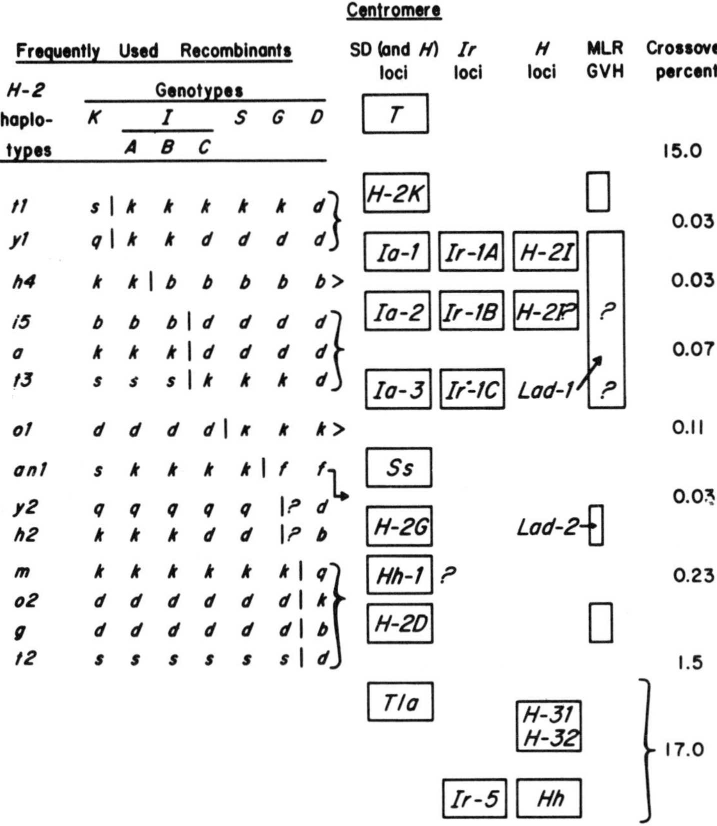


FIG. 6.3. Chromosome map of the *H-2* complex and some adjacent loci, with haplotypes and genotypes of some key recombinants also shown. The genotypes reveal the haplotypic origins of the *K*, *I-A*, *I-B*, *I-C*, *S*, *G*, and *D* regions of each recombinant. The location of the crossover that produced each recombinant is shown by a vertical line. Where two crossover events have occurred, as in *t1*, only the last to occur is marked. Columns 3 through 6 show (in boxes) the various loci in and adjacent to the complex. Column 3 shows the loci identified serologically (SD, serologically defined) and the histocompatibility (*H*) and hybrid histocompatibility (*Hh*) loci. Column 4 shows the immune response loci. Column 5 shows some additional *H* and *Hh* loci. Column 6 shows the loci that determine the mixed lymphocyte reaction (MLR) and the graft-versus-host (GVH) reaction. Whether the loci in the different columns are really different, or merely represent different manifestations of single loci, is uncertain.

as to the *Ia* subregion by which each is determined. This subject is still in its infancy, but some interesting points emerge. Inspection of the haplotype distribution in the nonrecombinant haplotypes at the top of the table suggests the existence of private and public specificities reminiscent of H-2. Specificities 2, 4, 10, and 14 have been found in

TABLE 6.7
THE *Ia* CHART[a]

| *H-2* haplotype | Parental haplotype | *Ia* specificity 1 | 2 | 3 | 4 | 5 | 6 | 7 | 8 | 9 | 10 | 11 | 12 | 13 | 14 | 15 | 16 | 17 |
|---|---|---|---|---|---|---|---|---|---|---|---|---|---|---|---|---|---|---|
| Nonrecombinant | | | | | | | | | | | | | | | | | | |
| *b* | | — | — | 3 | — | — | — | — | 8 | 9 | — | — | — | — | — | — | — | — |
| *d* | | — | — | — | — | — | 6 | 7 | 8 | — | — | 11 | — | — | — | 15 | 16 | — |
| | | 1 | — | — | — | 5 | — | — | — | — | — | — | — | 13 | 14 | — | — | — |
| *k* | | 1 | 2 | 3 | — | — | — | 7 | — | — | — | — | — | — | — | 15 | — | 17 |
| *p* | | — | — | — | — | 5 | 6 | 7 | — | — | — | — | — | 13 | — | — | — | — |
| *q* | | — | — | 3 | — | 5? | — | — | — | 9 | 10 | — | — | 13 | — | — | 16 | — |
| *r* | | — | — | — | — | 5 | 6 | 7 | — | 9 | — | — | 12 | — | — | — | — | 17 |
| *s* | | — | — | — | 4 | 5 | — | — | — | 9 | — | — | 12 | — | — | — | — | 17 |
| Recombinant | | | | | | | | | | | | | | | | | | |
| *a* | *d/k* | 1 | 2 | 3 | — | — | 6 | 7 | — | — | — | — | — | — | — | 15 | — | 17 |
| *g* | *b/d* | — | — | — | — | — | 6 | 7 | 8 | — | — | 11 | — | — | — | 15 | 16 | — |
| *h4* | *a/b* | 1 | 2 | 3 | — | — | — | — | — | — | — | — | — | — | — | — | — | 17 |
| *i5* | *a/b* | — | — | 3 | — | — | 6 | 7 | 8 | 9 | — | — | — | — | — | 15 | — | — |
| *t1* | *a1/s* | 1 | 2 | 3 | — | — | — | 7 | — | — | — | — | — | — | — | 15 | — | 17 |
| *t2* | *a/s* | — | — | — | 4 | 5 | — | — | — | 9 | — | — | 12 | — | — | — | — | 17 |
| *t3* | *s/t1* | — | — | — | 4 | 5 | — | 7 | — | 9 | — | — | 12 | — | — | — | — | 17 |
| *y2* | *a/q* | — | — | 3 | — | —? | — | — | — | 9 | 10 | — | — | 13 | — | — | 16 | — |
| *Ia* subregion | | A | A | B | A | A | C | C | A | A | ? | ? | ? | ? | ? | ? | ? | A |

[a] Abstracted from Shreffler and David (1975); David *et al.* (1975a); Sachs *et al.* (1975a); C. S. David, personal communication.

only one nonrecombinant haplotype. Inspection of the remaining specificities, which fall in the public class, suggests the possibility of allelic series comparable to H-2.1 and H-2.28. Thus, with the single exception of the joint presence of 8 and 9 in *H-2*$^b$, specificities 1, 8, and 9, all in subregion *A*, show a mutually exclusively relationship. Like some of the long public H-2 specificities, some of the Ia public specificities have diffuse limits because the antisera which define them, while similar in reaction patterns, are not identical.

### 4. *Cell and Tissue Distribution*

While it is clear from studies of the cell and tissue distribution of the Ia antigens that these antigens are present on at least some lymphocytes and some nonlymphoid tissues, there are curious contradictions in the various reports. These contradictions probably reflect our as yet very imperfect knowledge of a complex system.

The most striking contradictions concern the presence of Ia on T cells. Virtually all investigators have found it on B lymphocytes, but at least some antisera seem not to detect it on thymus-derived lymphocytes. One report indicates that it can be isolated from T lymphocytes, one that it cannot.

The difficulty of detecting Ia on T cells is reminiscent of the difficulty of detecting immunoglobulin on these cells. Perhaps in both cases this reflects the masking effect of the thick glycoprotein coat that is one of the features differentiating T from B lymphomcytes. But several investigators have suggested that it also reflects the diversity of Ia antigens. Chemical studies attest this diversity. Probably there are at least some differences in the Ia antigens of the different classes of lymphocytes. The outcome of a particular study would thus depend on the particular antisera employed. (Delovitch and McDevitt, 1975; Frelinger *et al.*, 197b; Gotze *et al.*, 1973; Hauptfeld *et al.*, 1974, 1975; Hess and Davies, 1974b; Lonai and McDevitt, 1974; Sachs *et al.*, 1975a,b; Sanderson and Davies, 1974.)

Besides their presence on lymphocytes, Ia antigens have been detected on fetal liver, macrophages, epidermal cells, and spermatozoa. They are not present on red cells, platelets, muscles, brain, or a variety of other tissues. (Hammerling *et al.*, 1975; Hauptfeld *et al.*, 1974; Sanderson and Davies, 1974.)

## C. The *H-2I* Locus

The availability of numerous recombinant *H-2* haplotypes makes possible a search for loci influencing graft rejection (*H* loci) in between

*H-2K* and *H-2D*. As can be seen from Fig. 6.3, donor–recipient pairs can be selected which differ at various internal regions or subregions of *H-2* but not at the two ends, long known for their *H* effect. Several investigators have carried out skin graft studies with recombinant pairs designed to take advantage of this fact. Results have generally been negative (review in Démant, 1973). However, Klein *et al.* (1974c), using one of the two known recombinants with an exchange at the far left of the *H-2* complex, appear to have located a third strong *H-2* locus.

The key recombinants in this study were $H\text{-}2^{t1}$, $H\text{-}2^{t2}$, and $H\text{-}2^{t3}$. Haplotype $H\text{-}2^{t1}$ is the product of two successive intra-*H-2* crossovers, and $H\text{-}2^{t3}$ probably of three such events. In the case of all three recombinants, $H\text{-}2^{s}$ was one of the parental haplotypes, and all three have the $H\text{-}2K^{s}$ allele at the far left and the $H\text{-}2D^{d}$ allele at the far right. The $H\text{-}2^{s}$ exchange which gave rise to $H\text{-}2^{t1}$ occurred at the far left between *H-2K* and *Ia-1*. $H\text{-}2^{t3}$ arose from $H\text{-}2^{t1}$ accidentally, while a line carrying the $H\text{-}2^{t1}$ haplotype was still segregating for $H\text{-}2^{s}$. The genotypes of the three recombinant haplotypes will be found in Fig. 6.3.

Klein *et al.* (1974c) found that grafts exchanged between recipient–donor pairs differing at $H\text{-}2^{t1}$ and $H\text{-}2^{t2}$ or $H\text{-}2^{t1}$ and $H\text{-}2^{t3}$ were rejected with median survival times ranging from 12 to 29 days. Sixteen days after grafting, antibodies with anti-Ia properties appeared in the recipients. Inspection of the genotypes of three the *H-2* complexes involved in these tests, as displayed in Fig. 6.3, shows that the incompatibility revealed by the tests is located in the *A* and/or *B* subregion of the *I* region. There thus appears to be an *H* locus, of strength comparable to *H-2K* and *H-2D*, in the *I-A* or *I-B* subregions of *H-2*. The symbol *H-2I* has been assigned.

## D. The *H-2G* Locus or Loci

While approximately one-half the map length of the *H-2* complex resides in the right half of the complex between *Ss* and *H-2D* (Fig. 6.3), genes comparable in number or ease of demonstration to those found in the left half are not known. However, there is now firm evidence for loci with CMAD properties within this right-hand end.

The best established locus in this region is *H-2G*, defined by specificity H-2.7. The recombinants which localize it can be inferred from Fig. 6.3. H-2.7 is unique among H-2 specificities in that it is much more abundant on red cells than on lymphocytes. Absorption with lymph node lymphocytes requires very large numbers of cells, and lymphocytes from thymus and spleen absorb even less effectively. Other tissues have not been tested. H-2.7 is present in four nonrecombinant haplotypes, *f, k, p,* and *s*. The density of the antigen determined by *k* is considerably less than for the other three, in fact $H\text{-}2^k$ was originally classed as 7-negative. No allelic specificities are known. (David *et al.*, 1975b; Klein *et al.*, 1975b.) The region defined by *H-2G* is called the *G* region.

While H-2.7 is not a cytotoxic specificity, a locus in the same general region has been tentatively identified by a cytotoxic antibody. The strain distribution of the two reactions are quite different. While this observation has not been confirmed, it suggests the possibility of the presence in the *G* region of additional CMAD loci, possibly analogous to the *Ia* loci. (Snell *et al.*, 1974.)

Evidence concerning the association of any histocompatibility effect with the *G* region is ambiguous. Recombinant pairs identical at *H-2D* but differing at *H-2G* show very weak skin graft rejections, but all pairs so far tested have differed at *I-C* and *S* as well as *G* (David *et al.*, 1975b; Klein *et al.*, 1975b). On the other hand, Blandova and Egorov (1974) have reported definite mapping of a histoincompatibility associated with haplotypes $H\text{-}2^b$ and $H\text{-}2^{bc}$ in the *G* region. They have tentatively assigned the symbol *H-2W*.

Loci determining a weak mixed lymphocyte response and the hybrid histocompatibility phenomenon may also be located in the *G* region (Chapter 8).

It is interesting to note that in the HLA as well as the *H-2* system there is a third locus with some resemblance to the two major CMAD loci (Chapter 9).

## IX. Comparisons of *H-2K* and *H-2D*

The availability of recombinants has made it possible to compare the effect of the two ends of *H-2* on a variety of immune processes. Numerous studies have shown that the *H-2K* region appears immunologically stronger than the *H-2D* region. Thus Démant (1970) found the *H-2K* region more efficacious in inducing graft-versus-host reactions than the *H-2D* region. McKenzie and Snell (1973, 1974) found that *H-2K* differences led to more rapid graft rejections and higher antibody titers than did *H-2D* differences. Curiously, despite the greater strength of the *K*-end barrier, greater passive enhancement of skin graft survival was obtained across this barrier than across *H-2D*. On the contrary, when rabbit anti-mouse lymphocyte serum (ALS) was used as the prolonging agent, *H-2D* differences responded better than *H-2K* differences (Němec *et al.*, 1973).

Most if not all of these differences between the *D* and *K* ends of *H-2* can now be explained in terms of *H-2K*-associated *Ia* and *H-2I* loci. Because of the rarity of recombinants between *H-2K* and these loci, the *H-2K* disparities always included disparities at these loci. Grafts with a *K*-end difference were thus being made across a double histoincompatibility. A second *H* locus may also be involved at the *D* end, but if so it is a weaker locus. The favorable role of *H-2K* in passive enhancement can be explained by the apparent importance of *Ia* in this phenomenon (Davies and Alkins, 1974; Section VIII,B,1).

## X. *H-2* Mutants and Minor Variants

Different *H-2* haplotypes in mice typically manifest multiple differences, presumably accumulated by mutation and recombination over a long period of time. By the use of appropriate recombinants, strain pairs can be obtained in which the degree of difference is substantially reduced. These strain pairs have contributed enormously to our understanding of the *H-2* complex. It is a reasonable assumption that strain pairs with a single difference could in some ways be even more informative. Such strain pairs are available through, and only through, mutation, although a somewhat analogous resource may be found in various minor variants of some of the widely used haplotypes.

### A. *H-2* Mutants

Studies of mutations at histocompatibility loci are reviewed in Chapter 3, Section IX. In the approximately 30,000 mice used in these studies in three different laboratories, more than 60 mutations have been found and reported (Kohn and Melvold, 1975). Nearly a third of these have been mutations at loci in the *H-2* complex, and of these *H-2* mutations, eight have now been analyzed in some detail. These tend to be mutations that occurred in inbred strains rather than $F_1$ hybrids, because mutations in inbred strains give rise immediately to the coisogenic lines that are essential for certain types of tests. The picture will become more complete when comparable studies of the mutants occurring in hybrids are available.

Table 6.8 is a condensation of some of the available information concerning the eight most thoroughly studied *H-2* mutants. It should be emphasized that all these mutations were discovered because they engendered a histoincompatibility; they are not a random sample of muta-

TABLE 6.8
SOME PROPERTIES OF EIGHT OF THE MORE THOROUGHLY TESTED *H-2* MUTANTS

| Symbol and/or haplotype | | Source | | | | | | |
|---|---|---|---|---|---|---|---|---|
| Mutant | | Strain | Haplotype | Mutant region | MLR[b] | CML[b] | Serological change | References[c] |
| B6.C-$H\text{-}2^{ba}$/By[a] | | (B6 × C) | $H\text{-}2^{b}$ | K | yes | yes | none? H-2.33? | 1,2,3,6,9,10,12,14 |
| B6(M505)/Eg | $H\text{-}2^{bd}$ | B6 | $H\text{-}2^{b}$ | K | yes | yes | none? H-2.33? | 6 |
| B6-$H\text{-}2^{bg1}$/Kh | | B6 | $H\text{-}2^{b}$ | K | yes | yes | none | 10,11,12 |
| B6-$H\text{-}2^{bg2}$/Kh | | B6 | $H\text{-}2^{b}$ | K | yes | yes | none | 10,11 |
| B6-$H\text{-}2^{bh}$/Kh | | B6 | $H\text{-}2^{b}$ | K | yes | yes | none | 10,11 |
| B10.D2(M504)/Eg | $H\text{-}2^{da}$ | B10.D2 | $H\text{-}2^{d}$ | D | yes | yes | yes H-2.4? | 5,7,13 |
| A.CA(M506)/Eg | $H\text{-}2^{fa}$ | (A.CA × A) | $H\text{-}2^{f}$ | | | | yes | 5 |
| CBA(M503)/Eg | $H\text{-}2^{ka}$ | CBA | $H\text{-}2^{k}$ | K | yes | yes | none | 8 |

[a] Mutants with the symbol By after the slash line were found by Bailey and co-workers, mutants marked Eg by Egorov and co-workers, mutants marked Kh by Kohn and co-workers.

[b] MLR, mixed lymphocyte reaction; CML, cell-mediated lysis.

[c] Key to references:

(1) Apt *et al.* (1975), (2) Bailey *et al.* (1971), (3) Berke and Amos (1973), (4) Dishkant *et al.* (1973), (5) Egorov (1974), (6) Forman and Klein (1975a), (7) Forman and Klein (1975b), (8) Klein *et al.* (1975a), (9) Klein *et al.* (1974b), (10) McKenzie *et al.* (1975), (11) Melief *et al.* (1975), (12) Nabholz *et al.* (1975), (13) Rychlíková *et al.* (1972), (14) Widmer *et al.* (1973).

tions within the *H-2* complex; also, five of them occurred in one strain, C57BL (B6), or one of its congenic partners, and a sixth (B6.C-$H\text{-}2^{ba}$) in a (B6 × C)$F_1$. There are indications that the *H-2* mutation rate is particularly high in strain B6. This again suggests that we may be dealing with a nonrepresentative, although not necessarily thereby an any less useful, sample.

The skin graft rejections engendered by the eight mutants in Table 6.8 were uniformly quite strong. Thus grafts from B6.C-$H\text{-}2^{ba}$ to B6 females were rejected with a median survival time of 12 days, from B6-$H\text{-}2^{bg2}$ to B6 females with a survival time of 26 days, and from B10.D2(M504) to B10.D2 (mixed sexes) with a survival time of 16 days. Grafts to males, as expected, showed a slightly longer average survival.

One of the first questions to be asked concerning the mutants is whether they are different or merely recurrences of apparently identical changes. The mutants B6-$H\text{-}2^{bg1}$ and B6-$H\text{-}2^{bg2}$ are identical—they accept each others grafts—and all the other mutations are different.

Another important question concerns the site of the mutation within the *H-2* complex. This can be answered by testing the ability of various recombinants, when crossed to the mutant, to complement the mutated region. The method may be illustrated with two complementation tests performed with mutant B6.C-$H\text{-}2^{ba}$. (1) Haplotype $H\text{-}2^d$ ($K^d$ $S^d$ $D^d$) did not complement, i.e., B6 skin did not grow on the $F_1$. (2) Recombinant $H\text{-}2^{i5}$ ($K^b$ $S^d$ $D^d$) did complement. Since test (1) proved that $S^d$ and $D^d$ are unable to complement, the complementation in test (2) must have been due to $K^b$. Thus the *K* region of B6 must have some factor which has been lost by this B6 mutant. This localizes the mutation in this region, or at least in the *K* end of *H-2*.

Such tests have shown that a surprising proportion of the mutants have occurred in the *K* region. In fact all 5 of the B6 mutants shown in Table 6.8 have occurred in this region. However, one mutation in B10.D2 was a *D* mutant. Complementation tests alone, even with the most favorable recombinants, cannot prove that the *K* mutants occurred in *H-2K* and the *D* mutants in *H-2D*. However, since all available evidence tends to associate strong histoincompatibilities with disparities at these loci, it is natural to assume that they are the site of the mutations.

Another question that has been asked is whether the mutants can engender mixed lymphocyte reactions (MLR) and cell-mediated lysis (CML). (See Chapter 8, Section I for a discussion of these phenomena.) Without exception, so far as tested, they have shown this capacity. This emphasizes the fundamental similarity of these *in vitro* phenomena to the actual process of graft rejection. Minor qualifications will be noted in Chapters 8 and 13.

The mutants in Table 6.8 have also all been subjected to serological analysis. The serologically demonstrable changes are far less pronounced than the histocompatibility changes, and probably because of this some of the reports are conflicting.

The most extensively tested mutant is $H\text{-}2^{ba}$. Bailey *et al.* (1971) and McKenzie *et al.* (1975) reported no serological change; Apt *et al.* (1975) and Klein *et al.* (1974b) reported a modest but seemingly unmistakable reduction in the ability of the mutant to absorb anti-33, the antibody that identifies the *K*-end private specificity of $H\text{-}2^{b}$. Nabholz *et al.* (1975) found a suggestion of a similar serological change.

Apt *et al.* and Klein *et al.* included mutant $H\text{-}2^{bd}$ in their serological analysis and report evidence of a change in specificity 33 very similar to that seen in $H\text{-}2^{ba}$. McKenzie *et al.* similarly included $H\text{-}2^{bg1}$, $H\text{-}2^{bg2}$, and $H\text{-}2^{bh}$ in their study, and again found that in their system no difference from $H\text{-}2^{b}$ was detectable.

Since a change in H-2.33 in two of the $H\text{-}2^{b}$ mutants has been observed in at least two separate studies, we probably must accept the evidence as valid. The negative results are possibly due to subtle differences in the antisera employed.

The clearest case of serological change in any of the mutants has occurred in $H\text{-}2^{da}$, the only *D*-end mutant that has received this degree of serological analyses. Antibodies were formed in both the $\text{H-2}^{\text{d}}$ anti-$\text{H-2}^{\text{da}}$ and in the reciprocal combination. Absorption analyses of these antisera demonstrated three new H-2 specificities, 40, 49, and 50. H-2.50 is a private specificity gained by $H\text{-}2^{da}$, 40 and 49 represent $H\text{-}2^{da}$ losses. There has also been a change in this mutant in private specificity H-2.4 of the $H\text{-}2D^{d}$ allele. $H\text{-}2^{fa}$ has also undergone a serological change demonstrable by reciprocal antisera made with mutant and parental strains. (Egorov, 1974.)

No serological change was found in $H\text{-}2^{ka}$. This further emphasizes the relative serological stability of the *K* end of *H-2*. (Klein *et al.*, 1975a.)

Nabholz *et al.* (1975) have used cell-mediated lysis (CML) with third-party target cells to analyze the nature of the change causing CML reactions between mutant $H\text{-}2^{ba}$ and its parent haplotype, $H\text{-}2^{b}$. By this approach, CML specificities can be demonstrated which can be compared with known serological specificities. There appears to have been more than one change, but the strongest reaction was against a specificity present in $H\text{-}2K^{b}$ and $H\text{-}2D^{k}$. Such a *K–D* cross-reaction is reminiscent of specificity H-2.36 (although the authors do not note this). Another reaction could be attributed to specificity 5. It is interesting that whereas the serological changes demonstrated in this mutant seem to involve a private specificity, the CML changes seem to involve public specificities, and moreover public specificities for which there is some ground for postulating a separate mutational site.

This brings us to the question of the precise site or sites at which these mutations have occurred. Beyond the point that there are both *K* end and *D* end mutants, there are no firm answers, but there is some suggestive evidence.

Since *H-2K* and *H-2D* are the classical determinants of serologically and histogenetically demonstrable *H-2* complex antigens, it is natural to assume that mutants determining *H-2*-associated histoincompatibilities and serological changes, seemingly associated with changes in H-2 specificities, are mutations at these loci. As we shall see in Chapter 8, however, while *H-2K* and *H-2D* play a major role in CML, strong mixed lymphocyte reactions (MLR) are typically associated with the *I* region of *H-2*. The strong MLR response engendered by the mutants is thus puzzling.

Rather direct evidence that the change in $H\text{-}2^{ba}$ is in *H-2K* comes from antiserum blocking experiments. Anti-H-2.33 sera were shown to completely abrogate specific cell lysis by appropriately sensitized $H\text{-}2^{ba}$ cells against $H\text{-}2^{b}$ targets, or of $H\text{-}2^{b}$ cells against $H\text{-}2^{ba}$ targets. Barring the possibility that the mutation is in a molecule in close physical association with the *H-2K* product, this is certainly rather direct proof of an *H-2K* locus mutation. (Nabholz *et al.*, 1975.)

This still leaves the puzzle of the major effect of the mutants on the MLR. Is it possible that these mutations, or at least some of them, are not simple point mutations, but involve some more complex change? The high *K* region mutation rate of the $H\text{-}2^{b}$ haplotype of strain B6 suggests the presence of some unusual genetic system; so it would perhaps not be surprising to find some unusual properties in the mutants. Indeed, complementation tests involving mutants $H\text{-}2^{ba}$ and $H\text{-}2^{bf}$, and strains C and B6.C-$H\text{-}2^{d}$, have indicated that mutations have occurred at two sites. One of these sites is shared by $H\text{-}2^{ba}$ and $H\text{-}2^{bf}$ and is within the introduced complex of B6.C-$H\text{-}2^{d}$; the other is outside this introduced complex. (D. W. Bailey and M. Cherry, personal communication.)

While the studies herein summarized clearly represent only a small beginning in exploitation of the informational potential of *H-2* mutants, it seems a safe assumption that future studies will do much to clarify the details of this small but fascinating chromosome region.

## B. Minor *H-2* Variants

The existence of minor variants of familiar *H-2* haplotypes has been suspected for a long time, but by the very nature of the case is often difficult to document. If such variants cause only very weak histoincompatibilities, tests to establish them are always open to the suspicion that rejections are due to contaminant genes. But minor variants are nevertheless interesting and deserving of study because they may represent types of change that are quite different from those detected as strong histocompatibility mutations.

Two well-documented minor variants are $H\text{-}2^{ja}$, a variant of $H\text{-}2^{j}$, and $H\text{-}2^{pa}$, a variant of $H\text{-}2^{p}$. In both cases the variants, although similar histogenetically and serologically to the type haplotypes, differ at the *Slp* locus. $H\text{-}2^{j}$ and $H\text{-}2^{ja}$ are of especial interest because their *H-2D* alleles resemble $H\text{-}2D^{b}$. However, there is evidence for minor differnces, both serological and histogenetic, between the *H-2D* genes of each of the three strains. (Snell *et al.*, 1953, 1973, 1974; G. D. Snell, unpublished.)

Another of the better-documented minor variants is $H\text{-}2^{bc}$, the $H\text{-}2^{b}$-like haplotype of strain 129. There is a moderately strong histoincompatibility determined by these haplotypes that maps between *Ss* and *H-2D* and hence in the *G* region. $H\text{-}2^{bc}$ also differs from $H\text{-}2^{b}$ in that it is associated with $Tla^{c}$ instead of $Tla^{b}$ and may therefore also differ at the weak histoincompatibilities closely linked to *Tla*. (Snell *et al.*, 1971c; Blandova and Egerov, 1974.)

Another category of *H-2* variants is indicated by the existence of what appear to be serological cross-reactions between the private specificities of certain haplotypes. Thus, as will be seen from Table 6.5, specificity 25 bridges private specificities 23 and K18, 38 bridges 15 and K16, and 55 bridges 30 and D21. There are a number of other bridging specificities not shown in our condensed *H-2* chart. Where such bridging specificities occur, the presence of one of the bridged private specificities in a recipient tends to weaken the serological response to the other. In one case there seems to be greater than average chemical similarities between the products of bridged alleles. The allelic differences in these cases cannot be classified as minor, but a phylogenetic relationship is perhaps indicated. (S. G. Nathenson, unpublished data; Snell *et al.*, 1973.)

## REFERENCES

Allen, S. L. 1955. Linkage relations of the genes histocompatibility-2 and fused tail, brachury and kinky tail in the mouse, as determined by tumor transplantation. *Genetics* **40**:627–650.

Amos, D. B. 1962. Isoantigens of mouse red cells. *Ann NY Acad Sci* **97**:69–82.

Apt, A. S., Z. Blandova, I. Dishkant, T. Shumova, A. A. Vedernikov, and I. G. Egorov. 1975 Study of *H-2* mutations in mice. IV. A comparison of the mutants M505 and Hz1 by skin grafting and serological techniques. *Immunogenetics* **1**:444–451.

Archer, J. R., D. A. Smith, D. A. L. Davies, and N. A. Staines. 1974. A skin-graft enhancing antiserum which recognizes two new B-cell alloantigens determined by the major histocompatibility locus of the mouse. *J Immunogen* **1**:337–344.

Bailey, D. W., G. D. Snell, and M. Cherry. 1971. Complementation and serological analysis of an *H-2* mutant. Pages 155–162 *in* A. Lengerová, and M. Vojtísková, eds. Immunogenetics of the *H-2* system. Karger, Basel.

Balner, H., A. van Leeuwen, W. v. Vreeswijk, H. Dersjant, and J. J. van Rood. 1971. Leukocyte antigens of Rehsus monkeys (RhL-A) and chimpanzees (ChL-A): Similarities with the human HL-A system. *Tissue Antigens* **1**:229–238.

Berke, G., and D. B. Amos. 1973. Cytotoxic lymphocytes in the absence of detectable antibody. *Nature (London), New Biol* **242**:237–238.

Blandova, Z. K., and I. K. Egorov. 1974. Analysis of slight differences in the main histocompatibility system *H-2* between the mouse strains C57BL/10 and 129. (In Russian, English summary.) *Genetika* **8**:171–173.

Čapcová, J., and P. Démant. 1972. Two new *H-2* specificities: H-2.44 and H-2.45. *Folia Biol (Praha)* **18**:231–236.

Čapcová, J., and P. Démant. 1974. Genetic studies of the *H-2* associated complement gene. *Folia Biol (Praha)* **20**:101–115.

Cohen, N., and W. H. Hildemann. 1968. Population studies of allograft rejection in the newt, *Diemictylus viridescens*. *Transplantation* **6**:208–217.

Colberg, J. E., B. Ribak, and C. Cohen. 1969. The role of tissue cells in anti-A hemagglutinin formation in rabbit skin allografts. *Transplantation* **8**:582–594.

Dausset, J., F. T. Rapaport, F. D. Cannon, and J. W. Ferrebee. 1971. Histocompatibility studies in a closely bred colony of dogs. III. Genetic definition of the DL-A system of canine histocompatibility, with particular reference to the comparative immunogenicity of the major transplantable organs. *J Exp Med* **134**: 1222–1237.

David, C. S., and D. C. Shreffler. 1972. Studies on recombination within the mouse *H-2* complex. II. Serological analysis of four recombinants, $H\text{-}2^{al}$, $H\text{-}2^{ol}$, $H\text{-}2^{tl}$, and $H\text{-}2^{th}$. *Tissue Antigens* **2**:241–249.

David, C. S., D. C. Shreffler, and J. A. Frelinger. 1973. New lymphocyte antigen system (Lna) controlled by the *Ir* region of the *H-2* complex. *Proc Natl Acad Sci USA* **70**:2509–2514.

David, C. S., J. A. Frelinger, and D. C. Shreffler. 1974. New lymphocyte antigens controlled by the *Ir-IgG* region of the *H-2* gene complex. *Transplantation* **17**:122–125.

David, C. S., T. H. Hansen, and D. C. Shreffler. 1975a. Studies on recombination within the mouse *H-2* gene complex. III. Further serological analysis of the *H-2* haplotypes. *Tissue Antigens* **6**:353–365.

David, C. S., J. H. Stimpfling, and D. C. Shreffler. 1975b. Identification of specificity H-2.7 as an erythrocyte antigen. Control by an independent locus, *H-2G*, between the S and *D* regions. *Immunogenetics* **2**:131–139.

Davies, D. A. L., and B. J. Alkins. 1974. What abrogates heart transplant rejection in immunological enhancement? *Nature (London)* **247**:294–296.

Delovitch, T. L., and H. O. McDevitt. 1975. Isolation and characterization of murine Ia antigens. *Immunogenetics* **2**:39–52.

Démant, P. 1966. Polymorphism of leukocyte antigens in rabbits. Pages 481–484 *in* Proc Xth European congress on animal blood groups and Biochemical polymorphism, Paris 1966. Institute National de la Recherche Agronomique, Paris.

Démant, P. 1970. Genetic requirements for graft versus host reactions in mouse. Different efficiency of incompatibility at *D*- and *K*-ends of the *H-2* locus. *Folia Biol (Praha)* **16**:273–275.

Démant, P. 1973. *H-2* gene complex and its role in alloimmune reactions. *Transplant Rev.* **15**:164–202.

Démant, P., G. D. Snell, and M. Cherry. 1971. Hemagglutination and cytotoxic studies of *H-2*. III. A family of 3-like specificities not in the C crossover region. *Transplantation* **11**:242–259.

Démant, P., G. D. Snell, M. Hess, F. Lemonnier, C. Neauport-Sautes, and F. Kourilsky, 1976. Separate and polymorphic genes controlling two types of polypeptide chains bearing the H-2 private and public specificities. *J Immunogenetics* **2**:263–271.

Dishkant, I. P., A. A. Vedernikov, and I. G. Egorov. 1973. Study of *H-2* mutations in mice. III. Serological analysis of the mutation 504 and its derived recombinant *H-2* haplotypes. (In Russian, English summary.) *Genetika* **9**:83–90.

Douglas, R., and H. G. Nieman. 1973. Application of the autoanalyser to *H-2* typing in the mouse. *Tissue Antigens* **3**:71–77.

Egorov, I. K. 1974. Genetic control of H-2 alloantigens as inferred from analysis of mutations. *Immunogenetics* **1**:97–107.

Forman, J., and J. Klein. 1975a. Analysis of *H-2* mutants: Evidence for multiple CML target specificities controlled by the $H\text{-}2K^b$ gene. *Immunogenetics* **1**:469–481.

Forman, J., and J. Klein. 1975b. Immunogenetic analysis of *H-2* mutants. II. Cellular immunity to the $H\text{-}2^{da}$ mutation. *J Immunol* **115**:711–715.

Frelinger, J. A., D. B. Murphy, and J. F. McCormick. 1974a. *Tla* types of *H-2* congenic and recombinant mice. *Transplantation* **18**:292–294.

Frelinger, J. A., J. E. Niederhuber, C. S. David, and D. C. Shreffler. 1974b. Evidence for the expression of Ia (*H-2*-associated) antigens on thymus-derived lymphocytes. *J Exp Med* **140**:1273–1284.

Gill, T. J., III. 1973. Antigenic determinants of synthetic polypeptides. Pages 136–169 *in* D. Pressman, T. B. Tomasi, Jr., A. L. Grossberg, and N. R. Rose eds. Specific receptors of antibodies, antigens, and cells. Karger, Basel.

Gorer, P. A. 1936. The detection of antigenic differences in mouse erythrocytes by the employment of immune sera. *Br J Exp Pathol* **17**:42–50.

Gorer, P. A. 1942. The role of antibodies in immunity to transplanted leukemia in mice. *J Pathol Bacteriol* **54**:51–65.

Gorer, P. A., and Z. B. Mikulska. 1959. Some further data on the *H-2* system of antigens. *Proc R Soc Lond [Biol]* **151**:57–69.

Gorer, P. A., and P. O'Gorman. 1956. The cytotoxic activity of antibodies in mice. *Transplant Bull* **3**:142–143.

Gorer, P. A., S. Lyman, and G. D. Snell. 1948. Studies on the genetic and antigenic basis of tumour transplantation. Linkage between a histocompatibility gene and "fused" in mice. *Proc R Soc Lond [Biol]* **135**:499–505.

Götze, D., R. A. Reisfeld, and J. Klein. 1973. Serological evidence for antigens controlled by the *Ir* region in mice. *J. Exp Med* **138**:1003–1008.

Hála, K., M. Vilhelmová, and J. Hartmanová. 1976. Probable crossing over in B blood group system of chickens. *Immunogenetics* **3**:97–103.

Hammerling, G. J., G. Mauve, E. Goldberg, and H. O. McDevitt. 1975. Tissue distribution of Ia antigens. Ia on spermatozoa, macrophages, and epidermal cells. *Immunogenetics* **1**:428–437.

Hauptfeld, V., and J. Klein, 1975. Molecular relationship between private and public H-2 antigens as determined by antigen redistribution method. *J Exp Med,* **142**:288–298.

Hauptfeld, V., D. Klein, and J. Klein. 1973. Serological identification of an *Ir*-region product. *Science* **181**:167–169.

Hauptfeld, V., M. Hauptfeld, and J. Klein. 1974. Tissue distribution of *I* region-associated antigens in the mouse. *J Immunol* **113**:181–188.

Hauptfeld, M., V. Hauptfeld, and J. Klein. 1975. Ia and H-2 antigens on blast cells. *Transplantation* **19**:528–530.

Hess, M., and D. A. L. Davies. 1974a. Basic structure of mouse histocompatibility antigens. *Eur J Biochem* **41**:1–13.

Hess, M., and D. A. L. Davies. 1974b. Membrane alloantigens controlled by the *I*-region of the *H-2* complex. Biochemical characterization using absorbed H-2 antisera. *Transplant Proc* **7**:209–212.

Hoecker, G., O. Pizarro, and A. Ramos. 1959. Some new antigens and histocompatibility factors in the mouse. *Transplant Bull* **6**:407–411.

Iha, T. H., G. Gerbrandt, W. F. Bodmer, D. McGary, and W. H. Stone. 1973. Cross-reactions of cattle lymphocytotoxic sera with HL-A and other human antigens. *Tissue Antigens* **3**:291–302.

Iványi, P. 1970. The major histocompatibility antigens in various species. *Curr Top Microbiol Immunol* **53**:1–90.

Iványi, P., and J. Forejt. 1974. Genetic factors closely associated with the major histocompatibility system: Structural and/or regulatory genes. Pages 143–152 *in* J. Libánský and L. Donner, eds. Present problems in hematology. Excerpta Med Found Amsterdam.

Iványi, P., and M. Micková. 1972. Testing of wild mice for "private" H-2 antigens. Cross reactions or nonspecific reactions? *Transplantation* **14**:802–804.

Ivašková, E., and P. Iványi. 1974. Cytotoxic effect of anti-H-2 sera on human lymphocytes: Association with HL-A7 and W27. *Folia Biol (Praha)* **20**:283–285.

Klein, J. 1973. List of congenic lines of mice. I. Lines with differences at alloantigen loci. *Transplantation* **15**:137–153.

Klein, J. 1974. Genetic polymorphism of the histocompatibility-2 loci of the mouse. *Annu Rev Genet* **8**:63–77.

Klein, J. 1975a. Biology of the mouse histocompatibility-2 complex. Springer-Verlag, Berlin and New York.

Klein, J. 1975b. Many questions (and almost no answers) about the phylogenetic origin of the major histocompatibility complex. *Adv Exp Med Biol* **64**:467–478.

Klein, J., and D. C. Shreffler. 1971. The *H-2* model for the major histocompatibility systems. *Transplant Rev* **6**:3–29.

Klein, J., F. H. Bach, F. Festenstein, H. O. McDevitt, D. C. Shreffler, G. D. Snell, and J. H. Stimpfling. 1974a. Genetic nomenclature for the *H-2* complex of the mouse. *Immunogenetics* **1**:184–188.

Klein, J., M. Hauptfeld, and V. Hauptfeld. 1974b. Serological distinction of mutants B6.C-H(zl) and B6.M505 from strain C57BL/6. *J Exp Med* **140**:1127–1132.

Klein, J., M. Hauptfeld, and V. Hauptfeld. 1974c. Evidence for a third, *Ir*-associated histocompatibility region in the *H-2* complex of the mouse. *Immunogenetics* **1**:45–56.

Klein, J., J. Forman, V. Hauptfeld, and I. K. Egorov. 1975a. Immunogenetic analysis of *H-2* mutations. III. Genetic mapping and involvement in immune reactions of the $H\text{-}2^{ka}$ mutation. *J Immunol* **115**:716–718.

Klein, J., V. Hauptfeld, and M. Hauptfeld. 1975b. Evidence for a fifth (*G*) region in the *H-2* complex of the mouse. *Immunogenetics* **2**:141–150.

Klein, J., M. Hauptfeld, and V. Hauptfeld. 1975c. Splitting of antigen H-2.9 and mapping of its genetic determinants. *Tissue Antigens* **6**:46–49.

Kohn, H. I., and R. W. Melvold. 1976. Divergent X-ray-induced mutation rates in the mouse for *H* and "7-locus" groups of loci. *Nature* (*Lond*) **259**:209–210.

Kolata, G. B. 1973. Repeated DNA: Molecular genetics of higher organisms. *Science* **182**:1009–1011.

Lemonnier, F., C. Neuport-Sautes, F. M. Kourilsky, and P. Démant. 1975. Relationships between private and public H-2 specificities on the cell surface. *Immunogenetics* **2**:517–529.

Lonai, P., and H. O. McDevitt. 1974. *I*-region genes are expressed on T and B lymphocytes. Studies of the mixed lymphocyte reaction (MLR). *J Exp Med* **140**:1317–1323.

Lyon, M. F., J. M. Butler, and R. Kemp. 1968. The positions of the centromeres in linkage groups II and IX of the mouse. *Genet Res* **11**:193–199.

McKenzie, I. F. C., G. Morgan, R. Melvord, and H. Kohn. 1976. Serological and complementation studies in four C57B46-*H-2* mutants. *Immunogenetics,* in press.

McKenzie, I. F. C., and G. D. Snell. 1973. Comparative immunogenicity and enhanceability of individual *H-2K* and *H-2D* specificities of the murine histocompatibility-2 complex. *J Exp Med* **138**:259–277.

McKenzie, I. F. C., and G. D. Snell. 1974. Immunogenicity and enhancement for the private specificities H-2.12, 16, 20, and 21. *Transplantation* **17**:328–330.

Melief, C. J. M., R. S. Schwartz, H. I. Kohn, and R. W. Melvold. 1975. Dermal histocompatibility and *in vitro* lymphocyte reactions of three new *H-2* mutants. *Immunogenetics,* **2**:337–348.

Micková, M., and P. Iványi. 1972. An estimate of the degree of heterozygosity at histocompatibility loci in wild populations of house mouse (*Mus Musculus*). *Folia Biol* (*Praha*) **18**:350–359.

Murphy, D. B., and D. C. Shreffler. 1975a. Cross-reactivity between *H-2K* and *H-2D* products. II. Identification of the cross-reacting specificities. *Transplantation* **20**:443–456.

Murphy, D. B., and D. C. Shreffler. 1975b. Cross-reactivity between *H-2K* and *H-2D* products. III. Effect of *H-2K–H-2D* cross sensitization on skin graft survival. *Transplantation,* **20**:38–44.

Nabholz, M., H. Young, T. Meo, V. Miggiano, A. Rijnbeek, and D. C. Shreffler. 1975. Genetic analysis of an *H-2* mutant, B6.C-$H\text{-}2^{ba}$, using cell-mediated lympholysis: T- and B-cell dictionaries for histocompatibility determinants are different. *Immunogenetics* **1**:457–468.

Nĕmec, M., K. Nouza, and P. Démant. 1973. Factors influencing different reactivity against H-2K and H-2D antigens in normal and ALS-suppressed mice. *Transplant Proc* **5**:275–279.

O'Brien, S. J. 1973. On estimating functional gene number in eukaryotes. *Nature* (*London*), *New Biol* **242**:52–54.

Ohno, S. 1972. So much "junk" DNA in our genome. Pages 366–370 *in* H. H. Smith, ed. Evolution of genetic systems. Gordon & Breach, New York.

Palm, J., and D. B. Wilson. 1973. The Ag-B locus of rats: A major histocompatibility complex? *Transplant Proc* **5**:1573–1577.

Pazderka, F., B. M. Longenecker, G. R. J. Law, and R. F. Ruth. 1975. The major histocompatibility complex of the chicken. *Immunogenetics* **2**:101–130.

Rychlíková, M., P. Démant, and I. K. Egorov. 1972. Mixed lymphocyte reaction caused by an *H-2D* mutation. *Folia Biol (Praha)* **18**:360–363.

Sachs, D. H., and J. L. Cone, 1973. A mouse "B" cell alloantigen determined by gene(s) linked to the major histocompatibility complex. *J Exp Med* **138**:1289–1304.

Sachs, D. H., S. E. Cullen, and C. S. David. 1975a. *Ir*-associated murine alloantigens. Serological and chemical definition of Ia specificities associated with the $H\text{-}2^b$ haplotype. *Transplantation* **19**:388–393.

Sachs, D. H., C. S. David, D. C. Shreffler, S. G. Nathenson, and H. O. McDevitt. 1975b. Ia antigens, proceedings of a workshop. *Immunogenetics* **2**:301–312.

Sanderson, A. R., and D. A. L. Davies. 1974. Genetic control of cell surface *Progr Immunol* **2**:364–367.

Shreffler, D. C. 1974. Genetic fine structure of the *H-2* gene complex. Pages 83–100 *in* G. M. Edelman, ed. Cellular selection and regulation in the immune response. Raven, New York.

Shreffler, D. C., and C. S. David. 1975. The *H-2* major histocompatibility complex. and the *I* immune response region: Genetic variation, function and organization. *Adv Immunol* **20**:125–195.

Shreffler, D. C., D. B. Amos, and R. Mark. 1966. Serological analysis of a recombination in the *H-2* region of the mouse. *Transplantation* **4**:300–322.

Slizynski, B. M. 1955. Chiasmata in the male mouse. *J Genet* **53**:597–605.

Snell, G. D. 1958. Histocompatibility genes of the mouse. II. Production and analysis of isogenic resistant lines. *J Natl Cancer Inst.* **21**:843–877.

Snell, G. D., and M. Cherry. 1972. Loci determining cell surface alloantigens. Pages 221–228 *in* P. Emmelot and P. Bentvelzen, eds. RNA viruses and host genome in oncogenesis. North-Holland Publ., Amsterdam.

Snell, G. D., and M. Cherry. 1974. Hemagglutination and cytotoxic studies of *H-2*. IV. Evidence that there are 3-like antigenic sites determined by both the *K* and *D* crossover regions. *Folia Biol (Praha)* **20**:81–100.

Snell, G. D., and J. H. Stimpfling. 1966. Genetics of tissue transplantation. Pages 457–491 *in* E. L. Green, ed. Biology of the laboratory mouse. McGraw-Hill, New York.

Snell, G. D., P. Smith, and F. Gabrielson. 1953. Analysis of the histocompatibility-2 locus in the mouse. *J Natl Cancer Inst* **14**:457–480.

Snell, G. D., G. Hoecker, D. B. Amos, and J. H. Stimpfling. 1964. A revised nomenclature for the histocompatibility-2 locus of the mouse. *Transplantation* **2**:777–784.

Snell, G. D., M. Cherry, and P. Démant. 1971a. Evidence that the H-2 private specificities can be arranged in two mutually exclusive systems possibly homologous with the two subsystems of HL-A. *Transplant Proc* **3**:183–186.

Snell, G. D., P. Démant, and M. Cherry. 1971b. Hemagglutination and cytotoxic studies of *H-2*. I. H-2.1 and related specificities in the *EK* crossover regions. *Transplantation* **11**:210–237.

Snell, G. D., R. J. Graff, and M. Cherry. 1971c. Histocompatibility genes of mice. XI. Evidence establishing a new histocompatibility locus, *H-12* and a new allele, $H\text{-}2^{bc}$. *Transplantation* **11**:525–530.

Snell, G. D., M. Cherry, and P. Démant. 1973. *H-2:* Its structure and similarity to HL-A. *Transplant Rev* **15**:3–25.

Snell, G. D., P. Démant, and M. Cherry. 1974. Hemagglutination and cytotoxic studies of *H-2*. V. The anti-27, 28, 29 family of antibodies. *Folia Biol (Praha)* **20**:145–160.

Sparrow, A. H., H. J. Price, and A. G. Unterbrink. 1972. A survey of DNA content per cell and per chromosome of prokaryotic and eukaryotic organisms: some evolutionary considerations. Pages 451–494 *in* H. H. Smith, ed. Evolution of genetic systems. Gordon & Breach, New York.

Staats, J. 1966. The laboratory mouse. Pages 1–9 *in* E. L. Green, ed. Biology of the laboratory mouse. McGraw-Hill, New York.

Staats, J. 1968. Standardized nomenclature for inbred strains of mice: Fourth listing. *Cancer Res* **28**:391–420.

Staats, J. 1972. Standardized nomenclature for inbred strains of mice: Fifth listing. *Cancer Res* **32**:1609–1646.

Staines, N. A., K. Guy, and D. A. L. Davies. 1974. Passive enhancement of mouse skin allografts. Specificity of the antiserum for major histocompatibility complex antigens. *Transplantation* **18**:192–195.

Stark, O., and V. Kren. 1969. Five congenic resistant lines of rats differing at the Rt *H-1* locus. *Transplantation* **8**:200–203.

Stimpfling, J. H., and O. Pizzaro. 1961. On the antigenic products of the $H\text{-}2^m$ allele in the laboratory mouse. *Transplant Bull* **28**:102–106.

Stimpfling, J. H., and A. Richardson. 1965. Recombination within the histocompatibility-2 locus of the mouse. *Genetics* **51**: 831–846.

Teisberg, P., B. Olaisen, T. Gedde-Dahl, Jr., and E. Thorsby. 1975. On the localization of the *Gb* locus within the *MHS* region of chromosome No. 6. *Tissue Antigens* **5**:257–261.

Vaiman, M., J. Haag, A. Arnoux, and P. Nizza. 1973. The histocompatibility complex SL-A in the pig. Possible recombination between regions governing MLR and serology, respectively. *Tissue Antigens* **3**:204–211.

van Leeuwen, A., H. R. E. Schuit, and J. J. van Rood. 1973. Typing for MLC (LD). II. The selection of non-stimulator cells for MLC inhibition tests using SD identical stimulator cells (MISIS) and fluorescent antibody. *Transplant Proc* **5**:1539–1542.

Widmer, M. B., B. J. Alter, F. W. Bach, M. L. Bach, and D. W. Bailey. 1973. Lymphocyte reactivity to serologically undetected components of the major histocompatibility complex. *Nature (Lond), New Biol* **242**:239–243.

Wolski, K. P., F. R. Schmid, and K. K. Mittal. 1975. Genetic linkage between the HL-A system and a deficit of the second component (C2) of complement. *Science* **188**:1020–1022.

CHAPTER 7

# IMMUNE RESPONSE GENES



It has been known for many years that there are individual and strain differences in antibody response, in ability to reject grafts, and in resistance to desease, and that these differences are at least partly heritable. It is only relatively recently, however, that there has been progress in unraveling the genetics of these phenomena. The key, as so often in biological research, was simplification. The typical antigen is complex—capable of inciting the formation of several or many antibodies. With the introduction of simple or *pauci-determinant* antigens, striking single locus effects on the immune response became apparent.

The first successes were achieved with synthetic polypeptides, but there are several other types of pauci-determinant antigens that have been used effectively. Alloantigens, though chemically complex, are simple with respect to a host of the same species. Denatured native proteins or native proteins with an attached hapten are effectively simple antigens. And complex antigens used in minimum quantity may stimulate only via one strong determinant.

This chapter deals primarily with three aspects of the rapidly growing body of information on immune response genes: (1) studies with mice, (2) the genetics of the immune response, and (3) the response to alloantigens. We shall touch only briefly on important work done with artificial antigens and on studies of mechanism. Valuable reviews will be found in Hildemann (1973), McDevitt and Landy (1973), Benacerraf and Katz (1975), Gasser and Silvers (1974), and McDevitt *et al.* (1974).

## I. *Ir-1*

### A. Genetics

The *Ir-1* (immune response-1) locus or complex was identified and shown to be *H-2*-linked through studies with the synthetic antigens (T,G)-A–L, (H,G)-A–L, and (P,G)-A–L. These antigens are made up of a poly-L-lysine backbone, with side chains consisting of specific, terminal amino acids, e.g., tyrosine and glutamic acid, attached to poly-DL-alanine.

The first step in genetic analysis was taken when McDevitt and Sela (1965), using (T,G)-A–L and (H,G)-A–L, showed that strain C57BL gave a high response to the first but not the second antigen and that strain CBA gave the reverse pattern. Tests in a backcross indicated that the capacity to respond was due to one major dominant gene with possible modifiers. McDevitt and Chinitz (1969) extended the study to many other strains and found a complete association with *H-2* haplotype. Thus all of 8 $H\text{-}2^b$ strains were high responders to (T,G)-A–L and all of 5 $H\text{-}2^k$ strains were low responders. In a backcross, response segregated with *H-2* type. The authors also included (P,G)-A–L in this study and showed that high and low response to this antigen had its own characteristic strain distribution pattern, distinct from that of the other two antigens. Thus strain DBA/1 ($H\text{-}2^q$) was a low responder to (T,G)- and (H,G)-A–L but a high responder to (P,G)-A–L.

These results raised the question whether *H-2* itself or some gene closely linked with it was the determinant of immune response. *H-2* recombinants (Chapter 6) provided the answer. In a series of studies, McDevitt and co-workers (1972, 1974) determined the response to the three copolymers of various recombinant haplotypes. The significance of these tests can be seen from an examination of Fig. 6.3. The lower half of the figure shows seven recombinants occurring between *Ss*, the S region marker, and *H-2D*, the D region marker. In every case, the immune response type stayed with *Ss*. The upper half of the figure shows seven recombinants between *H-2K*, the *K* region marker, and *Ss*. In five of these there was separation between immune response type and *Ss*; in two there was separation between immune response type and *H-2K*. These results place the immune response locus in a region between *H-2K* and *Ss*. The region was given the designation *I*, and the responsible locus the designation *Ir-1*.

It soon became apparent that *Ir-1* influences the immune response to many antigens besides the synthetic copolymers. Among the antibody responses found to be affected were those to mouse myeloma proteins. Alloantibodies against these proteins are the basis for distinguishing immunoglobulin allotypes. The strain distribution pattern of the responses correlated with the *H-2* haplotype, but with an interesting complication—high responses to IgA proteins sometimes went with low responses to IgG proteins, and vice versa. Taking advantage of this, and of the available recombinants, Lieberman *et al.* (1972) proved that the IgA and IgG responses are determined by separate *I* region loci. The key recombinant was *h4*. This responded to IgA according to its *K* end and to IgG according to its *D* end. This divided *I* into two parts, given the subregion designations *A* and *B*. *Ir-1* was divided into two loci: *Ir-1A* and *Ir-1B*.

Merryman and Mauer (1975), using synthetic terpolymers designated by the abbreviated symbol GLT, identified a third component of *Ir-1*. When tested in the CXB recombinant inbred strains, GLT gave the strain distribution pattern CBBCBB. Since this is the *H-2* pattern, association of the determining locus with *H-2* was indicated. Further studies, including tests with recombinants, placed the locus between *Ir-1B* and *Ss*. The symbol *Ir-1C* was assigned (Fig. 6.3).

There are thus three identified *Ir* loci in the *I* region of the *H-2* complex just as there are three identified *Ia* loci. Does this reflect the full complexity of the *I* region? Probably not, but only further studies can tell. We do not even know at the present whether the *Ir* and *Ia* gene products are identical, and one of the symbols therefore redundant, or different. The apparent identical or very similar positioning of the *Ir* and *Ia* effects may be spurious. Available evidence suggests such positioning, and this is reflected in Fig. 6.3, but new recombinants could alter the picture.

One complexity of the *Ir-1* system that is already apparent is the uniqueness of its influence on different antigens. Except for chemically very similar antigens, every antigen that has been studied shows a different pattern of association with *H-2* haplotype. This suggests that there must be numerous *Ir* alleles and/or loci (summarized in Shreffler and David, 1974).

Immune response effects associated with the MHC have been reported in rats, guinea pigs, rhesus monkeys, and man.

## B. Role of *Ir-1* in Response to Alloantigens and Autoantigens

There could be no more eloquent testimony to the ubiquity of *Ir-1* effects than the major influence of this locus on alloimmune responses. We have already mentioned its role in the response to immunoglobulin allotypes. It also modifies immune behavior to at least six membrane-bound alloantigens.

Despite certain obvious difficulties in demonstrating an effect of an *H-2*- associated *Ir* gene on the response to an *H-2* specificity, such an effect has been demonstrated. Hemaglutinin response to H-2.2, an *H-2D* private specificity, appears to be under the control of *Ir-1*. The key haplotypes are *i5*, a good responder, and *a*, a poor responder. Since, as will be seen from Fig. 6.3, the entire right end of these two haplotypes, including the *I-C*, *S*, and *D* regions, is identical, the implicated site must be at the left end, where *Ir-1* is located. It may be that there is a similar effect on other *H-2D* private specificities (Lilly *et al.*, 1973; Stimpfling and Durham, 1972; McKenzie, 1975).

The response to three other serologically demonstrated cell membrane alloantigens besides *H-2* has been shown to be influenced by *Ir-1*. Two of these, *Ea-1* and *Ea-2*, are erythrocyte antigens. Whereas $H\text{-}2^b$ carries a high responder allele to H-2.2, it carries a low responder allele to *Ea-1* and *Ea-2*. The antibody response to Thy-1.1, as measured by the number of plaque-forming cells, is also under *Ir-1* control, but shows interesting complexities to which we shall return later. (Gasser, 1972; Stimpfling, 1974; Fuji *et al.*, 1972.)

All *Ir-1* effects so far discussed are concerned with antibody response, but the *Ir-1* loci can also influence graft rejection and therefore, presumably, cell-mediated immunity. Several studies have shown that response to the male antigen, H-Y, is *Ir-1* influenced. Thus, when male skin was grafted to females of the CXB recombinant inbred strains, the strain distribution pattern for fast and slow rejections corresponded to the *H-2* pattern, CBBCBB. The *Ir-1* effect was also shown with transplants of male peritoneal exudate cells. In tests with *H-2* recombinants, haplotype *i5* was a responder like *b* and haplotypes *h2* and *h4* nonresponders like *a*. As will be seen from Fig. 6.3, this places the controlling locus in the *I* region and the *A* subregion. There is some evidence that different *H-2* haplotypes are associated with three levels of response; *b* and *s* appeared to be particularly good responders, and *a* and *f* particularly poor responders. The genetic background as well as the *H-2* haplotype influenced the rate of rejection, so other *Ir* loci besides *Ir-1* are involved in male graft rejection. (Bailey and Hoste, 1971; Stimpfling and Reichert, 1971; Wickstrand *et al.*, 1974.)

Wettstein and Haughton (1974), by using the ingenious device of double congenic strains, with a difference at *H-4* as well as *H-2*, were able to demonstrate a role of *H-2*, and hence presumably of *Ir-1*, in the rejection of skin grafts with an *H-4* disparity. $H\text{-}4^b$ skin was rejected by $H\text{-}4^a$ recipients in about 45 days when the genetic background was $H\text{-}2^b$ or $H\text{-}2^d$, in 75 days when the genetic background was $H\text{-}2^a$.

The induction of two experimental autoimmune diseases, autoimmune thyroiditis of mice and allergic encephalomyelitis of rats, has been shown to be influenced by the MHC haplotype. (Vladutiu and Rose, 1971; Williams and Moore, 1973.)

Another manifestation of cellular immunity, delayed-type hypersensitivity to picryl chloride, is also influenced by a gene or genes in the *H-2* complex. Contrary to the situation for the other antigens studied, there was evidence for an effect of the *D* as well as of the *K* end of *H-2*. The effect was complicated by the action of unidentified *Ir* loci (Shultz and Bailey, 1975).

## II. *Ir-2*

Gasser (1969) has demonstrated that antibody response to *Ea-1* is influenced by a locus linked to agouti (*a*) in chromosome 2. *H-13*, *H-3*, *Ly-4*, and *Ea-6* are in the same chromosome region. The symbol *Ir-2* has been assigned (Fig. 3.2). This locus may account for the observation of Snell *et al.* (1967) that either skin or marrow grafts with an *H-13* disparity are rejected by $H\text{-}3^a$ mice but accepted by $H\text{-}3^b$ mice. In the separation of *H-3* from *H-13* described in this study, *Ir-2* would have been expected to stay with *H-3*. If this effect is indeed due to *Ir-2*, it suggests that this locus, like *Ir-1*, influences cellular as well as humoral immunity. *Ir-2* is unusual among *Ir* loci in that responsiveness, at least to the Ea-1 antigen, is recessive. Nevertheless, it seems to operate as a true immune response locus; its influence is not due to the determination of shared or cross-tolerated antigens.

## III. *Ir-3*

Mozes *et al.* (1969) reported that when DBA/1 and SJL mice were immunized with the synthetic polypeptide, (P,G)-Pro–L, each strain produced a distinctive antibody. The DBA/1 antibody was reactive with the (P,G) part of the antigen, the SJL antibody with the Pro–L part. Responsiveness in each case was dominant. They showed, further, that the response of DBA/1 was *H-2*-linked, and the response of SJL not *H-2*-linked. The first response was presumably under the control of *Ir-1*; they postulated a new *Ir* locus, *Ir-3*, to account for the second response. No linkage information other than that relative to *H-2* resulted from this study, which leaves indeterminate the relation of *Ir-3* to most other *Ir* loci, but the authors did show that loci coding for the immunoglobulin heavy chains were not involved.

## IV. *Ir-4*

A fourth immune response locus has been demonstrated by studies of the response of mice to the antigenically potent enterobacterial lipopolysaccharides. Rank *et al.* (1969) used a purified enterobacterial antigen, lipoid A, which, in doses substantially above the level necessary to produce a specific response, induces antibodies that are cross-reactive with sheep red cells. Of the strains tested in this system, all were responders except C3H/HeJ. Strain C3H/DiSn and its congenic partner C3H.SW were among the responders (W.-R. Rank, personal communication), suggesting that the nonresponsiveness of C3H/HeJ was the result of mutation. Responsiveness was dominant.

Watson and Riblet (1974), using crude lipopolysaccharide as the immunogen and lipopolysaccharide-coated red cells as the test antigen, showed that the nonresponsiveness of C3H/HeJ mice segregated in a backcross as a unit factor independent of *H-2* and of immunoglobulin heavy chain allotype. In the same cross, the authors followed the characteristic ability of bacterial lipopolysaccharide to increase the maturation of antibody-forming cells nonspecifically. This was found to segregate with the specific response to the antigen.

Rank (1974) has suggested for the locus indicated by these studies the symbol *Ir-4*. No effect of *Ir-4* on alloimmune responses has been reported.

## V. *Ir-5*

As already noted (Section I,B), although *Ir-1* plays a major role in the antibody response to Thy-1.1, there are complications. Thus it was noted that the $F_1$ between low responding strains C57BL/6 and DBA/2 was a high responder. This suggests the complementary action of two loci, with responsiveness showing dominance. Zaleski and Klein (1974) analyzed this situation in backcrosses, in one of which the *T* locus as well as *H-2* was used as a marker, and showed that the results could be explained by postulating a second locus, *Ir-5*, in chromosome 17. *Ir-5* is about 19 crossover units from *H-2*, on the side away from *T* (Fig. 3.2).

## VI. A Sex-Linked *Ir* Locus

Three studies in mice have indicated the existence of a sex-linked *Ir* locus. Amsbaugh *et al.* (1972) found a high antibody response to type III pneumococcal polysaccharide in strain BALB/c and a very low response in strain CBA/HN. $F_1$ males from the cross ♀ CBA/HN × ♂ BALB/c were low responders, and $F_1$ females high responders, as expected in the case of a sex-linked gene. Similar results were reported by Scher *et al.* (1973), using a synthetic double-stranded RNA as an antigen. CBA/HN formed no antibody to this antigen, strains C3H/He and C57BL/6 were weak responders, and strain AL/N was a strong responder. The major determinant of the difference between CBA/HN and AL/N was sex-linked. Mozes and Fuchs (1974) reported similar determination of the antibody response to denatured DNA. Sex-linked responsiveness shows dominance in $F_1$ females.

## VII. An Immune Response Locus Linked to the Immunoglobulin Heavy Chain Loci

According to current evidence, the various mammalian immunoglobulins are derived from the products of three, independent gene complexes. One contains loci that code for the heavy chain constant and variable regions, the other two code, respectively, for the kappa ($\kappa$) and lambda (λ) light chain constant and variable regions. (See Hildemann, 1970, for additional details.) The mouse heavy chain constant region (allotype) locus, designated *Ig-1,* is linked to the prealbumin (*Pre*) locus (Taylor *et al.,* 1975a). Neither of these loci has as yet been placed in the chromosome map, but recombinant inbred strain patterns have been determined; these should facilitate localization. The murine κ light chain complex seems to be linked to *Ly-3* in chromosome 6 (Gottlieb, 1974). The λ light chain complex has not been located in the mouse. Several authors have reported an immune response effect associated with *Ig-1.*

Blomberg *et al.* (1972) studied the antibody response of inbred and recombinant inbred mice to α-1,3-dextran. Four inbred strains, including C, gave a high response and produced antibodies with λ light chains; six inbred strains, including B, gave a low antibody response and produced antibodies with κ light chains. $(C \times B)F_1$ responded at a level only a little below the C parent. In the CXB recombinant inbred strains, the pattern of response was BBCBBCB. This is unlike the *H-2* pattern, CBBCBBB; the responsible locus therefore is not *H-2*-associated and cannot be *Ir-1.* The pattern, however, is identical with that of the cluster of loci, *Ig-1, Ig-2,* etc., which control immunoglobulin heavy chain constant region allotype. The authors suggest that the observed variations in the immune response are determined by different alleles at a variable region locus (or loci) in this same gene cluster. Riblet *et al.* (1975) have shown that the postulated locus, given the provisional symbol $V_H$-dex, shows 0.3% recombination with *Ig-1.*

McKenzie (1975) has shown that the antibody response to *H-2* specificity H-2.32, besides being subject to the influence of *Ir-1,* is also subject to influence by an *Ig-1* linked locus. As in the case of α-1,3-dextran, the CXB pattern was BBCBBCB. Association with *Ig-1* was confirmed by showing that the nonresponsiveness of strain B had been introduced along with the *Ig-1* allele of strain B into a C.B-*Ig-1* congenic line.

Taylor *et al.* (1975b) have studied the genetics of the natural antibodies to chicken erythrocytes which are found in normal mouse serum. Strain C has a high natural level of antibody, and strain B has a low level. The pattern of response in the CXB strains was BBCBBBB. This is similar but not identical to that for *Ig-1.* A pattern similar to that of *Ig-1* was also found in the AKXL recombinant inbred strains. At least one other gene with an effect on agglutinin levels has segregated in the AKXL cross. Whether the complicating influence of other loci accounts for the apparent separation of immune response type and allotype seen in some lines in this study, or whether the separation indicates action of a locus distinct from but linked to the *Ig-1* complex, is not yet clear.

## VIII. Other Immune Response Loci

The immune mechanism of mammals is extraordinarily complex, and this must be reflected in the complexity of the genetic systems that produce it. Probably mutations at almost any one of the loci concerned with the development of the lymphoid, myeloid, and reticuloendothelial systems could have some effect on the immune response. We may assume, therefore, that many more *Ir* loci will be discovered. The list we have given here, based on work with mice, could be considerably extended by adding investigations with man. Thus the hereditary agammaglobulinemias modify immune responses, though less specifically than the *Ir* loci.

There have been numerous studies with mice showing strain differences in antibody response or in resistance to disease or tumor development. With a few notable exceptions, these have not contributed to our knowledge of individual loci; in any case they are of little relevance to histocompatibility. There are, however, two additional immune response effects that deserve mention.

The widely used strain C57BL (B), instead of switching from IgM to IgG production following a second immunization, tends to keep on producing IgM. At least three loci are involved (Silver *et al.*, 1972). In a quite unrelated study, Goodman and Koprowski (1962), by the production of a congenic line and the use of cultured macrophages, showed that susceptibility of mice to arbovirus B is substantially influenced by a single locus that controls the ability of macrophages to inhibit intracellular virus multiplication. These studies suggest the potential diversity of *Ir* effects and *Ir* mechanisms.

## IX. Mechanisms

According to much but not all of the available evidence, the *Ir-1* loci act at the level of T helper cells in their role as collaborators with B cells in the generation of the secondary response. Nonresponders fail to recognize the carrier part of the antigen in the way that responders do. Responders and nonresponders make equal IgM primary responses but unequal secondary IgG responses. In athymic animals, difference between the two *Ir-1* types is abolished. (Benacerraf and Katz, 1975; McDevitt *et al.*, 1974.)

The *Ir* effect associated with the immunoglobulin heavy chain loci would be expected to be expressed at the level of the B cells, and available evidence is in accordance with this presumption.

The sex-linked *Ir* locus, which influences antibody production to synthetic RNA, acts at the B cell level, and probably at the level of the primary, IgM response. Thymectomy does not alter its action, and if the synthetic RNA is coupled to an appropriate carrier, nonresponders can make a late response. The B cells of unresponsive strain CBA/HN are either seriously defective or lacking (Scher *et al.*, 1973, 1975).

## REFERENCES

Amsbaugh, D. F., C. T. Hansen, B. Prescott, P. W. Stashak, D. R. Barthold, and P. J. Baker. 1972. Genetic control of the antibody response to type III pneumococcal polysaccharide in mice. I. Evidence that an X-linked gene plays a decisive role in determining responsiveness. *J Exp Med* **136**:931–949.

Bailey, D. W., and J. Hoste. 1971. A gene governing the female immune response to the male antigen in mice. *Transplantation* **11**:404–407.

Benacerraf, B., and D. H. Katz. 1975. The histocompatibility-linked immune response genes. *Adv Cancer Res* **21**:121–173.

Blomberg, B., W. R. Geckeler, and M. Weigert. 1972. Genetics of the antibody response to dextran in mice. *Science* **177**:178–180.

Fuji, H., M. Zaleski, and F. Milgrom. 1972. Genetic control of immune response to θ-AKR alloantigen. *J Immunol* **108**:223–230.

Gasser, D. L. 1969. Genetic control of the immune response in mice. I. Segregation data and localization to the fifth linkage group of a gene affecting antibody production. *J Immunol* **103**:66–70.

Gasser, D. L. 1972. Involvement of *H-2* locus in a multigenetically determined immune response. *Nature (Lond), New Biol* **235**:155–156.

Gasser, D. L., and W. K. Silvers. 1974. Genetic determinants of immunological responsiveness. *Adv Immunol* **18**:1–66.

Goodman, G. T., and H. Koprowski. 1962. Macrophages as a cellular expression of inherited natural resistance. *Proc Natl Acad Sci USA* **48**:160–165.

Gottlieb, P. D. 1974. Genetic correlation of a mouse light chain variable region marker with a thymocyte surface antigen. *J Exp Med* **140**:1432–1436.

Hildemann, W. H. 1970. Immunogenetics. Holden-Day, San Francisco, California.

Hildemann, W. H. 1973. Genetics of immune responsiveness. *Annu Rev Genet* **7**:19–36.

Lieberman, R., W. E. Paul, W. Humphry, Jr., and J. H. Stimpfling. 1972. *H-2* linked immune response (*Ir*) genes; Independent loci for *Ir-IgG* and *Ir-IgA* genes. *J Exp Med* **136**:1231–1240.

Lilly, F., H. Graham, and R. Coley. 1973. Genetic control of the antibody response to the H-2.2 alloantigen in mice. *Transplant Proc* **5**:193–196.

McDevitt, H. O., and A. Chinitz. 1969. Genetic control of the antibody response: Relationship between immune response and histocompatibility (*H-2*) type. *Science* **163**:1207–1208.

McDevitt, H. O., and M. Landy, eds. 1973. Genetic control of immune responsiveness. Academic Press, New York.

McDevitt, H. O., and M. Sela. 1965. Genetic control of the antibody response. I. Demonstration of determinant-specific differences in response to synthetic polypeptide antigens in two strains of inbred mice. *J Exp Med* **122**:517–531.

McDevitt, H. O., B. D. Deak, D. C. Shreffler, J. Klein, J. H. Stimpfling, and G.D. Snell. 1972. Genetic control of the immune response. *J Exp Med* **135**:1259–1278.

McDevitt, H. O., K. M. Bechtol, and G. T. Hämmerling. 1974. Histocompatibility-linked genetic control of specific immune responses. Pages 101–120 *in* G. M. Edelman, ed. Cellular selection and regulation in the immune response. Raven, New York.

McKenzie, I. F. C. 1975. The genetic control of the humoral immune response to *H-2D* alloantigenic specificities. *Immunogenetics* **1**:529–530 (abstr).

Merryman, C. F., and P. H. Maurer. 1975. Characterization of a new *Ir-GLT* gene and its location in the *I*-region of the *H-2* complex. *Immunogenetics* **1**:549–559.

Mozes, E., and S. Fuchs. 1974. Linkage between immune response potential to DNA and the X chromosome. *Nature (Lond)* **249**:167–169.

Mozes, E., H. O. McDevitt, J.-C. Jaton, and M. Sela. 1969. The genetic control of antibody specificity. *J Exp Med* **130**:1263–1278.

Rank, W.-R. 1974. *Mouse News Letter* **51**:27.

Rank, W.-R., V. Flügge, and R. di Pauli. 1969. Inheritance of the lipoid A-induced 19 S-plaque-forming-cell-response in mice: Evidence for three antigen-recognition-mechanisms. *Behringwerk-Mitt* **49**:222–229.

Riblet, R., M. Cohn, and M. Weigert. 1975. Linkage analysis of the dextran response gene. *Immunogenetics* **1**:525–526 (abstr).

Scher, I., M. M. Franz, and A. D. Steinberg. 1973. The genetics of the immune response to a synthetic double-stranded RNA in a mutant CBA mouse strain. *J Immunol* **110**:1396–1401.

Scher, I., A. Ahmed, D. M. Strong, A. D. Steinberg, and W. E. Paul. 1975. X-linked B-lymphocyte immune defect in CBA/HN mice. I. Studies of the function and composition of spleen cells. *J Exp Med* **141**:788–803.

Shreffler, D. C., and C. S. David. 1974. The *H-2* major histocompatibility complex and the *I* immune response region: Genetic variation, function and organization. *Adv Immunol* **20**:125–195.

Shultz, L. D., and D. W. Bailey. 1975. Genetic control of contact sensitivity in mice: Effect of *H-2* and non-*H-2* loci. *Immunogenetics* **1**:570–583.

Silver, D. M., I. F. C. McKenzie, and H. J. Winn. 1972. Variations in the response of C57BL/10J and A/J mice to sheep red blood cells. I. Serological characterization and genetic analysis. *J Exp Med* **136**:1063–1071.

Snell, G. D., G. Cudkowicz, and H. P. Bunker. 1967. Histocompatibility genes of mice. VII. *H-13,* a new histocompatibility locus of the fifth linkage group. *Transplantation* **5**:492–503.

Stimpfling, J. H. 1974. The *Ea-2* (*H-14*) cellular antigen system in the mouse. *Transplantation* **18**:350–356.

Stimpfling, J. H., and T. Durham. 1972. Genetic control by the *H-2* gene complex of the alloantibody response to an H-2 antigen. *J Immunol* **4**:947–951.

Stimpfling, J. H., and A. E. Reichert. 1971. Male-specific graft rejection and the *H-2* locus. *Transplantation* **12**:527–530.

Taylor, B. A., D. W. Bailey, M. Cherry, R. Riblet, and M. Weigert. 1975a. Genes for immunoglobulin heavy chain and serum prealbumin protein are linked in the mouse. *Nature* (*Lond*), **256**:644–646.

Taylor, B. A., M. Cherry, D. W. Bailey, and L. S. Shapiro. 1975b. Genetic control of levels of natural antibodies to chicken erythrocytes in mouse serum: Association with the *Ig-1* locus. *Immunogenetics* **1**:529 (abstr).

Vladutiu, A. O., and N. R. Rose. 1971. Autoimmune murine thyroiditis relation to histocompatibility-2 (*H-2*) type. *Science* **174**:1137–1138.

Watson, J., and R. Riblet. 1974. Genetic control of responses to bacterial lipopolysaccharides in mice. I. Evidence for a single gene that influences mitogenic and immunogenic responses to lipopolysaccharides. *J Exp Med* **140**:1147–1161.

Wettstein, P. J., and G. Haughton. 1974. Production, testing, and utility of double congenic strains of mice. I. B10-$H\text{-}2^{a}H\text{-}4^{b}p$/Wts and B10-$H\text{-}2^{d}H\text{-}4^{b}p$/Wts. *Transplantation* **17**:513–517.

Wickstrand, C. J., G. Haughton, and D. W. Bailey. 1974. The male antigen. II. Regulation of the primary and secondary responses to H-Y by *H-2* associated genes. *Cell Immunol* **10**:238–247.

Williams, R. M., and M. J. Moore. 1973. Linkage of susceptibility to experimental allergic encephalomyelitis to the major histocompatibility locus in the rat. *J Exp Med* **138**:775–783.

Zaleski, M., and J. Klein. 1974. Immune response of mice to Thy-1.1 antigen: Genetic control by alleles at the *Ir-5* locus loosely linked to the *H-2* complex. *J Immunol* **113**:1170–1177.

CHAPTER 8

# ALLOGENETIC CELL INTERACTIONS UNIQUELY DEPENDENT ON *H-2*



The subject of this chapter is a group of experimentally induced cell interactions whose unifying property is the unique role played by the major histocompatibility complex (MHC). Some of them run counter to the usual immunologic and histogenetic tenets. Most of them are *in vitro* reactions, and most of them depend on lymphocytes; but hybrid resistance and radiation resistant graft refection are *in vivo* phenomena, although with *in vitro* counterparts, and allogeneic inhibition can be observed in the absence of lymphoid cells or products.

Much of our information concerning these phenomena comes from the mouse, and in this chapter we shall limit ourselves, with a few exceptions, to murine studies.

## I. The Mixed Lymphocyte Reaction and Cell-Mediated Lysis

Allogeneic lymphocytes of certain genotypes when cultured together undergo DNA and RNA synthesis, blast cell formation, and cell division. After several days of culture, effector cells are generated which can destroy, either *in vitro* or *in vivo,* cells isogeneic with those with which they were cocultivated. The first of these phenomena, known as the *mixed lymphocyte reaction* or *MLR,* can be quantitated by measuring the uptake of radiolabeled thymidine added shortly before the cells are harvested. This serves as an indicator of DNA synthesis. To limit the response to one of the two genotypes in the mixture, DNA synthesis can be prevented in one of the cell types by X-irradiation or treatment with mitomycin C. This makes it possible to draw a sharp distinction between the *stimulating cell* and the *responding cell.* The response peaks at about 3 days, and the cells are usually harvested at this time.

The second of the two phenomena, when studied *in vitro,* is known as *cell-mediated lysis* or CML. It follows the MLR sequentially, potent *effector cells* being generated after about 5 days of mixed culture. At this point, the cultured cells are combined with radiolabeled target cells, and cell destruction is determined by the release of label. As targets, various cell types, e.g., spleen cells stimulated to blast transformation by phytohemagglutinin, leukemia cells, peritoneal macrophages, and cultured fibroblasts, have been employed. Both $^{51}$Cr and $^{125}$IUdR have been used as labels. (Berke and Amos, 1973; Brondz *et al.*, 1975; Cerottini and Brunner, 1974; Forman and Möller, 1974; Nabholz *et al.*, 1975.)

The determinants of the MLR are sometimes referred to as *lymphocyte defined,* or *LD,* determinants. This is in contradistinction to the *serologically defined,* or *SD,* determinants discussed in earlier chapters. We now turn to a consideration of the genetics of the LD determinants.

The basic data that we start with in genetic studies of the MLR is that a strain pair with a defined, and in the best cases a severely restricted, difference shows or does not show stimulation. If the cells from one of the strains have been treated to inhibit cell division, we have the further information that one strain is acting as the stimulator (the inactivated strain) and the other as the responder. Presumably the stimulating and responding cells have specific cell surface components that determine their respective roles. However, is the genetic disparity that we use to localize the MLR effect a disparity in the stimulating determinant, or the responding determinant, or in both? By analogy with graft rejection, we tend to assume that we are localizing the stimulating determinant and that the responding determinant is some sort of antibody produced by genes at which the strain pair need not differ. However, we must not forget that there is no firm proof of this.

## A. The Role of *H-2*

The major role played by *H-2* in the MLR was shown in studies by Dutton (1966a,b). Congenic strain pairs with an *H-2* difference generally displayed strong stimulation; several strain pairs matched at *H-2* but with multiple non-*H-2* differences gave weak stimulation; congenic strain pairs with *H-1*, *H-7*, *H-8*, and *H-9* differences failed to give significant stimulation. The results suggested an even more disparate role for *H-2*, as compared with non-*H-2* loci, than that seen in graft rejection. While more refined methods used subsequently have revealed stimulation due to defined non-*H-2* incompatibilities, the unique importance of *H-2* in the MLR remains unchallenged.

As the complexity of the *H-2* region became increasingly apparent, the next step for investigators concerned with the genetics of the MLR was, clearly, to localize the MLR *H-2* locus or loci more precisely.

### 1. *Information from Recombinants and Mutants*

Investigators seeking to pinpoint within the *H-2* complex the precise genetic determinants of the MLR naturally turned to *H-2* recombinants. Strain pairs were selected, all on a strain B background, which differed by defined segments of the *H-2* complex. The nature of the tests and the information that they yielded can be seen from a few representative examples taken from the studies of Bach and co-workers, and Meo and co-workers (summarized in Shreffler and David, 1975). The genotype of each tested pair and, hence, the regions of indentity and of difference, can be seen in Fig. 6.3. Haplotypes *i5* and *a* differ by a region to the left of a crossover between *I-B* and *I-C*. Haplotypes *i5* and *b* differ by a region to the right of this same crossover. Both pairs showed stimulation. Hence, there are LD determinants in both ends of *H-2*. Haplotypes *t1* and *t3*, differing only in *I-A* and *I-B* gave strong stimulation. This localized a major *K*-end determinant in the *I* region. However, *y1* and *a*, with a *K* difference only, also stimulated, although very weakly, so *K* itself, and perhaps specifically *H-2K*, has some LD effect. Other tests have localized minor LD effects in the *G* and *D* regions. There thus appear to be at least four LD determinants associated, respectively, with *K*, *I*, *G*, and *D*. The strongest LD effect is associated with *I*. This *I* determinant has been called *Lad-1*, the *G*-region determined *Lad-2*. There is some uncertainty as to the role of the different subregions of *I*. The *t1* versus *t3* test already cited shows that a strong effect is determined by subregions *A* and/or *B*. Other tests emphasize the role of *A*. Tests with haplotypes differing at *I-C* and S, (*G* undetermined), gave very weak to moderately strong responses. Perhaps the stronger response was due to an *I-C* plus a *G* difference. Since, as we shall see, there are immune response effects associated with the manifestation of the MLR, this could account for some of the instances of weak or negative results. Positive cases are thus more significant than negative ones. The information concerning LD determinants is summarized in Fig. 6.3 in the column headed MLR.

One of the major discoveries concerning the MLR and CML is that, although the two phenomena are generated under identical conditions of an *in vitro* cultivation, their genetic requirements are different. This has been shown with both human and mouse lymphocyte cultures. While there are some inconsistencies in the mouse data, presumably due to different sensitivities of the methods used, the essential conclusion of the studies is that while incompatibilities at the *I* region of the *H-2* complex generate the strongest MLR's, it is *K* or *D* incompatibilities that are necessary for the expression of CML.

Examples from the study of Nabholz *et al.* (1974) will serve to illustrate the nature of the evidence. These authors, by making use of recombinants, tested the effect on CML of various restricted areas of *H-2* incompatibility. A responder cell was activated by a stimulator cell with incompatibility at several *H-2* regions and tested against a target cell that might share only one or two of these regional incompatibilities.

In one test, haplotype *t2* was stimulated by haplotype *a* and reacted against haplotype *t1*. As can be seen from Fig. 6.3, the effector cell had been activated against the *K*, *I*, and *S* regions, but the target cell shared with the stimulator only the *I-A* and *I-B* regions. There was no cytolysis; hence, *I-A* and *I-B* gene products are presumably not effective in CML. This and other similar tests led to the conclusion that *I* region incompatibilities alone cannot generate CML.

In another test, haplotype *a* was stimulated by haplotype *s* (all regions are *s*) and reacted against haplotype *t1*. The effector cells had been stimulated by incompatibilities in all *H-2* regions but was tested against cells having only a *K* difference. Cell-mediated lysis did occur. This and other similar tests have led to the conclusion that CML does not occur unless there are *K* and/or *D* region differences.

While the need for a *K* and/or *D* region incompatible target for the expression of CML appears established, there remain questions as to whether an *I* region LD difference is also necessary, at least in the generation phase of the process. Nabholz *et al.* (1974) point out that although only one incompatibility was known in their combinations, others could have been present. Schendel and Bach (1974), using two stimulator genotypes and specialized methods of inactivation, found that CML stimulation requires both LD and SD differences. However, *H-2K* mutants, paired with the genotype from which they arose, did produce CML. Barring the eventuality that two loci were changed, an eventuality that could be regarded as highly unlikely were it not for some peculiarities of *H-2* mutants, this result rules out the need for differences at LD loci. (Forman and Klein, 1975; Nabholz *et al.*, 1975; Rychlíková *et al.*, 1972; and others.)

### 2. *Private versus Public H-2 Specificities in CML*

Brondz *et al.* (1975), Forman and Möller (1974), and Nabholz *et al.* (1975) have investigated the specificity of CML by reacting effector cells against targets of an *H-2* haplotype different from that of the stimulator. By the use of a variety of haplotypes, including recombinants, the effect of private versus public and *K*-end versus *D*-end specificities could be distinguished. There were a number of differences in methods, but the results are probably generally comparable.

In two of the studies, the conclusion was reached that CML is directed only against H-2 private specificities, the public specificities playing no role. Both H-2K and H-2D private specificities were active, and each antigen generated its own population of effector cells. In a third study, definite cross-reactions between different H-2K and, indeed, between H-2K and H-2D antigens were observed. Whether these were cross-reactions in the strict sense of the term, or were the product of a second, public antigenic site is not clear

### 3. *In Vitro $F_1$ versus Parent Reactions*

Adler *et al.* (1970), Katz-Heber *et al.* (1973), and Gebhardt *et al.* (1974) have reported a slight but clearly significant response of $F_1$ spleen cells to inactivated cells of the parental strains. This heterodox phenomenon was noted in congenic combinations differing only at *H-2*, as well as in combinations with multiple disparities. The strongest reactions occurred in combinations where the stimulating parent cells were $H\text{-}2^b$, a result of interest in connection with the phenomenon of hybrid resistance (Section II,C). Other authors have not noted this phenomenon, but one may assume technical variations can make some test systems more sensitive than others.

$F_1$ versus parent reactions are contrary to the usual laws of histocompatibility. There is no obvious explanation of the phenomenon. It has been shown that mitomycin-treated cells can release a blastogenic factor (Kennedy and Ekpaha-Mensah, 1973b) that can nonspecifically stimulate responding cells, but Gebhardt *et al.* were unable to detect such a factor in their culture supernatants. Perhaps more conclusive, they showed that elimination of the responding $F_1$ cell population prevented response to the same parent genotype when readded, but not to the other parent genotype. An explanation in terms of a stimulating factor released by the parental cells is also of doubtful applicability to an MLR of $F_1$ versus parent red cell stroma reported by Adler *et al.* (1970). An oddity of this observation is that since red cells lack the Ia antigens, the reaction would have had to be against either H-2 itself or some non-H-2 antigen.

### 4. *The Secondary MLR and CML Responses*

Human studies suggest an altogether unique role for the major LD region (equals the mouse *I* region) in the induction of the secondary MLR and CML responses.

Lymphocytes primed *in vitro* against allogeneic lymphocytes with an LD difference showed an accelerated MLR response when challenged 14 days later either with the same cells or with third-party cells. The only requirement for secondary induction was that the inducing cells be LD-disparate to the responding cells; the disparity did not have to be the same as that carried by the original inducers. The secondary responses generated by third-party cells, although always accelerated, tended to be weaker than those incited by the original inducers, although not significantly so.

Tests of secondary CML induction likewise indicated that any LD-disparate lymphocytes, even when HLA compatible, could trigger a strong CML response against the original stimulator. Third-party cells were fully as efficient as the priming cell in inducing the accelerated appearance of cytotoxic effectors specific for the priming cell. The effectors thus induced showed little or no CML activity against the third-party cells. (Mawas *et al.*, 1975; Charmot *et al.*, 1975.)

If these results are applicable to the murine system, they imply an extraordinarily important role for *I* region disparities in triggering the secondary MLR or CML responses. Moreover, *any* disparity, whether like or unlike that carried by the original inducer, apparently can trigger the secondary CML response.

### B. The Role of Non-*H-2* Loci

A great deal of information has now been added to the initial observation of Dutton (1966b) that multiple non-*H-2* differences can stimulate an MLR. Probably the effects observed by Dutton can be attributed to a locus, designated *Mls,* which was identified and analyzed by Festenstein and co-workers (Festenstein and Démant, 1973; Abbasi and Festenstein, 1973; Festenstein, 1974). It has four known alleles. The strain distribution of three of these is shown in Table 5.2. Alleles $Mls^a$ and $Mls^d$ are the strongest stimulators. The locus has at most a very weak histocompatibility effect as tested with skin and heart transplants. The MLR response due to *Mls* incompatibility does not lead to the generation of effector cells capable of causing CML. Recombinant inbred strain patterns obtained in the AKXL and BXD lines indicate that *Mls* is linked with *ald* and *Dip-1* in chromosome 1 (B. A. Taylor and H. Festenstein, personal communication).

Some of the known non-*H-2* histocompatibility and lymphocyte alloantigen loci appear to be able to cause MLR, but the responses are weak, and in some cases have been demonstrated only through the use of special techniques.

Mangi and Mardiney (1971) have reported weak but consistent stimulation with congenic pairs differing at *H-1, H-3* + *H-13* (and as we now know, also *Ly-4*), and *H-4.* Differences at the very weak *H* loci *H9, H-10,* and *H-11* did not incite an MLR. Adler *et al.* (1970) and Smith (1972) have also reported low but consistent responses attributable to an *H-3* + *H-13* difference, and Smith to an *H-7* difference. Ramseier and Lindemann (1972), using an unusual modification of the MLR technique (the PAR assay), found activity due to the Y-linked locus, *H-Y.* Peck and Click (1973) found an MLR with congenic pairs differing at *Thy-1* (and hence, as indicated by Fig. 3.2, perhaps also the closely linked *H-25*). This manifestation of MLR was unusual in that it occurred only in a serum-free medium and peaked at 4 instead of at 3 days. Rychlíková and Iványi (1969) failed to find an MLR in congenic pairs with *H-1* or *H-3* + *H-13* differences. Smith (1972) has emphasized that the culture conditions may be the limiting factor in the demonstration of mixed lymphocyte stimulation due to most alloantigen determining loci other than *H-2*.

## C. Immune Response Effects in the MLR

Rychlíková *et al.* (1973) have shown that the *H-2* halotype present in strain pairs matched at *H-2*, but differing at *Mls* and other non-*H-2* loci, can influence the intensity of the non-*H-2* response. For example, the strain pair B10.A and A, with multiple non-*H-2* differences but both $H\text{-}2^a$, gave an MLR, but the pair B10 and A.BY, with the same non-*H-2* differences but both $H\text{-}2^b$, gave no response. Thus there is an immune response effect on the mixed lymphocyte reaction quite comparable to the major immune response effects on antibody production, and since this effect is associated with the *H-2* complex, it may very well be due to one of the *Ir-1* loci (Chapter 7).

The *graft-versus-host* (GVH) reaction, in which transplanted lymphocytes attack an allogeneic host, shows genetic and other parallels to the MLR and CML (Festenstein and Démant, 1973; Klein and Park, 1973). Because of the greater complexity of the *in vivo* situation, it is generally less informative than its *in vitro* counterpart, and we shall not discuss it here.

## D. Mechanisms

### 1. The Stimulator Cell

If a variety of histoincompatibilities can induce the mixed lymphocyte reaction, we might expect the spectrum of cell types capable of acting as stimulator cells to be as broad as the distribution of histocompatibility antigens. Actually, this seems not to be the case. Thus, Lane and Ling (1973) found no stimulation with dissociated rat kidney, brain, or thyroid cells, although all these cell types possess Rt H-1 antigen. There may be a number of reasons for this. The strongest MLR's are associated with *I*-region incompatibilities, and hence presumably with the Ia antigens that are expressed only on a few cell types (Chapter 6, Section VIII,B). It is possible that some mixed culture techniques are insufficiently sensitive to pick up other incompatibilities. Also, in the preparation of cells from solid tissues, trypsinization is usually used, and this could remove or damage potentially stimulating antigens.

While some cell types seem not to stimulate, it has been shown that stimulator potential is not confined to lymphocytes. Thus cell preparations from both skin and vascular endothelium have been shown to stimulate (Lane and Ling, 1973; Vetto and Burger, 1972). It is of interest to note that skin contains Ia antigens; the presence of these antigens on vascular endothelium has not been determined. As to lymphocytes themselves, reports are not entirely consistent. Generally typical, however, is the finding of Plate and McKenzie (1973) that B cells prepared from lymph nodes by treatment with anti-Thy-1 stimulate better than T cells separated by treatment with anti-Ly-4. Again there is a possible correlation with the presence or concentration of Ia.

Lozner *et al.* (1974) have noted a correlation between the distribution of certain Ia specificities and the MLR. Perhaps the most convincing evidence that Ia functions as an MLR antigen is the observation that anti-Ia specific for the stimulator cell can block the reaction (Sanderson and Davies, 1974; Meo *et al.*, 1975). Of course this does not rule out the possibility that *H-2* itself stimulates when the disparity is at *K* or *D* rather than *I*. In the case of *Mls* locus incompatibility, B cells stimulate but thymus cells do not (Click, 1974).

### 2. *The Responder Cell*

As shown by the studies of Plate and McKenzie (1973) and others, a responder cell population competent to mount an MLR must include mature T cells. More specifically, it probably must include T helper cells. While, however, there is some disagreement as to details, there is evidence that this cell type alone cannot make an effective response. The following two studies illustrate some of the complexities.

Bach *et al.* (1971) used leukocytes from human blood and techniques designed to separate the lymphocytes from the monocytes and polymorphonuclear leukocytes. The purified lymphocytes did not respond to allogeneic cells, but their responsiveness could be restored by adding some of the phagocytes or a supernatant from a culture of phagocytes.

Dyminski and Smith (1975) used a method of density gradient centrifugation to separate from mouse thymus two populations of cells, TH-1 and TH-2, which represent, respectively, the T effector and the T helper cell. When *H-2* incompatible TH-2 cells were mixed, no MLR resulted. However, the addition of 1 part in 10 of spleen cells isogenic with the responder TH-2 population fully restored the response capability. The effective agents were shown to have the properties of B cells. It should be noted that the stimulators in this study were mitomycin-treated T cells, not B cells. B cells were avoided because of evidence that, even when present as inactivated stimulators, they could supply the missing ir gredient.

The results of these two studies must be regarded either as contradictory or as indicating that two distinct cell types can provide to the responding cell a second stimulus necessary to potentiate the primary stimulus provided by allogeneic confrontation.

Immunologically, the MLR–CML responder cells have the properties of the cells known to function in graft rejection. In both cases, the active cells are T cells. In both cases, functional capacity is lacking at birth and matures gradually. Another important similarity is the restriction of the capacity to respond to a given alloantigen to a single cell clone or small group of clones. This has been demonstrated in the case of the MLR by allowing the cells reactive with one MHC genotype to incorporate a lethal dose of radioactive thymidine. The remaining cells are then found to have lost their capacity to respond to the original genotype, but to retain the capacity to respond to other genotypes. Evidence of the clonal nature of the MLR is also provided by tolerance studies. Cells from rats rendered tolerant at birth to a particular MHC haplotype do not respond to this haplotype in mixed culture. This does not apply when tolerance is induced in adult animals, and even in rats rendered tolerant at birth there may be exceptions in the case of CML, but these phenomena are principally of interest in connection with the multiplicity of mechanisms that can cause unresponsiveness. (Adler *et al.*, 1971; Bernstein and Wright, 1975; Kilshaw *et al.*, 1975; Salmon *et al.*, 1971.)

An unusual aspect of the clonal nature of the MLR is the high percentage of lymphocytes involved. The responding clones must be either unusually large or unusually numerous. The phenomenon has been noted by a number of authors. In various studies, the observed values have ranged from 1 to 6% of the total lymphocyte population. This value is high, both in terms of the percent of cells responding to nonallogeneic antigens and of the many thousands of clones presumed to exist of which only a small fraction should, according to conventional theory, react with one antigen. This phenomenon is perhaps partly explained by the fact that the MHC determines not one, but several or many, antigens. Immunization is said not to increase the proportion of responding cells. (Wilson *et al.*, 1972; Lonai *et al.*, 1973.)

In contrast to the effective stimulation induced by allogeneic cells with an MHC disparity, xenogenic cells, according to most but not all observers, stimulate poorly. This contrasts also with their effectiveness as antibody inducers (Wilson *et al.*, 1972).

## II. Hybrid Resistance, Radiation Resistant Graft Rejection, and Allogeneic Inhibition

### A. Early Studies

According to the usually accepted laws of transplantation, grafts from an inbred strain to an $F_1$ hybrid, of which the inbred strain is one parent, are accepted. The phenomenon of *hybrid resistance* is an exception. The phenomenon was first noted with transplants of leukemias of thymic origin. In addition to its genetic uniqueness, it was also shown that hybrid resistance, unlike the resistance to allogeneic grafts, was not increased by prior immunization and could be largely overcome by the use of large cell doses (Snell, 1958; Snell and Stevens, 1961).

Hybrid resistance was soon demonstrated for a variety of other cell types that are transplantable as single-cell suspensions. Different criteria of survival had to be used for different types of grafts, but, by the employment of appropriate methods, the phenomenon was shown to occur with spleen cells, sarcoma and carcinoma cells, and bone marrow cells. What may be hybrid resistance was also seen with grafts of B10 peritoneal exudate cells to (B10 × B10.D2) recipients. Results with skin were conflicting. (Boyse, 1959; Hellström, 1964; Popp, 1961; Haughton and Cooper, 1973.) While a possible role of the X-linked histocompatibility locus was not adequately controlled in the early experiments, it is clear that this was not the cause of graft failure in most instances.

One of the most useful methods of studying hybrid resistance was introduced by Cudkowicz (1965). The method uses the uptake of a radioactive label, $^{131}$IUdR, in the spleen as the measure of growth of transplanted marrow. Recipient mice are heavily irradiated (700–900 R) and given about $10^6$ bone marrow cells i.v. 2 hours thereafter. Five days later $^{131}$IUdR is injected, the mice killed 18 hours later, and the radioactivity of the spleen determined.

Using this method, and appropriate backcross and *H-2* recombinant mice, Cudkowicz and Stimpfling (1964a,b) found hybrid resistance to be almost wholly determined by *H-2* or a closely linked gene. The determinant(s), moreover, appeared to be at the *D*-end of *H-2*. While an *H-2* disparity was a necessary requirement for the manifestation of hybrid resistance, it was not a sufficient requirement; although B10 grafts failed to grow in a (B10 × C3H)$F_1$ or its reciprocal, C3H grafts grew almost as well as in an isogenic recipient. B10 skin grafts were accepted by the $F_1$.

Although Cudkowicz and Stimpfling and some other observers have failed to see hybrid resistance of skin grafts, Eichwald *et al.* (1965) did observe rejections or crisis in 87% of female parent to female $F_1$ grafts. One parent in their cross was B6, a strain favorable to the manifestation of hybrid resistance. These authors, however, did note 7% of crises or rejections in their controls. (See Chapter 2, Section II, for possible significance of rejections of isografts.)

As an explanation of hybrid resistance, Cudkowicz and co-workers suggested the existence of *H-2*-linked recessive histocompatibility genes. Such genes would generate an antigen or antigens in each parent which would be lacking in the $F_1$, provided the $F_1$ was heterozygous at the postulated locus. Cudkowicz has called the proposed loci *hybrid* (or *hemopoietic*) *histocompatibility* or *Hh* loci.

It should be noted that Cudkowicz's postulate is a very unusual one. In the typical Mendelian recessive, each allele of a heterozygote, according to the usual assumption, produces an end product, but only one product, that of the dominant allele, is phenotypically expressed. In the case of codominance, which is typical of ordinary *H* genes, both alleles produce end products and both are phenotypically expressed. The unusual feature of the postulated *Hh* loci is that, although they produce a demonstrable product when homozygous, they produce, when heterozygous, either no end product, or products neither of which is phenotypically expressed.

McCulloch and Till (1963) and Lengerová *et al.* (1973) measured hybrid resistance to marrow transplants by counting the colonies that form in the spleen following infusion of marrow cells into irradiated recipients. In the method of Lengerová *et al.*, the interval from transplantation to the determination of cell survival was 9 or 10 instead of 5 days, as in the $^{131}$IUdR method.

Besides the suppression by irradiated $F_1$ of parental grafts, it was soon shown that growth of allogeneic marrow was suppressed by homozygous irradiated recipients. In both situations, the immune capacity of the recipients was presumably severely limited or virtually destroyed. We shall refer to this phenomenon, whether seen in $F_1$ versus parent or allogeneic combinations, as *radiation resistant graft rejection.* It is apparently limited to lymphoid cells, possibly to marrow cells. That hybrid resistance is also radiation resistant adds another dimension to its oddity.

Although hybrids suppress the growth of parental marrow, they apparently do not entirely eliminate the parental cells. After about 2 weeks, substantial growth of the transferred cells may occur (Goodman *et al.*, 1970).

An important feature of hybrid resistance to marrow grafts is that it is not subject to an alternative interpretation that may apply to some parent to $F_1$ tumor grafts. It is well known that many and perhaps all tumors have tumor-specific antigens. It has been suggested that hybrids may react to these antigens better than homozygotes. More favorable immune response alleles might be present in the $F_1$ than in a pure strain (Sanford and Soo, 1971). This explanation of hybrid resistance may not apply to all tumor transplants; it certainly does not apply to marrow transplants.

The discovery of hybrid resistance *in vivo* naturally led to a search for *in vitro* counterparts, and, indeed, death of cells exposed to either $F_1$ or homozygous allogeneic antigen in a variety of forms was shown to occur. In one test system, cultured sarcoma monolayers were exposed to cell homogenates or extracts. Survival of the sarcoma cells was determined by dye exclusion or other appropriate methods. In another system, embryonic monolayers with added phytohemagglutinin (PHA), a substance predisposing to cell adhesion, were exposed to intact spleen or lymph node cells. In some cases, the lymphoid cells were heavily irradiated. Death of target cells was indicated by the appearance of cell-free plaques where the lymphoid cells had been added. Both systems led to the death of *H-2* incompatible targets. These *in vitro* phenomena were given the name of *allogeneic inhibition.* (Hellström *et al.*, 1964; Hellström and Hellström, 1967; Möller and Möller, 1965.)

Since allogeneic inhibition could be induced by heavily irradiated cells or cell extracts, it evidently did not require the active intervention of effector cells. On the contrary, it appeared that confrontation with allogeneic compounds induced some sort of self-destruction. This led to a controversy as to whether the mechanism in the *in vivo* phenomena of hybrid resistance and radiation resistant rejection is also a self-destruction of the transplant or whether host cells actively destroy the graft.

### B. Terminology

Because of the complexities and uncertainties concerning the agent in these phenomena, the terms target cell and effector cell used in MLR studies are not appropriate here. We shall, instead, refer to the cell whose survival or death is under observation as the *test cell.* The allogeneic, semiisogeneic, or isogeneic cell or cell extract with which the test cell is confronted we shall refer to simply as the *effector.*

### C. Genetic Studies

#### 1. *H-2-Associated Incompatibilities*

The numerous genetic studies of hybrid resistance, radiation resistant graft rejection, and allogeneic inhibition establish a major role for *H-2* in these phenomena. They also reveal obvious complexities, at least one important discrepancy, and some role for non-*H-2* loci. Because most of them were done before the widespread use of *H-2* recombinants, the part played by individual *H-2* regions is imperfectly known, but crossover studies implicate several chromosome 17 loci.

Genetic data from a number of different studies are summarized in Table 8.1. The studies providing these data used a variety of techniques,

TABLE 8.1
INHIBITION OR DESTRUCTION OF TEST CELLS IN SYSTEMS WHERE THE CELL DAMAGE IS PRESUMABLY NOT ATTRIBUTABLE TO ORDINARY IMMUNE REACTIONS

| | Classification of incompatibilities | | | Test systems | | | |
|---|---|---|---|---|---|---|---|
| | | Genetic combination | | *In vivo* (marrow grafts) | | *In vitro* | |
| Case No. | Locus or loci | Test cell | Effector (host or antigen) | $^{125}$IUdR uptake[a] | Colony counts[b] | Effector a living cell | Effector an antigen preparation |
| 1 | Control | *xx* | *xx* | ++++ | ++++ | ++++ | ++++ |
| 2 | *H-2K* + *D* | *xx* | *yy* | —[c] | — | —,[c,d,e] +[e,f,g] | +[e,h] |
| 3 | | *xx* | *xy* | —[c] | ++ | —,[d,e] ++,[e,f] +[c,g] | ++[e,h] |
| 4 | | *xy* | *xx* | ++++ | + to +++ | —,[d,e] +++[e,j] | +++,[h] ++[e,i] |
| 5 | | *xy* | *yz* | + to ++++ | | | |
| 6 | | *xy* | *ww* or *wz* | ++++ | | | |
| 7 | | *xy* | *xx* + *yy* | | ++++ | ++++[e,j] | ++++[e,i] |
| 8 | *H-2K* | *xx* | *yy* | +++ | +++ | | |
| 9 | | *xx* | *xy* | +, ++++[e] | | | |
| 10 | *H-2D* | *xx* | *yy* | | + | —[d] | |
| 11 | | *xx* | *xy* | —[e] | | —[d] | |
| 12 | *H-1* + others | *xx* | *yy* | ++++ | | —[k] | +++[h] |
| 13 | *H-1* | *xx* | *yy* | | + | | |
| 14 | | *xx* | *xy* | ++++ | | | |
| 15 | *H-3* + *H-13* | *xx* | *yy* | —[l] | + | | |
| 16 | | *xx* | *xy* | ++++ | | | |

[a] Data from Cudkowicz and Stimpfling (1964a,b), Cudkowicz (1964), Cudkowicz and Bennett (1971a), Bennett (1972), Lotzová and Cudkowicz (1973). Marrow cells [about $10^6$ to $2 \times 10^6$ ($4 \times 10^7$ in case 12)] injected i.v. into X-irradiated hosts (600–800 R). Proliferation in spleen determined 4–5 days later by $^{125}$IUdR uptake.

[b] Data from Lengerová and Zeleny (1968), Lengerová *et al.* (1973). Marrow cells ($0.7 \times 10^5$ to $1.4 \times 10^5$) injected i.v. into 3–4 subgroups of $\gamma$-irradiated mice (850 R) at increasing doses. Proliferation in spleen determined 9–10 days later by colony count.

[c] Some exceptions.

[d] Data from Möller and Möller (1965). Untreated or X-irradiated (1500 R) lymph node cells (effectors) layered on cultured mouse embryo cells (test cells) with added PHA. Destruction of test cells demonstrated by the appearance of relatively cell-free plaques from 1 to 6 days later.

[e] Strains congenic; disparities were *H-2* only.

[f] Data from Hellström *et al.* (1969). Dilute suspensions of sarcoma (test) cells plated in petri dishes and overlayed with intact lymph node (effector) cells plus PHA. Inhibition measured by reduction in number of sarcoma colonies as compared with controls.

[g] Data from Mayhew and Bennett (1971). Lymph node cells incubated with adherent fiberblasts, usually from an established cell line, for 20–24 hours. No PHA added. Lymph node cells irradiated in some experiments. Cytotoxicity index based on number of remaining adherent cells.

[h] Data from Hellström *et al.* (1969). Same as footnote *f* except that effector was disintegrated lymph node cells.

[i] Data from Lengerová *et al.* (1973). Bone marrow (test) cells exposed for 1 hour to spleen cell extracts, then injected into irradiated, isogeneic hosts and spleen colonies counted.

[j] Data from Lengerová *et al.* (1973). Bone marrow (test) cells exposed for 1 hour to irradiated (5000 R) lymph node cells (effectors) in 100-fold excess, then injected into irradiated isogeneic hosts and spleen colonies counted.

[k] Data from Möller and Möller (1966). Sarcoma (test) cells mixed with irradiated (3000–10,000 R) lymph node (effector) cells plus PHA. Viability tested by inoculation into isogeneic mice. In another study, similar results were seen with human fiberblasts and lymphocytes.

[l] Data from Snell *et al.* (1967). Same as footnote *a*, except that recipient mice were preimmunized with three injections of donor thymus. Rejection possibly was due to antibody remaining from immunization. This study also included one group of mice conforming to case number 16, but preimmunized like the case number 15 group. All case 16 mice, whether preimmunized or not, accepted the marrow grafts.

and the data in the original papers appear in a variety of forms. In the table we have reduced them to a single scale. Four plus signs (++++) indicate growth at the control level, a minus sign (−) complete inhibition of growth, the symbols +++, ++, and + various intermediate levels of growth. Our transformation of the original data to this scale is, of necessity, somewhat arbitrary.

The original studies, again, used a great variety of *H-2* haplotypes and strains. We have reduced these to a limited number of basic allelic or phenotypic combinations. Thus, case 1, test cell *xx*–effector *xx*, includes all isogeneic control combinations; case 2, test cell *xx*–effector *yy*, all simple allogeneic combinations; case 3, test cell *xx*–effector *xy*, all semi-isogeneic or $F_1$ versus parent combinations. Case 4 is the reciprocal of case 3. Case 5 is an experimental combination used only by one author; it will be explained when we discuss this case. The genetic data thus telescoped convey much of the essential information established by the tests, but obscure some details which will be mentioned in the text. Footnotes to the table briefly describe the technical details of the four listed test systems.

All combinations, other than control, showed inhibition in at least some of the studies and some of the strain pairings, but there were complexities and exceptions requiring comment. Table 8.1 does not give information as to the influence of strain background on the inhibition produced by *H-2* incompatibilities, but the studies of Cudkowicz and co-workers show it to be extremely important. Thus, DBA/2 ($H\text{-}2^d$) marrow grew normally in 129 ($H\text{-}2^b$) recipients but was strongly inhibited in B10 (also $H\text{-}2^b$) and (B10 × 129)$F_1$ recipients. Growth was normal in B10-$H\text{-}2^d$ congenic mice, so the B10 background without an *H-2* difference was incompetent to induce resistance. Background was equally important in semiisogeneic combinations. An important role for modifying genes is indicated.

The one major discrepancy between different studies is revealed by case 4 in Table 8.1, heterozygous test cells confronted with a homozygous effector. Cudkowicz and co-workers and Hellström *et al.* (1969) report no inhibition in this combination. Other workers, including Lengerová *et al.*, saw inhibition in their marrow transplant tests. Possibly the difference between the Cudkowicz and Lengerová studies is due to the different periods of observation. If rejection does occur in this combination, it cannot be due to a recessive antigen.

Other tests relevant to the recessive *Hh* gene hypothesis are summarized in cases 5 and 6 in Table 8.1. Here the test cells are heterozygous and, hence, can carry an *Hh* gene product only when their two *H-2* haplotypes happen to have the same *Hh* allele at some *Hh* locus or loci. The effectors are either heterozygous or homozygous, but carry one or more *H-2* haplotypes lacking in the test cell. In these combinations, resistance, according to the *Hh* gene hypothesis, can occur frequently only if there are several *Hh* loci and few *Hh* alleles. Resistance was observed in both groups of marrow transplant experiments, but Cudkowicz and co-workers stress its rarity.

Case 7 in Table 8.1 summarizes experiments by Lengerová *et al.* (1973) in which heterozygous test cells were exposed to a simulated identically heterozygous and, hence, "isogeneic" effector. This was done *in vivo* by creating radiation chimeras repopulated simultaneously with $H\text{-}2^x$ and $H\text{-}2^y$ fetal liver cells, and then challenging in the usual fashion with $H\text{-}2^x/H\text{-}2^y$ bone marrow. The same genetic situation was created *in vitro* by using cell or antigen mixtures as the effector. In all cases, test cells grew normally provided the two effector genotypes were present in equal proportions. If the proportions were distinctly unequal, e.g., 1:5, some inhibition occurred.

The *in vitro* experiments indicate that the test cell is responding to the total genetic milieu, and not to its individual components. This is true even when the effectors are living cells with which the test cells must make individual contact. In some way the test cells accumulate and react to the sum of their individual experiences. The interpretation of the *in vivo* experiments must be conditioned by the well-established ability of allogeneic lymphoid cells to live together peaceably in chimeras. Although their genotype is such that, according to the aggressor host cell hypothesis, they should attack the graft, they have lost their ability to do so. Nevertheless if hybrid resistance is interpreted as merely an extension of allogeneic inhibition, the *in vivo* and *in vitro* tests can be regarded as mutually confirmatory.

Studies of the number and position of the loci in the *H-2* complex which influence hybrid resistance and radiation resistant graft rejection have been carried out by the use of *H-2* recombinants and backcrosses. Cases 8 through 11 (Table 8.1) summarize the results with recombinants. They point to active loci—*Hh* loci in the terminology of Cudkowicz—at both ends of *H-2*. As originally reported by Cudkowicz and Stimpfling (1964a), and confirmed by other authors, *D*-end disparities are more conducive to rejection than disparities at the *K* end. When all genes are on a C57BL background, only *D*-end disparities may be active. But some *K*-end disparities are also effective. Thus, substantial resistance was seen in the combination $H\text{-}2^d$ into $(H\text{-}2^{i5} \times H\text{-}2^d)$, which has differences only in the *K*, *I-A*, and *I-B* regions. Cudkowicz has designated the *D*-end locus *Hh-1*.

Insofar as *D*-end disparities are more important than disparities involving *K*, this represents another unusual feature of hybrid resistance, since the reverse is usually the case.

The information on *Hh* loci from linkage studies carried out by Cudkowicz and co-workers is summarized in Cudkowicz and Lotzová (1973). Besides the *K*-end effect and *Hh-1* in the *D* region, evidence has been found for three loci to the right of *Hh-1* at distances, respectively, of 4, 16, and 31 crossover units from *H-2D* (Fig. 3.2). This maps these three loci next to, respectively, *H-31* and *H-32, Ir-5,* and *Gv-1.* Does this possibly mean that there are other *H-2*-like clusters in chromosome 7 besides *H-2* itself? All we can be sure of at the present is that there is much of interest to be learned about the right-hand end of this chromosome.

In mapping *Hh* loci, homozygous grafts and heterozygous recipients have been used. It is not a foregone conclusion that these same *Hh* loci determine resistance in homozygous allogeneic combinations.

While the recessive *H* gene hypothesis may be open to question, the determination of hybrid resistance by multiple loci in the *H-2* complex seems well established. We shall refer to these as *Hh* loci without implying any commitment as to their genetic nature.

2. *Non-H-2 Incompatibilities*

There has been no really adequate study of the role of non-*H-2* incompatibilities in allogeneic inhibition or marrow graft rejection, but several authors have run small scale tests. In several of the tests, congenic lines with *H-1* or *H-3* + *H-13* differences were used. The results of this group of studies are summarized in Table 8.1, cases 12–16. They seem to say that simple allogeneic disparities lead to rejection, but that heterozygous effectors do not damage homozygous parent cells. Case 12 (allogeneic mismatch at multiple non-*H-2* loci) shows in the *in vivo* tests, an apparent exception. However, the mice in this group received $4 \times 10^7$ cells, whereas the mice in the comparable case 15 received $10^6$ cells. In no case is hybrid resistance seen. If valid, this difference in the consequence of hybrid and allogeneic non-*H-2* disparities is most interesting, and for want of clear contradictory evidence we shall accept it, but we must emphasize the imperfections in the evidence.

While hybrid resistance was not seen with *H-1* or *H-3* + *H-13* disparities, Cudkowicz and Rossi (1972) have shown that, in at least one strain combination, a weak non-*H-2* hybrid effect can be demonstrated. Using a (B6 × D2) ×D2 backcross, they found that there was segregation for an *H-2* effect as expected, but also for a weak non-*H-2* effect. In some experiments, there was also considerable resistance in the parent to

$F_1$ combination, D2 → (C × D2), where both strains are *H-2*$^d$ so that no *H-2* disparity was present.

It is noteworthy that, in both these combinations, the parent strains had the *Mls* alleles *Mls*$^a$ and *Mls*$^b$, which lead to the strongest MLR's of any *Mls* allelic pair. Indeed, Pena-Martinez *et al.* (1973) have shown that marrow grafts with homozygous *Mls* differences are resisted by irradiated recipients. Unfortunately, there have as yet been no tests with congenic *Mls* lines or any real comparisons of the rejection of parental as compared with homozygous allogeneic grafts. If, indeed, it turns out that, after *H-2, Mls* is the other important locus in both the MLR and in hybrid resistance, this will convey an important suggestion of some fundamental similarity in the phenomena.

### D. Mechanisms

If we are to explain the histocompatibility reactions that we have been examining in this section, two major questions must be answered. (1) Is damage to the test cell a passive process—a form of self-destruction or suicide in the face of effector alloantigen—or is it an active process involving production of cytotoxin by the effector under the inductive influence of the histoincompatible target? Experimental differentiation between these alternatives may not be easy, especially since both may be at work, separately or in combination. (2) If and insofar as cell destruction in the unusual $F_1$ versus parent combination is an active process, is it explained by the uniqueness of the parent strain antigen or by the uniqueness of the $F_1$ effector cell? In either case, it violates the usual laws of transplantation and seemingly must depend on hitherto unrecognized mechanisms. We shall not attempt here to answer question (2)—a possible answer will be proposed in a forthcoming paper (Snell, 1976)—but we do give some relevant evidence in the reminder of this chapter.

We turn now to the consideration of the first alternative under question (1): cell self-destruction in the face of an allogeneic mismatch.

#### 1. Allogeneic Inhibition

Cell self-destruction as an explanation of $F_1$ versus parent reactions is least likely in the case of the *in vivo* systems. If an active aggressor cell is at work anywhere, it should be here. Cell self-destruction is most likely, in fact, an almost necessary postulate, in the *in vitro* systems where cell damage occurs in the face of incompatible cell homogenates or extracts. It is a probable explanation where the effector cell is very heavily irradiated, as in the experiments of Möller and Möller (1965,

1966). In one experiment of these authors, even nonlymphoid tumor cells treated with 10,000 R were shown to be competent effectors. It must be noted, however, that while three groups have seen cell damage in these systems (Table 8.1), other investigators (Granger and Kolb, 1968; G. Cudkowicz, personal communication) have failed to see it. In at least one of these negative studies, the homogenates were from cells prepared by trypsinization, a treatment that might remove *H*-2 antigen. Granger and Kolb did see inhibition in the living cell system with added PHA.

While the function of PHA was originally supposed to be simply inducing cell adhesion, it was subsequently shown to play an active role in the generation of aggressor cells capable of releasing cytotoxin. The cytotoxin acted nonspecifically, killing both effector and test cells. The systems involving PHA may, therefore, be a special case (Granger and Kolb, 1968; Möller and Lundgren, 1969).

But even in the *in vitro* living cell systems not employing PHA, it is possible that cell death is a form of test cell suicide. If cell products can indeed cause allogeneic inhibition, it is not unreasonable to suppose that alloantigens on or secreted by the living cell can cause it. One of the few confirmatory bits of evidence comes from the experiments of Lengerová *et al.*, summarized in case number 8, Table 8.1, and, more specifically, the *in vitro* experiment with living effector cells. A mixture of $xx + yy$ effectors failed to damage $xy$ test cells, just as a mixture of $xx + yy$ extracts failed to damage them. And yet $xx$ and $yy$ effector cells or extracts used separately did cause damage, though rather slight, especially in the experiment with cells (case number 4). It is hard to explain this in terms of active aggression by the effector cells. However, one might postulate that the effector cells turned their aggression against each other, while the test cells escaped undamaged. This, however, would seem to exclude a mechanism based on the release of cytotoxin. Since the difference between cases 4 and 7 was not great, this experiment would certainly bear with independent confirmation.

A possible clue as to the mechanism of allogeneic inhibition is the observation, made with both human and mouse material, that fibroblasts exposed to allogeneic lymphocyte homogenates or extracts show chromosomal abnormalities, including hyperploidy and chromosome breaks and bridges not seen in autogeneic or isogeneic controls. PHA was not used in these studies (Fialkow, 1967; Hellström *et al.*, 1969).

Möller and Möller (1966) and Hellström and Hellström (1967) have suggested that allogeneic inhibition may serve the useful function of eliminating certain types of mutant and, hence, perhaps potentially cancerous cells. This hypothesis presupposes that cell surface components, and perhaps particularly components determined by the *H-2* complex, are somehow concerned with the regulation of cell growth.

### 2. *Cytotoxic Effector Cells*

If a cytotoxic lymphocyte is the active agent in hybrid resistance and the related phenomena that we have been considering, it must have unusual properties. Hybrid resistance occurs in heavily irradiated animals; the more familiar effector cell types would not function after this degree of irradiation. Hybrid resistance is not increased by immunization; the familiar effectors are more effective in immunized animals, and, finally, no effector whose recognition system consists of cell-bound immunoglobulin would manifest (barring the existence of recessive *H* genes, and one other very special qualification we need not go into here) an $F_1$ versus parent reaction.

While the well-known lymphoid effectors seem not to qualify as agents of hybrid resistance, a cell type that does qualify has recently been identified. Most of the evidence comes from a murine *in vitro* system developed by Mayhew and Bennett (1971) in which lymphoid cells are cultured with target fibroblasts without added PHA. The active cells have been given the designation *M cells.* Some of the properties that characterize M cells are summarized below (Bennett, 1973; Cudkowicz and Bennett, 1971a,b; Mayhew and Bennett, 1974; Möller *et al.*, 1969).

M cells appear to be of bone marrow, not thymic, origin. Cells active in the *in vitro* system are found in bone marrow, spleen, and lymph nodes. Thymocytes are not active, and, in fact, they depress the activity of other lymphocytes. Similar evidence comes from the *in vivo* system. Thymectomized animals retain normal hybrid resistance and, indeed, added thymocytes depress just as they do *in vitro*. Also, an anti-host non-H-2 antiserum, probably containing anti-Ly-4 which is specific for B cells, was shown to abrogate hybrid resistance (Gregory *et al.*, 1972; McKenzie and Snell, 1975).

That the M cell, although of bone marrow origin, is not the same as the familiar antibody precursor or B lymphocyte is indicated by experiments with $^{89}$Sr, a radioactive bone-seeking isotope. Mice injected with $^{89}$Sr showed a severely depleted marrow and had lost the ability to reject marrow allografts. Nevertheless, the spleen contained near-normal numbers of antibody-forming precursors and erythropoietic progenitor cells. Although M cells were destroyed, B cells were not.

Tests in the *in vitro* system revealed complications not shown by the *in vivo* system. Although *in vivo*, anti-host serum and $^{89}$Sr treatment both eliminated hybrid resistance, neither completely eliminated *in vitro* activity. In fact, node and spleen cells from $^{89}$Sr-treated mice were normally cytotoxic. But when these cells were treated with antiserum, activity was abolished. The authors suggest as a possible explanation that two effector cell types may have been active *in vitro*. Possibly, also, cell death occurred due to both cell self-destruction and effector cytotoxicity.

In the *in vivo* system there is evidence that macrophages play a role. Hybrid resistance in this system was abolished by silica particles, which act as a macrophage inhibitor (Lotzomá and Cudkowicz, 1974). However, since macrophages are reported as being resistant to both anti-Ly-4 and host treatment with $^{89}$Sr, they presumably are not the *in vitro* synergistic cell.

The M cell shows the expected radiation resistance. Both the M cell and the *in vivo* effector, moreover, have been shown to come from a radiation-sensitive precursor.

Shearer and Cudkowicz (1975) have reported an *in vitro* method of demonstrating hybrid resistance quite different in its technical details from that developed by Mayhew and Bennett (1971). The procedure is essentially that used in studies of cell-mediated lysis (CML). Spleen was the source of both effector cells and of irradiated stimulating cells. These were cultured together for 5 days. Cytotoxic activity was then assayed by another 4 hours of culture with $^{51}$Cr-labeled target cells. These were ascites tumors, either leukemias or a mastocytoma.

The properties of this *in vitro* reaction were studied in tests run in parallel with comparable tests using the standard Cudkowicz *in vivo* system. Both allogeneic and $F_1$ versus parent combinations were used. The same combinations showed activity in both systems. Thus, in both systems, when (B6 $\times$ C3H) hybrids were tested against the separate parent types, B6 test cells were inhibited but C3H test cells were not. In the *in vitro* as in the *in vivo* system, multiple prior injections of the test hybrid with B6 cells specifically destroyed the capacity of the hybrid's cells to inhibit targets of the B6 genotype. One of the most significant tests concerned the age at which cells with effector capacity appear. Previous studies had shown that in the *in vivo* system the capacity for both hybrid and allogeneic radiation resistant rejection develops quite abruptly between the ages of 20 and 24 days. In the *in vitro* system, hybrid resistance was not demonstrable until 24 days, but allogeneic resistance was demonstrable at 20 days. The existence of two different effector cells in the latter system is indicated. Since the method employed was essentially the standard CML technique, we must assume that in the allogeneic combination the active cell was the T effector. In the hybrid combinations, the authors attribute activity to the combined action of macrophages and marrow-derived lymphocytes. The latter could be the M cell.

While the two *in vitro* test systems seemed to give similar results, there were major technical differences. Mayhew and Bennett used a single cell type instead of different cells as stimulator and target, they cocultivated 24 hours instead of 5 days, and their targets were fibroblasts instead of leukemias.

Möller *et al.* (1969), using the PHA *in vitro* system, have established an important property of the effector cell in this system—an important property, at least, if we make the assumption that the effector plays an active rather than a passive role. Lymphoid cells from mice with induced tolerance to skin grafts were cytotoxic to donor cells *in vitro.* Strain A mice were rendered unresponsive by the injection at birth of (A $\times$ CBA)$F_1$ spleen cells. Tolerance was confirmed by skin grafting. Spleen and node cells from these mice, known to be chimeras, whose hemopoietic and lymphopoietic systems are largely of $F_1$ origin, were then tested against CBA and $F_1$ fibroblasts. Cell destruction was seen in both combinations.

This test is subject to various qualifications. It is not certain that the effector in the PHA system, if indeed an active agent, is the same as the M cell of the Mayhew–Bennett system. The combinations used involved allogeneic rather than, or as well as, parent versus $F_1$ confrontation. Most important, there is now some question as to whether tolerance induced at birth is due to clonal deletion or to blocking factors in the serum, although the A–CBA combination used by Möller *et al.* was standard with Medawar and co-workers and is the least suspect of several combinations that have been tested. The results do at least suggest that the activity of M cells is not subject to clonal deletion, but further evidence would certainly be desirable.

While conventional tolerance possibly does not extend to the *in vitro* hybrid resistance system, unresponsiveness in the *in vivo* system can be induced by multiple injection of spleen cells. The phenomenon is *H-2*-specific; unresponsiveness to marrow of one $H\text{-}2^b$ strain can be induced by spleen injections from another $H\text{-}2^b$ strain (Cudkowicz and Bennett, 1971b). The phenomenon may be related to the dose effect noted by Snell (1958).

We turn now to the genetics of the phenomena under examination. One point of interest is the similarity between the *in vitro* and *in vivo* systems. Thus, in both systems, C3H $\times$ B10) effectors attack test cells from the B10 parent but not from the C3H parent. Additional insight concerning the genetics of resistance comes from experiments with marrow chimeras. Srain 129 is susceptible to D2 marrow grafts, strain B10 resistant. Since both strains are *H-2*$^b$ (129 may have a minor variant of *H-2*$^b$), the difference is presumably due to modifying genes. When chimeras, made by reciprocal B10 ⇄ 129 marrow grafts to irradiated hosts, were challenged in the usual manner with D2 marrow, resistance correlated with the genotype of the transferred marrow. This observation appears more compatible with an active than a passive role of the recipient's lymphocytes in graft rejection.

Besides its other peculiarities, radiation resistant rejection shows the unusual property of greater strength in males than in females. For ordinary immune reactions, the reverse is true.

A number of studies of the effect of various physiologically active compounds on the *in vivo* and *in vitro* allogeneic and $F_1$ versus parent phenomena have been reported. Perhaps the most important conclusion to emerge from these studies is that M cell activity does not require DNA synthesis but does require a brief period of protein synthesis. This is in keeping with the concept that a cytotoxin is elaborated, although no such cell product has yet been identified. Alternatively, it may be that the necessary cell binding is contingent on active cell metabolism or that the metabolic processes lead to release of *H-2* complex products, which then act indirectly by the allogeneic inhibition method.

In separate studies, it has been reported that alloantisera can block both test and the effector cells. While the antisera used in these studies leave much to be desired, there is at least the implication that *H-2* complex products are the active agents on both cell types. If valid, this is a most important conclusion (Möller, 1967; Mayhew and Bennett, 1974).

One of the normal functions of M cells may be protection against leukemogenesis. Resistance to malignant erythropoiesis induced by the Friend spleen focus-forming virus is under genetic control, and the active cell is not a thymocyte. Kumar *et al.* (1974), moreover, have presented evidence that the cell has the properties of the M lymphocyte. The *Fv-2* locus in chromosome 9 (Fig. 3.2), one of the genes controlling Friend virus expression, may function through an influence on M cell activity (M. Bennett, personal communication).

## III. The Influence of *H-2* on Cell Collaboration

The production of antibody to most antigens requires the collaboration of three different cell types—T helper lymphocytes, B lymphocytes, and macrophages. While the process requires recognition of and response to antigen by both T and B cells, the two cell types respond to different parts of the antigen molecule. In experimental situations, where the antigen is a complex of a relatively simple synthetic molecule and a protein, the B cell may respond to the former and the T cell to the latter. The B cell is then said to react with the *hapten* and the T cell with the *carrier*. Antibody will be formed against the hapten. What may turn out to be an important clue to *H-2* function is the discovery that the *H-2* complex, and to a lesser degree the *Mls* locus, influence this collaborative process.

### A. T–B Cell Collaboration

It has been shown, both in *in vivo* and *in vitro* systems, that T–B cell collaboration requires compatibility at *H-2*. The *in vivo* system made use of genetically athymic mice, presumably incompetent to reject allogeneic grafts. *H-2* compatible but not *H-2* incompatible thymocyte transfusions restored immune competence. Only the *H-2* compatible tranfused T cells appeared to be able to collaborate with the recipient B cells. Non-*H-2* incompatibilities did not interfere with collaboration.

This experiment is open to the objection that genetically athymic mice can, in fact, reject *H-2* incompatible marrow grafts, presumably through the agency of M cells. Possibly they can also reject thymocytes (G. Cudkowicz, personal communication).

The *in vitro* system was more complex, and we shall not describe the details, but it was not open to objections that apply to the *in vivo* system. The results obtained with it strongly suggest that *H-2* compatibility is necessary for T–B collaboration. It has, however, been suggested that the failure of antibody production in the incompatible systems is due to the killing of B cells by the incompatible T cells (Heber-Katz and Wilson, 1975).

The results in the two systems did differ in one significant respect. In the *in vivo* system, $F_1$ T cells combined with parental strain B cells showed some impairment of collaboration, a phenomenon reminiscent of hybrid resistance. In the *in vitro* system, the $F_1$–parental cell combination functioned normally.

When cell interactions involving *H-2* are demonstrated, the question immediately arises, what part of *H-2* is involved? By the use of appropriate recombinants it was shown in the *in vitro* system that T–B cell collaboration requires only an *I* region match. The *K*, *S*, and *D* regions appear to be irrelevant. (Kindred and Shreffler, 1972; Katz *et al.*, 1975.)

### B. T Cell–Macrophage Collaboration

At least one function of macrophages in the three-cell collaboration required for antibody production is the appropriate presentation of antigen to T cells. In a system using two inbred strains of guinea pigs, incompatible at the MHC of this species, it has been shown that this T cell–macrophage interaction is dependent of MHC compatibility. The role of the MHC was further emphasized by showing that alloantisera, directed presumably against the MHC, could block collaboration in an otherwise compatible, parent-plus-$F_1$ system. The antibody was effective only when it was directed against the haplotype shared by both cell types (Rosenthal and Shevach, 1973).

### C. The Allogeneic Effect

In a curious inverse of the need for MHC compatibility in cell collaboration, an MHC incompatibility can, in some situations, be substituted for the usual immunological contribution of the T cell. Thus, in one experiment, spleen cells from strain CBA, primed to hapten A carrier B, were challenged with hapten A carrier C. The cells, unaided, made no antibody response. However, a response could be evoked either by adding compatible cells primed to C, or simply incompatible cells. In another experiment, it was shown that supernatants from 20 hour cultures of incompatible cells restored the antibody response of spleen cells from genetically athymic mice. (Kennedy and Ekpaha-Menash, 1973a; Kettman and Skorvall, 1974; Rajewsky *et al.*, 1972.)

Further genetic analysis has shown that, in mice, a *K*-end incompatibility (which could include an *I* region incompatibility) is a much more effective inducer than a *D*-end incompatibility, and that *Mls* incompatibility also has an inductive effect.

The allogeneic effect in T–B cell collaboration is reminiscent of the induction of secondary MLR and CML responses by MHC allogeneic disparities (Section I,A,4). There is no generally accepted interpretation of the allogeneic effect, but one possibility is that B cell triggering requires not only interaction with antigen but also a second stimulus. This normally comes from a T cell interaction with the same antigen, but it can also come from confrontation with an MHC incompatibility.

## IV. Role of *H-2* in Cytotoxicity against "Weak" Cell Surface Antigens

Another group of studies has revealed a major role of the *H-2* complex in the reaction of cytotoxic effector cells against cell surface antigens known to be, or which can be plausibly interpreted as, weak (Bevan, 1975a,b; Shearer, 1974; Ilfeld *et al.*, 1975; Zinkernagel, 1974; Zinkernagel and Doherty, 1974; Blanden *et al.*, 1975; Gardner *et al.*, 1975; Koszinowski and Thomssen, 1975; Koszinowski and Ertl, 1975). The antigens used were cells with multiple, non-*H-2* disparities, cells whose surface structure had been modified with trinitrophenyl (TNP), autoantigens of mouse embryo fibroblasts, cells infected with *Listeria monocytogenes,* or cells infected with lymphocytic choriomeningitis virus, ectromelia virus, or vaccinia virus. Immune effector cells against these antigens were obtained by *in vivo* immunization of mice and/or *in vitro* coculture. In the typical experiment, immune spleen cells were harvested and tested for cytotoxicity against $^{51}$Cr labeled target cells, either identical with the immunizing cell, or with the same weak disparity but with an added *H-2* disparity. Targets matching the immunogen were always strongly lysed. Targets matching the immunogen but with an added *H-2* disparity, although presumably bearing a full complement of the antigen or antigens against which immunity was directed, showed very little more lysis than negative controls. Appropriate tests showed that the cytotoxic effector cells were T cells.

Because both plan and outcome of the genetics in all systems were remarkably similar, it will surface to illustrate a typical experiment, as described above, and some experiments with more complex implications, with examples from the non-*H*-2 system of Bevan. Some key tests are shown in Table 8.2.

The strains used were C (*H-2$^d$*), B (*H-2$^b$*), B.D (*H-2$^d$* on a B background), B.BR (*H-2$^k$* on a B background), D (*H-2$^d$*), and C.B (*H-2$^b$* on a C background). Two $F_1$ hybrid combinations involving these strains were also used. In all experiments, three types of cells were involved, effector cells, immunizing cells, and target cells. The immunizing cells were always so selected that immunization could occur only against non-H-2 alloantigens. Three experiments are shown in the table. In the first (cases 1–6), strain C was the source of the effector cells; in the second (cases 7–9), strain C.B; in the third (cases 10–12), a $(C \times C.B)F_1$. The first line in each group is the negative control, the second the positive control in which immunizing cell and target cell are identical.

Cases 3 and 4 of the first experiment illustrate the point, already made, that target cells with the full non-*H-2* complement against which the effector cells were immune, but carrying also an *H*-2 disparity, are not lysed. Case 5 adds the information that as long as the *H*-2 match is retained, substantial lysis will occur even with only a partial non-*H*-2 match. Case 6, and also case 9 of experiment 2, where the target cells are $F_1$ in genotype, show that the roles played by both the non-H-2 alloantigens and the H-2 alloantigens display dominance. Only one set of non-H-2 alloantigens of the target has to match the immunizing alloantigens and only one set of H-2 alloantigens has to match the effector

TABLE 8.2
THE ROLE OF *H-2* MATCH IN CYTOLYSIS BY EFFECTOR T CELLS IMMUNIZED AGAINST MULTIPLE NON-*H-2* DISPARITIES[a]

| Case no. | Source of effector cells[b] | Immunizing cells[b] | Target cells[b] | Lysis |
|---|---|---|---|---|
| 1 | C (*d*) | B.D (*d*) | C (*d*) | − |
| 2 | | | B.D (*d*) | ++ |
| 3 | | | B (*b*) | − |
| 4 | | | B.BR (k) | − |
| 5 | | | D (*d*) | + |
| 6 | | | (C × B) (*d*/*b*) | ++ |
| 7 | C.B (*b*) | B (*b*) | C.B (*b*) | − |
| 8 | | | B (*b*) | ++ |
| 9 | | | (C × B) (*d*/*b*) | ++ |
| 10 | (C × C.B) (*d*/*b*) | B.D (*d*) | (C × C.B) (*d*/*b*) | − |
| 11 | | | B.D (*d*) | ++ |
| 12 | | | B (*b*) | − |

[a] Condensed from Bevan (1975a,b, and personal communication).
[b] *H-2* haplotype of each strain given in parentheses. Immunizations were done by priming the effector cell donors with an intraperitoneal injection of living non-*H-2* mismatched but *H-2* matched stimulating cells, and 18–40 days later removing the spleens and boosting for 4 days *in vitro* with irradiated stimulating cells. Target cells were spleen (B) cells induced to blast transformation with LPS and labeled with $^{51}$Cr.

cell H-2 surface structure. Moreover, the significant *H-2* and non-*H-2* products can be determined by genes that entered in coupling (case 9) or in repulsion (case 6).

This type of result suggests what Zinkernagel and Doherty (1974) have called the *intimacy* interpretation. The weak non-*H-2* disparities, even though multiple, lead to a binding of effector to target of itself too weak to induce lysis. Some further binding force is necessary. This is provided by some *H-2* product or products, so long as these come from identical haplotypes.

This interpretation fits well with concepts that we shall develop in Chapter 13, where we suggest that the "weakness" of non-H-2 antigens may be the result of an inaccessible location in the cell membrane, making antibody binding difficult. But additional, quite similar experiments reported by both Zinkernagel and Doherty (1974) and Bevan (1975b) raise problems.

The nature of the problems, as manifest in the non-*H-2* system employed by Bevan, is illustrated by the third experiment in Table 8.2. Here the effector is an $F_1$, homozygous for the non-*H-2* genotype of strain C, but heterozygous at *H-2* ($H\text{-}2^d/H\text{-}2^b$). The immunizing cell is B.D, with the non-*H-2* genotype of strain B, and with an *H-2* type ($H\text{-}2^d$) matching one of the effector's parents. When, in this experimental context, target cells were the same as immunizing cells (case 11), strong lysis occurred. But when the target cells were from strain B, still with the full complement of necessary non-*H-2* genes, but with an *H-2* type which, although represented in the effector, *was unlike that of the immunizer,* no lysis occurred. Here there would appear to have been all the necessary conditions for lysis. The non-H-2 immune receptors of the effector could find their full complement of antigens on the target, and there was an *H-2* match to provide the intimacy effect. Yet the expected lysis did not occur.

An entirely comparable result was observed by Zinkerhagel and Doherty (1974) in the lymphocytic choriomeningitis virus system. These authors have suggested, as an explanation, that the antigenic change in the cell surface produced by the virus is actually a change in some *H-2* component. For the sake of simplicity, we can illustrate this in the experimental context of experiment 3, Table 8.2, although the actual strains used by Zinkerhagel and Doherty were in part different. The assumption, then, is that a *d/b* effector immunized to virus-infected *d* cells, would actually be immune to a virus-modified antigen, dV. Such an effector could effectively lyse dV cells, but if the target cells were *b/b*, the antigen would be bV. Even though *b* haplotype products were present in the membrane of effector cells, permitting the intimacy effect, if this were relevant, lysis would not occur simply because the target antigen was not present.

This is an attractive hypothesis. We know of no evidence against it, and it certainly must be entertained as a possibility. However, an attempt to apply it to the non-*H-2* system leads to serious complications.

We might assume, as one possibility, that there is a non-*H-2* locus that modifies the structure of some *H-2* complex product. Thus, in the context of experiment 3, Table 8.2, some $H\text{-}2^d$ product might be antigentically different in strain B.D than in strain C. There are two objections to this assumption: (1) There is no histogenetic or serological evidence for such a non-*H-2* effect on *H-2;* (2) even if a modified $H\text{-}2^d$ product in B.D led to a response that would find no corresponding antigen in strain B, there would still be some 30 shared non-H-2 antigens against which cytotoxicity could occur.

Another alternative, suggested by Bevan, is that *H-2* modifies non-*H-2*. However we have to assume, in the context of experiment 3, that the great majority of some 30 non-H-2 antigens in the presence of $H\text{-}2^d$ are so unlike the same gene products in the presence of $H\text{-}2^b$ as to be unrecognized by the anti-B.D effector cells. This not only seems inherently improbable, but is unsupported by any histogenetic experiment, e.g., from cross-immunization in the presence of different *H-2* alleles.

Is there any alternative? If the $F_1$ effector cell in experiment 3 could in some way "remember" that the immunizing cell was $H\text{-}2^d$, even though unable to respond immunologically to the $H\text{-}2^d$ antigens, the nonresponse to strain B might be explained. We suggest as one way in which such "memory" might occur the following admittedly speculative hypothesis.

The *d*-determined antigens of the *d*/*b* effectors find a match in the homozygous *d* immunizers, but the *b*-determined antigens do not. We suggest that certain *d*-determined antigens respond by undergoing a relative increase, while the corresponding *b*-determined antigens undergo a relative decrease. Such consequences of use and disuse are not uncommon in nature. The changes could occur relatively rapidly because of the high rate of turnover of *H-2* products in the cell membrane (Chapter 11, Section VII). If the process continued until the H-$2^b$ on the surface of the effector cells had largely disappeared, the result would be that the effectors would have lost their ability to show the intimacy effect with the B target cells of case number 12 in the table. They would have lost, phenotypically, the H-2 cell surface components necessary for binding to the $H\text{-}2^b$ genotype.

This same interpretation is applicable to the Zinkernagel virus system. The details are more complicated. Suffice it to say that in the $F_1$ versus parent experiment, the immune effector cells were passed through immunosuppressed, virus-infected recipients, in which the postulated surface modification could take place, before being used in the *in vitro* cytotoxic test.

Studies of the virus system have established one more important point. Using appropriate recombinants, Blanden *et al.* (1975) have shown that the components of the *H-2* complex which must be matched to permit lymphocytotoxic destruction of infected cells are at the *K* and *D* ends. The *I* region appears relatively unimportant. Preliminary evidence for Bevan's non-*H-2* system points in the same direction. Tests by Koszinowski and Ertl (1975) of the blocking effect of H-2 antisera on the lysis of vaccinia virus infected cells also point to *H-2K* and *H-2D* as active agents in potentiating the lysis. However, the antisera in these experiments, or at least the anti-H-2K, could have contained anti-Ia.

Studies by Ilfeld *et al.* (1975) of cytotoxicity determined by an autoantigen of cultured mouse embryo fibroblasts, although showing the same basic requirements for an *H-2* match as the non-*H-2* and lymphocytic choriomeningetis virus systems, also showed significant differences. A *D* end match between effector lymphocytes and target fibroblasts did not permit cytotoxicity; a *K* and/or *I* match was required. Also in combinations using $F_1$ targets, one of which was comparable to cases 6 and 9 of Table 8.2, lysis did not occur. No combination comparable to case 12 of Table 8.2 was included.

## V. Summary and Conclusions

The cell interaction phenomena that we have been considering in this chapter, show a number of peculiarities that set them apart from familiar allograft and immune responses. One aspect that they have in common is the predominant role played by the *H-2* complex, and to a lesser degree the *Mls* locus. The $F_1$ versus parent reaction may be entirely contingent on these loci. That the *Mls* locus is, at most, a very weak *H* locus emphasizes the unique role that it plays. It is important to add that the non-*H-2* loci do evoke responses, although weakly.

While any interpretation of these phenomena in the present state of our knowledge must remain speculative, they suggest the possibility that both a special class of marrow-derived lymphocyte, the M cell, and the T helper cell possess a recognition system(s) distinct from classical immunoglobulin. We would also note that the T cell seems to have recognition potentials that are not possessed by the M cell. They also suggest that the role of the products of the *H-2* complex is the regulation of lymphoid cell interactions and perhaps more generalized cell interactions, with the induction or inhibition of mitosis as one end product.

## REFERENCES

Abbasi, K., and H. Festenstein. 1973. Antigenic strength investigated by cell-mediated lympholysis in mice. *Eur J Immunol* 3:430–435.

Adler, W. H., T. Takiguchi, B. Marsh, and R. T. Smith. 1970. Cellular recognition by mouse lymphocytes *in vitro*. II. Specific stimulation by histocompatibility antigens in mixed cell culture. *J Immunol* **105**:984–1000.

Adler, W. H., T. Takiguchi, and R. T. Smith. 1971. Effect of age upon primary alloantigen recognition by mouse spleen cells. *J Immunol* **107**:1357–1362.

Bach, M. L., B. Alter, D. Zoschke, and F. H. Bach. 1971. Soluble adherent cell activity permitting purified lymphocyte response. *Transplant Proc* **3**:844–847.

Bennett, M. 1972. Rejection of marrow allografts. Importance of *H-2* homozygosity of donor cells. *Transplantation* **14**:289–298.

Bennett, M. 1973. Prevention of marrow allograft rejection with radioactive strontium: Evidence for marrow-dependent effector cells. *J Immunol* **110**:510–516.

Berke, G., and D. B. Amos. 1973. Mechanism of lymphocyte-mediated cytolysis. The LMC cycle and its role in transplantation immunity. *Transplant Rev* **17**:71–107.

Bernstein, I. D., and P. W. Wright. 1975. Immunologic reactivity in tolerant rats. *Transplant Proc* **7**:389–391.

Bevan, M. J. 1975a. Interaction antigen detected by cytotoxic cells with the major histocompatibility complex as modifier. *Nature* (*Lond*) **256**:419–421.

Bevan, M. J. 1975b. The major histocompatibility complex determines susceptibility to cytotoxic T cells directed against minor histocompatibility antigens. *J Exp Med* **142**:1349–1364.

Blanden, R. V., P. C. Doherty, M. B. C. Dunlop, I. D. Gardner, R. M. Zinkernagel, and C. S. David. 1975. Genes required for cytotoxicity against virus infected target cells in *K* and *D* regions of the *H-2* complex. *Nature* (*Lond*) **254**:269–270.

Boyse, E. A. 1959. The fate of mouse spleen cells transplanted into homologous and $F_1$ hybrid hosts. *Immunology* **2**:170–181.

Brondz, B. D., I. G. Egorov, and G. I. Drizlikh. 1975. Private specificities of *H-2K* and *H-2D* loci as possible selective targets for effector lymphocytes in cell-mediated immunity. *J Exp Med* **141**:11–26.

Cerottini, J. C., and K. T. Brunner. 1974. Cell-mediated cytotoxicity, allograft rejection and tumor immunity. *Adv Immunol* **18**:67–132.

Charmot, D., C. E. Mawas, and M. Sasportes. 1975. Secondary response of *in vitro* primed human lymphocytes to allogeneic cells. II. Role of HL-A mixed lymphocyte reaction stimulating products and non-specific mitogens in the generation of secondary cytotoxic effectors by *in vitro* primed lymphocytes. *Immunogenetics* **2**:465–483.

Click, R. E. 1974. Immune responses *in vitro*. IX. Absence of the mixed leukocyte stimulation, *M*-locus product from thymus cells. *J Exp Med* **139**:1628–1632.

Cudkowicz, G. 1964. Hybrid resistance to parental hemopoietic cell grafts: Implications for bone marrow chimeras. *Exp Hematol* **7**:34.

Cudkowicz, G. 1965. The immunological basis of hybrid resistance to parental marrow grafts. Pages 37–56 *in* J. Palm, ed. Isoantigens and cell interactions. Wistar Institute Press, Philadelphia, Pennsylvania.

Cudkowicz, G., and M. Bennett. 1971a. Peculiar immunobiology of bone marrow allografts. I. Graft rejection by irradiated responder mice. *J Exp Med* **134**:83–102.

Cudkowicz, G., and M. Bennett. 1971b. Peculiar immunobiology of bone marrow allografts. II. Rejection of parental grafts by resistant $F_1$ hybrid mice. *J Exp Med* **134**:1513–1528.

Cudkowicz, G., and E. Lotzová. 1973. Hemopoietic cell-defined components of the major histocompatibility complex of mice: Identification of responsive and unresponsive recipients for bone marrow transplants. *Transplant Proc* **5**:1399–1405.

Cudkowicz, G., and G. B. Rossi. 1972. Hybrid resistance to parental DBA/2 grafts: Independence from the *H-2* locus. I. Studies with normal hematopoietic cells. *J Natl Cancer Inst* **48**:131–140.

Cudkowicz, G., and J. H. Stimpfling. 1964a. Hybrid resistance controlled by *H-2* region: Correction of data. *Science* **147**: 1056.

Cudkowicz, G., and J. H. Stimpfling. 1964b. Deficient growth of C57BL marrow cells transplanted in $F_1$ hybrid mice. Association with the histocompatibility-2 locus. *Immunology* **7**:291–306.

Dutton, R. W. 1966a. Spleen cell proliferation in response to homologous antigens studied in congenic resistant strains of mice. *J Exp Med* **123**:665–671.

Dutton, R. W. 1966b. Symposium on *in vitro* studies of the immune response. II. Significance of the reaction of lymphoid cells to homologous tissue. *Bacteriol Rev* **30**:397–407.

Dyminski, J. W., and R. T. Smith. 1975. Evidence for a B-cell-like helper function in mixed lymphocyte culture between immunocompetent thymus cells. *J Exp Med* **141**:360–373.

Eichwald, E. J., B. Wetzel, and E. C. Lustgraff. 1965. On the hybrid effect in skin grafting. *Transplantation* **3**:764–766.

Festenstein, H. 1974. Pertinent features of *M*-locus determinants including revised nomenclature and strain distribution. *Transplantation* **18**:555–557.

Festenstein, H., and P. Démant. 1973. Workshop summary on genetic determinants of cell-mediated immune reactions in the mouse. *Transplant Proc* **5**:1321–1327.

Fialkow, P. J. 1967. The induction of chromosomal aberrations *in vitro* by allogeneic lymphocyte extract. *Transplantation* **5**:989–995.

Forman, J., and J. Klein. 1975. Analysis of *H-2* mutants: Evidence for multiple CML target specificities controlled by the $H\text{-}2K^b$ gene. *Immunogenetics* **1**:469–481.

Forman, J.. and G. Möller. 1974. Generation of cytotoxic lymphocytes in mixed lymphocyte reactions. II. Importance of private and public *H-2* alloantigens on the expression of cytotoxicity. *Immunogenetics* **1**:211–225.

Gardner, I. D., N. A. Bowern, and R. V. Blanden. 1975. Cell-mediated cytotoxicity against ectromelia virus-infected cells. III. Role of the *H-2* gene complex. *Eur J Immunol* **5**:122–127.

Gebhardt, B. M., Y. Nakao, and R. T. Smith. 1974. Clonal character of $F_1$ hybrid lymphocyte subset recognition of parental cells in one-way mixed lymphocyte culture. *J Exp Med* **140**:370–382.

Goodman, J. W., F. B. Martin, and C. C. Congdon. 1970. Histology of poor growth of parental marrow cells in $F_1$ hybrid mice: Absence of cellular immune response. *Arch Pathol* **89**:226–234.

Granger, G. A., and W. P. Kolb. 1968. Lymphocyte *in vitro* cytotoxicity: Mechanisms of immune and non-immune small lymphocyte mediated target L cell destruction. *J Immunol* **101**:111–120.

Gregory, C. J., E. A. McCulloch, and J. E. Till. 1972. Repressed growth of C57BL marrow in hybrid hosts reversed by antisera directed against non-H-2 alloantigens. *Transplantation* **13**:138–141.

Haughton, G., and M. Cooper. 1973. Specific immunosuppression by passive antibody. IV. Mechanism of reversal by spleens or peritoneal exudate cells from immune animals. *Cell Immunol* **8**:384–394.

Hellström, K. E. 1964. Growth inhibition of sarcoma and carcinoma cells of homozygous origin. *Science* **143**:477–478.

Hellström, K. E., and I. Hellström. 1967. Allogeneic inhibition of transplanted tumor cells. *Progr Exp Tumor Res* **9**:40–76.

Hellström, K. E., I. Hellström, and G. Haughton. 1964. Demonstration of syngeneic preference *in vitro*. *Nature* (*Lond*) **204**:661–664.

Hellström, K. E., I. Hellström, and D. Motet. 1969. *In vitro* studies on allogeneic inhibition. Pages 155–166 *in* R. T. Smith and R. A. Good, eds. Cellular recognition. Appleton, New York.

Ilfeld, D., C. Carnaud, and E. Klein. 1975. Cytotoxicity of autosensitized lymphocytes restricted to the *H-2K* end of targets. *Immunogenetics* **2**:231–240.

Katz, D. H., M. Graves, M. E. Dorf, H. Dimuzio, and B. Benacerraf. 1975. Cell interactions between histoincompatible T and B lymphocytes. VII. Cooperative responses between lymphocytes are controlled by genes in the *I* region of the *H-2* complex. *J Exp Med* **141**:263–268.

Katz-Heber, E., A. B. Peck, and R. E. Click. 1973. Immune responses *in vitro*. II. Mixed leukocyte interaction in a protein-free medium. *Eur J Immunol* **3**:379–385.

Kennedy, J. C., and J. A. Ekpaha-Mensah. 1973a. Genetics of stimulation of *in vitro* hemolytic plaque-forming cell responses by irradiated allogeneic spleen cells. *J Immunol* **110**:1108–1117.

Kennedy, J. C., and J. A. Ekpaha-Mensah. 1973b. Histocompatibility recognition reactions by irradiated or mitomycin-treated parental cells against hybrid spleen cells produces hybrid cell proliferation and illusion of reaction of hybrid against parent. *J Immunol* **111**:1639–1652.

Kettman, J., and H. Skorvall. 1974. The allogeneic effect: Bystander effect in the primary immune response *in vitro*. *Eur J Immunol* **4**:641–645.

Kilshaw, P. J., L. Brent, C. G. Brooks, R. R. C. New, and M. Pinto. 1975. Studies on the mechanism of specific unresponsiveness to skin allografts in mice. *Transplant Proc* **7**:385–387.

Kindred, B., and D. C. Shreffler. 1972. *H-2* dependence of cooperation between T and B cells *in vivo*. *J Immunol* **109**:940–943.

Klein, J., and J. M. Park. 1973. Graft-versus-host reaction across different regions of the *H-2* complex of the mouse. *J Exp Med* **137**:1213–1225.

Koszinowski, U., and H. Ertl. 1975. Lysis mediated by T cells and restricted by H-2 antigen of target cells infected with vaccinia virus. *Nature* (*Lond*) **255**:552–554.

Koszinowski, U., and R. Thomssen. 1975. Target cell-dependent T cell-mediated lysis of vaccinia virus-infected cells. *Eur J Immunol* **5**:245–250.

Kumar, V., M. Bennett, and R. J. Eckner. 1974. Mechanisms of genetic resistance to Friend virus leukemia in mice. I. Role of $^{89}$Sr-sensitive effector cells responsible for rejection of bone marrow allografts. *J Exp Med* **139**:1093–1109.

Lane, J. T., and N. R. Ling. 1973. Rat thymocytes. The allogeneic response and syngeneic effects in mixed culture with tissue cells from various organs. *Transplantation* **16**:602–609.

Lengerová, A., and V. Zelený. 1968. Syngeneic host requirement of bone marrow cells for their maximum spleen colony-forming capacity to be manifested. *Folia Biol* (*Praha*) **14**:101–114.

Lengerová, A., V. Matousek, and V. Zelený. 1973. Analysis of deficient colony-forming performance of bone marrow cells in non-syngeneic cell milieu—The impact of non-immune interactions on the behavior of pleuripotent stem cells and the role of *H-2* gene products. *Transplant Rev* **15**:89–122.

Lonai, P., A. Eliraz, H. Wekerle, and M. Feldman. 1973. Depletion of specific graft-versus-host reactivity following absorption of nonsensitized lymphocytes on allogenic fibroblasts. *Transplantation* **15**:368–374.

Lotzová, E., and G. Cudkowicz. 1973. Resistance of irradiated $F_1$ hybrid and allogeneic mice to bone marrow grafts of NZB donors. *J Immunol* **110**:791–800.

Lotzová, E., and G. Cudkowicz. 1974. Abrogation of resistance to bone marrow grafts by silica particles. Prevention of the silica effect by the macrophage stabilizer poly-2-vinylpyridine *N*-oxide. *J Immunol* **113**:798–803.

Lozner, E. C., D. H. Sachs, G. M. Shearer, and W. D. Terry. 1974. B-cell alloantigens determined by the *H-2* linked *Ir* region are associated with mixed lymphocyte culture stimulation. *Science* **183**:757–759.

McCulloch, A. E., and J. E. Till. 1963. Repression of colony-forming ability of C57BL hematopoietic cells transferred into non-isologous hosts. *J Cell Comp Physiol* **61**:301–308.

McKenzie, I. F. C., and G. D. Snell. 1975. Ly-4.2: A cell membrane alloantigen of murine B lymphocytes. I. Population studies. *J Immunol* **114**:848–855.

Mangi, R. J., and M. R. Mardiney, Jr. 1971. The mixed lymphocyte reaction. *Transplantation* **11**:369–373.

Mawas, C. E., D. Charmot, and M. Sasportes. 1975. Secondary response of *in vitro* primed human lymphocytes to allogeneic cells. I. Role of the HL-A antigens and mixed lymphocyte reaction stimulating determinants in secondary *in vitro* proliferative response. *Immunogenetics* **2**:449–463.

Mayhew, E., and M. Bennett. 1971. An *in vitro* reaction between lymphoid cells and target fibroblastic cells: A possible model for *in vivo* rejection of haemopoietic allografts. *Immunology* **21**:123–136.

Mayhew, E., and M. Bennett. 1974. Metabolic and physiologic studies of nonimmune lymphoid cells cytotoxic for fibroblast cells *in vitro*. *Cell Immunol* **13**:41–51.

Meo, T., C. S. David, A. M. Rijnbeek, N. Nabholz, V. Miggiano, and D. C. Shreffler. 1975. Inhibition of mouse MLR by anti-Ia sera. *Transplant Proc* **7**:127–129.

Möller, E. 1967. Cytotoxicity by nonimmune allogeneic lymphoid cells. Specific suppression by antibody treatment of the lymphoid cells. *J Exp Med* **126**:395–405.

Möller, E., W. Lapp, and L. Lindholm. 1969. Allogeneic inhibition in tolerant animals. *Transplant Proc* **1**:543–547.

Möller, G., and G. Lundgren. 1969. Aggressive lymphocytes and sensitive target cells: two pathways for cytotoxicity. Pages 177–190 *in* R. T. Smith and R. A. Good, eds. Cellular recognition. Appleton, New York.

Möller, G., and E. Möller. 1965. Plaque-formation by non-immune and X-irradiated lymphoid cells on monolayers of mouse embryo cells. *Nature* (*Lond*) **208**:260–263.

Möller, G., and E. Möller. 1966. Growth inhibition by interaction between allogeneic cells. *Ann Med Exp Biol Fenn* **44**:181–190.

Nabholz, M., J. Vives, H. M. Young, T. Meo, V. Miggiano, A. Rijnbeck, and D. C. Shreffler. 1974. Cell-mediated cell lysis *in vitro:* Genetic control of killer cell production and target specificities in the mouse. *Eur J Immunol* **4**:378–387.

Nabholz, M., H. Young, T. Meo, V. Miggiano, A. Rijnbeek, and D. C. Shreffler. 1975. Genetic analysis of an *H-2* mutant, B6.C-$H\text{-}2^{ba}$, using cell-mediated lympholysis. T- and B-cell dictionaries for histocompatibility determinants are different. *Immunogenetics* **1**:457–468.

Peck, A. B., and R. E. Click. 1973. Immune responses *in vitro*. VIII. Mixed leukocyte culture reactivity induced by $\theta$ antigen. *Transplantation* **16**:339–342.

Peña-Martinez, J., B. Huber, and H. Festenstein. 1973. The influence of *H-2* and non-*H-2 M* locus on spleen colony formation after allogeneic bone marrow transplantation in irradiated mice, assayed by $^{59}$Fe uptake and colony counting. *Transplant Proc* **5**:1393–1397.

Plate, J. M. D., and I. F. C. McKenzie. 1973. "B" cell stimulation of allogeneic T-cell proliferation in mixed lymphocyte culture. *Nature* (*Lond*) (*New Biol*) **245**:247–249.

Popp, R. A. 1961. Regression of grafted bone marrow in homologous irradiated mouse chimeras. *J Natl Cancer Inst* **26**:629–640.

Rajewsky, K., G. E. Roelants, and B. A. Askonas. 1972. Carrier specificity and the allogeneic affect in mice. *Eur J Immunol* **2**:592–598.

Ramseier, H., and J. Lindenmann. 1972. Alliotypic antibodies. *Transplant Rev* **10**:57–96.

Rosenthal, A. S., and E. M. Shevach. 1973. Function of macrophages in antigen recognition by guinea pig T lymphocytes. I. Requirement for histocompatible macrophages and lymphocytes. *J Exp Med* **138**:1194–1212.

Rychlíková, M., and P. Iványi. 1969. Mixed lymphocyte cultures and histocompatibility antigens in mice. *Folia Biol* (*Praha*) **15**:126–135.

Rychlíková, M., P. Démant, and I. K. Egorov. 1972. Mixed lymphocyte reaction caused by an *H-2D* mutation. *Folia Biol* (*Praha*) **18**:360–363.

Rychlíková, M., P. Démant, and P. Iványi. 1973. The mixed lymphocyte reaction in *H-2K, H-2D,* and non-*H-2* incompatibility. *Biomedicine* **18**:401–407.

Salmon, S. E., R. S. Krakauer, and W. F. Whitmore. 1971. Lymphocyte stimulation: Selective destruction of cells during blastogenic response to transplantation antigens. *Science* **172**:490–492.

Sanderson, A. R., and D. A. L. Davies. 1974. Genetic control of cell surface antigens. *Progr Immunol* **2**:364–367.

Sanford, B. H., and S. F. Soo. 1971. Resistance to transplants of recent spontaneous parental line tumors by $F_1$ hybrid hosts. *J Natl Cancer Inst* **46**:95–101.

Schendel, D. J., and F. H. Bach. 1974. Genetic control of cell-mediated lympholysis in mouse. *J Exp Med* **140**:1534–1546.

Shearer, G. M. 1974. Cell-mediated cytotoxicity to trinitrophenyl-modified syngeneic lymphocytes. *Eur J Immunol* **4**:527–533.

Shearer, G. M., and G. Cudkowicz. 1975. Induction of $F_1$ hybrid antiparent cytotoxic effector cells: An *in vitro* model for hemopoietic histoincompatibility. *Science* **190**:890–893.

Shreffler, D. C., and C. S. David. 1975. The *H-2* major histocompatibility complex and the *I* immune response region: Genetic variation, function, and organization. *Adv Immunol* **20**:125–195.

Smith, R. T. 1972. Specific recognition reactions at the cellular level in mouse lymphoreticular cell subpopulations. *Transplant Rev* **11**:178–216.

Snell, G. D. 1958. Histocompatibility genes of the mouse. II. Production and analysis of isogenic resistant lines. *J Natl Cancer Inst* **21**:843–877.

Snell, G. D. 1976. Recognition structures determined by the *H*-2 complex. *Transplant Proc,* in press.

Snell, G. D., and L. C. Stevens. 1961. Histocompatibility genes of mice. III. *H-1* and *H-4,* two histocompatibility loci in the first linkage group. *Immunology* **4**:366–379.

Snell, G. D., G. Cudkowicz, and H. P. Bunker. 1967. Histocompatibility genes of mice. VII. *H-13,* a new histocompatibility locus in the fifth linkage group. *Transplantation* **5**:492–503.

Vetto, R. M., and D. R. Burger. 1972. Endothelial cell stimulation of allogeneic lymphocytes. *Transplantation* **14**:652–654.

Wilson, D. B., J. C. Howard, and P. C. Nowell. 1972. Some biological aspects of lymphocytes reactive to strong histocompatibility alloantigens. *Transplant Rev* **12**:3–29.

Zinkernagel, R. M. 1974. Restriction by *H-2* gene complex of transfer of cell-mediated immunity to *Listeria monocytogenes. Nature* (*Lond*) **251**:230–233.

Zinkernagel, R. M., and P. C. Doherty. 1974. Immunological surveillance against altered self components by sensitized T lymphocytes in lymphocytic choriomeningitis. *Nature* (*Lond*) **251**:547–548.

CHAPTER 9

# THE HLA COMPLEX: SEROLOGY AND GENETICS



Men, like mice, possess a short chromosome segment that carries not only the genes determining the major transplantation antigens but also a whole series of other genes, currently the subject of intensive study, which seem to play an important role in immune processes. Although our knowledge of the genetics of the *H-2* complex is still greater than that of the *HLA complex*, its human equivalent, our understanding of the latter is undergoing extraordinary expansion.

Of the known genes in the mouse *H-2* complex, only the equivalents of those governing the products that are serologically definable on cell surfaces and those governing the response of lymphocytes in contact with allogeneic cells in culture, known as lymphocyte-defined, have as yet been found in man. But in Chapter 12 it will be shown that the many associations between HLA antigens and diseases suggest also the presence of immune response (*Ir*) genes in HLA as in *H-2*. Other antigens detected mainly on mouse B lymphocytes (Ia antigens) also have their equivalent in man.

Although the *H-2* system was and is a model for the HLA system, the latter, because of the intensive study of large and diverse populations has made, and will continue to make, its own unique contributions.

We shall relate, successively, the means of detection, the genetics, and the nature of the different gene products, of the HLA region.

## I. Historical Background

The first stages in the serology of the human system were not, in fact, inspired by the work on mice, since it did not seem that humans possessed erythrocyte histocompatibility antigens detectable by hemagglutination as in mice. The procedure was quite different.

Between 1920 and 1950 many publications appeared, especially from the Italian school, trying to prove the existence of leukolytic substances in the blood of leukopenic patients. It was in this spirit that Dausset and Nenna (1952) and Moeschlin and Wagner (1952) independently described the first leukoagglutination reactions of immunological origin. It is now known that whereas Moeschlin's leukoagglutinins were in fact allergic autoantibodies induced by amidopyrin, Dausset's were the first anti-leukocyte alloantibodies to be observed. This interpretation became obvious in 1953 when it was found that the antibodies were inactive against the serum donor's own leukocytes but active on only a small proportion of group O unrelated individuals (Dausset, 1954; Miescher and Fauconnet, 1954). A systematic study of antibodies developed after blood transfusions was undertaken using the leukoagglutination technique (Payne, 1957), and the first HLA leukocyte specificity, Mac, was detected using six sera that reacted in a similar, but not identical way (Dausset, 1958). A role for antigens of this kind in transplantation was thereby suggested, since Amos (1953) has proved that H-2 antigens could be detected on mouse leukocytes by leukoagglutination.

In spite of this first opening, the uncertainty of the techniques used and the extreme complexity of the genetic situation slowed progress in the immunogenetics of leukoplatelet antigens. Shulman made a brilliant contribution when, through the development and use of the technique of quantitative complement fixation on platelets, he was able to describe the $Pl^A$ system and other platelet specificities that are now known to belong to the HLA system (reviewed in Shulman *et al.*, 1964).

An important step was taken in 1958 when Van Rood *et al.* (1958) and Payne and Rolfs (1958) independently discovered the extreme frequency of anti-leukocyte antibodies in the sera of multiparous women.

The introduction of the computer to help unravel the apparently inextricable tangle of serological reactions enabled Van Rood and Van Leeuwen (1963) to describe two entities, 4a and 4b, which behave more or less like alleles. Nevertheless, as confirmed by other studies, there were too many heterozygotes, the significance of which is still unknown. Meanwhile, Payne *et al.* (1964), working with the sera of multiparous women, described two specificities in a first or LA series, LA1 and LA2 (identical to Mac), which behaved in the population and segregated in families like alleles.

One of the turning points in the history of histocompatibility antigens was the beginning, in 1964, of an intensive international collaboration that has continued to this day. It would appear that such a united effort is unique in biological science. The permanent exchange of biological material, techniques and ideas has considerably speeded up discoveries. Although it would be highly desirable to quote all those who contributed to this collaborative work with the same enthusiasm, they are unfortunately far too numerous, and the reader is referred to the series of volumes that mark the various stages (Dausset, 1956; Walford, 1960, 1969; Russell *et al.*, 1965; Balner *et al.*, 1965; Curtoni *et al.*, 1967; Svejgaard, 1969; Kissmeyer-Nielsen and Thorsby, 1970; Terasaki, 1970; Dausset and Colombani, 1973; Kissmeyer-Nielsen, 1975).

It was B. Amos who organized the First Workshop and Conference on Histocompatibility in 1964, where the research teams' sera and techniques were compared in the first common "on the bench" study. The results were so discordant that they could not really be published.

The second Workshop, held in 1965 (directed by J. J. Van Rood) enabled the different specificities described by the various teams to be compared. This time the results were coherent. Specificities emerged clearly, and the genetic analysis of specificities was possible. Because of the positive and negative associations demonstrable between these specificities, Dausset *et al.* (1965) postulated that they all belonged to a single, complex immunogenic system analogous to the *H-2* system. They suggested the name *Hu-1 system.* The 4 series of antigens was extended by Bodmer and Payne (1965) by the addition of specificities 4c and 4d. Van Rood *et al.* (1965) described three series of specificities, 7, 8, and 9. Terasaki and his collaborators (Vredovoe *et al.*, 1966) classified the reactions of the sera they studied into six groups, probably belonging to the same system.

Simple associations between specificities were not sufficient to prove membership in a single system. Family studies were necessary, and this was the objective set by R. Ceppellini for the Third Workshop. The study of 11 families using the best sera available in the world led to the concept of a single system being generally accepted. No recombination was found between any of the specificities in any of the families (Ceppellini *et al.*, 1967). Soon a sufficient number of informative families had been studied to prove the allelic transmission of the first (Bodmer *et al.*, 1966) and second segregant series of specificities (Dausset *et al.*, 1968; Kissmeyer-Nielsen *et al.*, 1968; Singal *et al.*, 1968).

It then became possible to evaluate the distance between the two loci using families in which there were recombinations (reviewed by Weitkamp *et al.*, 1973). Also many new specificities were described in the two allelic series.

By means of the analysis of a study of 300 families with the same reagents, the Fourth Workshop (1970), organized by Terasaki, firmly established the concept of a system containing two closely linked, polyallelic loci. However, even then the possibility of a third locus, identified by a serum (AJ), was suggested (Kissmeyer-Nielsen *et al.*, 1971; Sandberg *et al.*, 1970). The existence of this third allelic series has since been confirmed.

In 1972, serological and genetic progress in the HLA system was sufficient to allow a vast anthropological investigation to be undertaken. This was the object of the Fifth Workshop directed by J. Dausset (Dausset and Colombani, 1973). In this way it was possible to confirm that the genetic concept, as established for Caucasians, was valid for all other populations, in spite of the great diversity of gene frequencies in the various peoples. The Sixth Workshop was mainly devoted to the first steps of HLA-D typing and the recent description of human Ia equivalents (Kissmeyer-Nielsen, 1975).

Despite the extensive data already accumulated, our knowledge of HLA immunogenetics is still incomplete. The existence of multiple antigenic sites on the product of a single gene, postulated in 1965 (Dausset *et al.*, 1965; Iványi and Dausset, 1966), is now accepted. Some of these sites are probably the human equivalent of the short and long "public" specificities of the *H-2* system. Public specificities are shared by two or more allelic products, each bearing one private specificity.

Public specificities common to the end products of the first two HLA loci (interlocus) have been described (Legrand and Dausset, 1975a).

One of the main obstacles encountered in reading the early literature on HLA is the extraordinary variety of names given to the specificities. These are mostly composed of numbers preceded by an abbreviation of the author's name or of the town in which the discovery was made. Fortunately the WHO commission rapidly instituted standardized nomenclature. The region is called HLA (A stands for the first system). Each specificity that is well established has a number preceded by the sign A, B, C, D, etc., designating the locus. Some specificities are not yet firmly established, and these are still designated by W (Workshop) followed by a number. The most recently discovered specificities are still known by the name given them by their discoverers. The equivalents of the various symbols are given in Tables 9.1–9.4. *Phenotypes* are written with the specificities indicated in any order (e.g., HLA-Al,2; B7,12; Cw4,w5; Dw2,w4), *Genotypes* have the specificities, in this case used as indicative of alleles, in the order of their occurrence on each chromosome (e.g., HLA-Al,B7,Cw4,Dw2/A2,B12,Cw5,Dw4). The *haplotype* refers to the genes on one chromosome (e.g., HLA-A1,B7,Cw4,Dw2).

## II. HLA Antibodies and Serological Methods

### A. Sources of Antibodies

It is apparently well established that natural anti-HLA antibodies do not exist. Since 1952, systematic studies have shown that sera from nontransfused men do not contain this kind of antibody, at least detectable by normal leukoagglutination techniques. Since then, thousands of normal sera have been used as controls for the various lymphocytotoxicity or platelet complement fixation techniques, with the same results. However, Collins *et al.* (1973) discovered an anti-B8 in the serum of a nontransfused individual. It is the first example of an anti-HLA antibody appearing under these conditions and suggests the possibility of immunization by an outside agent with a similar or identical structure. Another natural antibody, detecting almost only the A2 homozygous individuals, was found by Lepage and Dausset (in Kissmeyer-Nielsen, 1975).

On the other hand, anti-HLA antibodies are frequent in women immunized by pregnancy. At first it was thought that several stimuli were necessary for the appearance of these antibodies and that they could be developed by multiparous women only. In fact, they may appear

TABLE 9.1
COMPARATIVE TERMINOLOGY OF SPECIFICITIES DETERMINED BY THE HLA-A LOCUS (FIRST OR LA LOCUS)[a]

| HL-A official or workshop designation New | Old | | | | | | Kiss-meyer-Nielsen | | | | |
|---|---|---|---|---|---|---|---|---|---|---|---|
| HLA- | HL-A | Amos | Batch-elor | Bodmer and Payne | Cep-pel-lini | Dausset and Colombani | and Thorsby | Terasaki | Van Rood | Walford | Others |
| A1 | 1 | Ao19 | Bt1 | LA1 | To8 | Da11 | | Te1 | | Lc-1 | |
| A2 (Mac) | 2 | Ao1 | Bt5 | LA2 | To9 | Mac, Da1 | | Te2 | | Lc-2 | |
| A2 + A28 | | | | | | Da2 | Ba | Te16 | 8a | | PlGrLy[B1] |
| A3 | 3 | <Ao4 | <Bt18 | <LA3 | To10 | <Da12 | | <Te8 | | <Lc-3 | |
| A3 + A11 | | | | | | Da12 | ILN | | | | |
| A9 | 9 | Ao35 | Bt9 or 21 | LA4 | To12 | Da16 | Stewart | Te4 | | Lc-11 (Hunt B) | |
| Aw23 (9.1) | W23 | | | | | 9′(Da27) | | | | Lc-11 (Hunt C) | |
| Aw24 (9.2) | W24 | Ao82 | | | | 9″(Da32) | | | | | |
| A10 | 10 | | Bt8 | | | Da17 | KH | Te12 | | | |
| Aw25 (10.1) | W25 | <Ao28 | | | To31 | 10″(Da29) | | | | | |
| Aw26 (10.2) | W26 | | | | To40 | 10′(Da28) | | | | | |
| A11 | 11 | Ao45 | | | To26 | Da21 | ILN*, EA | Te13 | | | GE20 |
| A19 | W19 | | | | | | Li | Te19 | | ≃Thompson | GE33 |
| A29 (19.1) | W29 | Ao77 | Bt15 | | | Da22 | | Te63 | | | |
| (19.2) | W30+31 | | | | | Da25 | | | | | |
| Aw30 (19.3) | W30 | | | | | Da25′(Da26) | | Te66 | | Lc-21 | |
| Aw31 (19.4) | W31 | | | LA-W | | Da25″(Da33) | | | | Lc-26.1 | |
| Aw32 (19.5) | W32 | Ao28 | | | To30 | | | Te59 | | | GE32 |
| Aw33 (19.6) | | | | | | | | | | | >Fe55 |
| A28 | W28 | Ao5 | | | | $1^B$ or Da15 | Ba* | Te28 or 40 | | Lc-17 | Bg[c] |
| Aw34 | | | | | | | | | | | Malay or HLA10.3 |
| Aw36 | | | | | | | | | | | Mo*, LT |
| Aw43 | | | | | | | | | | | BK |

[a] From Dausset and Colombani (1973) where the first publication of each specificity is reference (and modified from Kissmeyer-Nielsen, 1976).

TABLE 9.2

Comparative Terminology of Specificities Determined by the HLA-B Locus (Second or Four Locus)[a,b]

| HL-A official or workshop designation New | Old | | | | | | | | | | |
|---|---|---|---|---|---|---|---|---|---|---|---|
| HLA- | HL-A | Amos | Batch-elor | Bod-mer and Payne | Cepel-lini | Daus-set and Col-om-bani | Kiss-meyer-Nielsen and Thorsby | Terasaki | Van Rood | Walford | Others |
| B5 | 5 | Ao12 | Bt25 | <4c | To5 | Da5 | MH | Te11 (old) | (1)[c] | <Lc-19 | |
| B7 | 7 | Ao2 | <Bt4 | 4d | | Da10 | | | <7c = 6c,6b | Lc-8 | Bg[a] |
| B8 | 8 | | Bt2 | | To7 | Da8 | | | 7d | Lc-7 | |
| B12 | 12 | Ao15 | >Bt6 | 4a11 | To11 | Da4 | T12 | Te9 | (1) | Merrit-A | |
| B13 | 13 | HK | Bt23 | | To21 | | HN | Te26 | <6b(1) | | |
| Bw35 | W5 | Ao13 | | <4c* | | Da20 | R* | Te5 or 50 | (1) | >Lc-16 | GE11 |
| Bw40 | W10 | | | | To23 | | BB | Te10 or 60 | <6b | | GE23 |
| B14 | W14 | | | | | Da18 | | Te14 or 54 | | | MaKi |
| Bw15 | W15 | | >Bt26 | | | Da23 | LND | Te15 or 55 | <7a(1) | Lc-25 | |
| Bw16 | W16 | Ao81 | | | | | U18 | Te64 | (1) | | |
| Bw38 | W16.1 | | | | | Da31 | | | | | |
| Bw39 | W16.2 | | | | | | | | | | |
| Bw17 | W17 | Ao70 | Bt12 | | | | SL-MaPi | Te17 or 57 | Orlina (1) | | Bg[b], MaPi |
| B18 | W18 | | Bt20 | <4c* | | | CM | Te18 or 58 | (1) | | GE28 |
| Bw21 | W21 | | | | | Da24 | ET | Te61 | 7be (1) | | |
| Bw22 | W22 | | | | To28 | | AA | | <7c | | GE22 |
| (22.1) | | | Bt22 | | | | | Te22 or 51 | | | |
| (22.2) | | | | | | Da30 | | | | | |
| B27 | W27 | <Ao10 | | | | | FJH | Te27 or 52 | <7c | | |
| Bw37 | | | | | | | | | | | Ty |
| Bw41 | | | | | | Da34 | | | | | Sabell, LK |
| Bw42 | | | | | | | | | | | MWA |
| Bw4 | W4 | Ao27 | | | <To2 | Da3 | | | 4a | | |
| Bw6 | W6 | Ao72 | | | To6 | Da7 | | | 4b | | |

[a] From Dausset and Colombani (1973) where the first publication of each specificity is reference (and modified from Kissmeyer-Nielsen, 1976).
[b] Some *B* locus symbols without equivalents and not shown in the table are 407*, TT*; JA = KSO*; HR; Hs = Sin2; 6a; 7b.
[c] (1), Cross-reacting with 7b.

TABLE 9.3
COMPARATIVE TERMINOLOGY OF SPECIFICITIES DETERMINED BY THE HLA-C LOCUS (THIRD OR AJ LOCUS)

| Workshop designation HLA- | Svejgaard *et al.* (1973) | Mayr *et al.* (1973) |
|---|---|---|
| Cw1 | AJ | T1 |
| Cw2 | 170, Sa 532 | T2 |
| Cw3 | UPS | T3 |
| Cw4 | RH315 | T4 |
| Cw5 | | T5 |
| | | T6 |

during the first pregnancy. In most cases, a multiparous woman will have had the opportunity to become immunized against the paternal specificities on one or both HLA haplotypes, depending on which haplotype the father has transmitted to each child. Accordingly, she will often possess a mixture of antibodies, which makes the identification of their respective specificities somewhat difficult. The incidence of leukocyte antibodies in parous women has been the subject of several studies (Payne, 1957, 1962; Van Rood *et al.*, 1958; Ahrons, 1971; Nymand, 1974). The frequency of occurrence increases with the number of pregnancies (Fig. 9.1). However, it does not appear that parity has any influence, although fetuses aborted very early are unable to give an antigenic

TABLE 9.4
COMPARATIVE TERMINOLOGY OF SPECIFICITIES DETERMINED BY THE HLA-D LOCUS (MLR OR LD LOCUS)

| Workshop designation HLA- | Most investigators[a] | Others[a] |
|---|---|---|
| Dw1 | LD-W5a | j, Pf, XVII |
| Dw2 | LD-7a | S, Pi, V |
| Dw3 | LD-8a | Sr, XI |
| Dw4 | LD-12a | L, XVIII |
| Dw5 | LD-16a | IV |
| Dw6 | LD-15a | XIV |
| | LD-107 | XII |
| | LD-108 | Co |

[a] See Kissmeyer-Nielsen (1976).

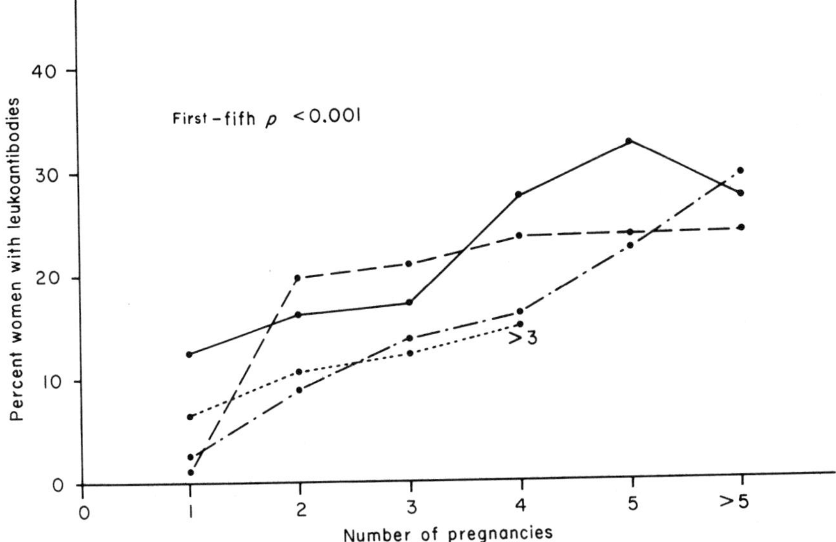


FIG. 9.1. Percentage of anti-leukocyte immunizations in relation to the number of pregnancies, regardless of previous transfusions. Dashed line, leukoagglutination on defibrinated blood (Payne 1962); dot-dashed line, leukoagglutination on defibrinated blood (Jensen, 1966); dotted line, lymphocytotoxicity (Ahrons, 1971); solid line, lymphocytotoxicity (J. Vives, personal communication). Leukoagglutination on defibrinated blood has a similar sensitivity to lymphocytotoxicity. Leukoagglutination on blood treated with Sequestrene, however, gives only 6% immunization after five pregnancies (Van Rood, 1962).

stimulus. The serological techniques used to detect antibodies have a great influence: Lymphocytotoxic antibodies are frequent (20% of the sera tested); platelet complement-fixing antibodies are rare (about 2%). ABO and rhesus fetomaternal incompatibility does not have a significant influence. However, leukoantibodies are more frequent in sera that contain antibodies against erythrocyte blood groups than in those that do not (32% versus 6%) (Salmon and Schwartz, 1960).

Antibodies appear at varying times in pregnant women. In primiparous women, antibodies are found in about 10% at delivery (Overweg and Engelfriet, 1969) and sometimes as early as in the sixth month (Nymand, 1974). In multiparous women, a distinction should be made as to whether the current pregnancy is a restimulation of an immunization caused by an earlier pregnancy or whether it is a new stimulus. Should it prove to be the former, a relatively powerful antibody is seen to reappear rapidly; in the latter case, the response will be weak or absent, but sometimes antibodies directed against the other haplotype reappear or increase in titer, although the fetus does not possess this haplotype.

The persistence of antibodies in maternal serum is extremely variable. The controlling factors are still largely unknown. Sometimes a relatively powerful antibody will be found in the serum after several months or even years (these are often leukoagglutinins); sometimes, and more usually, the antibodies disappear rapidly, sometimes within 1 month of parturition, depending on the initial titer.

In the vast majority of cases antibodies are composed of molecules capable of passing through the filter formed by the placenta and reaching the corresponding antigens of the fetus. Antibodies are found in cord sera from about 20% of the cases where the mother becomes immunized (Jensen, 1966; Payne, 1964). Nevertheless, in spite of the substantial antigenic mass of the fetus, circulating antibodies are present in the mother throughout the pregnancy. The antibodies are usually harmless to the fetus (see Nymand, 1974).

Immunization by transfusion is extremely frequent. In women it is added to immunization by pregnancy and is therefore even more frequent. The frequency of immunization naturally depends on the number of transfusions (Fig. 9.2) and the frequency in the population of the HLA specificities that the patient does not possess. The most striking

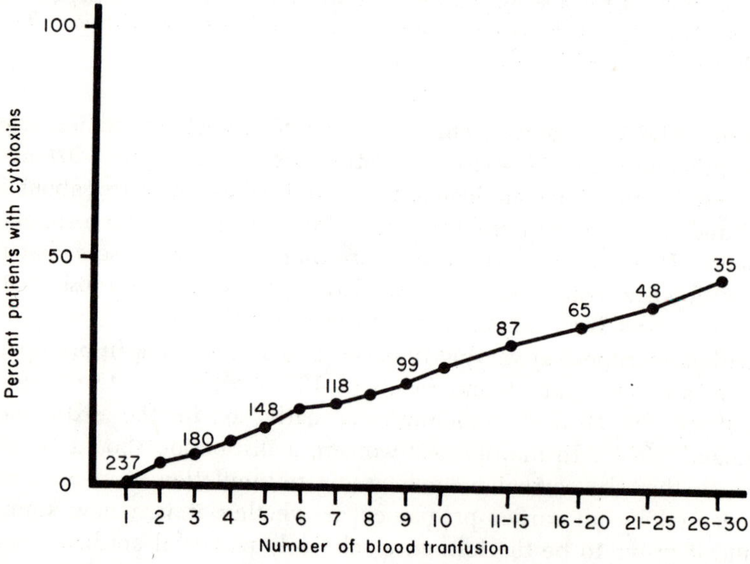


Fig. 9.2. Percentage of patients developing lymphocytotoxins in relation to the number of blood transfusions. (From Opelz *et al.*, 1973, courtesy of *Transplantation*.)

example is that of the specificity A2, which is present in approximately 50% of Caucasoid individuals. Accordingly, half the blood given to an A2-negative patient will contain the incompatible antigen. On the other hand, the chances of encountering a low-frequency specificity, such as B13, present in approximately 5% of the population, are much smaller. Obviously then the frequency of appearance of antibodies directed against relatively widespread specificities (20–50%) is high. Inasmuch as these conditions are nearly always fulfilled, polytransfused patients regularly develop antibodies and their sera rapidly become polyspecific. Without special treatment, these sera are unsatisfactory reagents. Nevertheless, they can be used by isolating one of the antibody populations by absorption–elution or, when one of the antibodies has a far higher titer than the others, simply by dilution.

Multiparous women and polytransfused patients have provided and continue to provide most of the sera used. However, there have also been cases of patients who received blood from a single donor (Marchal *et al.*, 1958). It was from sera obtained in this way that the first specificity, Mac, was described. Nevertheless, because of the extreme complexity of the genetic and serological situations, there is increasing recourse to provoked, and therefore planned, immunizations. Healthy volunteers are immunized, after taking all possible medical and ethical precautions. The best results have been obtained from immunizations between related individuals, differing by only one HLA haplotype. The father is usually the recipient. It occasionally happens that the father differs from one of his children by a single HLA antigen only. This is the ideal situation in which to obtain an immunization that is maximally specific.

In multiparous women, as well as in immunized patients or volunteers, it has been noted that no matter how many stimuli may have been administered, a certain percentage of individuals do not develop antibodies, or they disappear after a very brief appearance. A considerable percentage of multiparous women who have been pregnant more than five times (65–70%) have not developed any antibodies detectable by the usual techniques. This high percentage cannot be explained by the mother and child having identical specificities, since the polymorphism of the HLA system is so great that this situation is rare. About 50% of patients receiving hemodialysis were reported to have failed to produce lymphocytotoxins, although they had received up to 30 transfusions (Opelz *et al.*, 1973). This apparent resistance to immunization could be caused in various ways: The existence of very frequent so-called *cross-reactions* between specificities at the same locus and the existence of blocking antibodies that cannot fix complement have been proved. Moreover, by analogy with mice, it is possible to envisage that HLA immunization requires the presence of an appropriate immune response (*Ir*) allele for each determinant.

Perhaps this apparent inability to respond usually reflects an inadequate dose of immunogens. After a single massive transfusion prior to heart surgery, 96% of patients develop leukoantibodies. In mice and rats, where there is no restriction on antigen dose, anti-H-2 lymphocytotoxic antibodies are almost always obtainable, although some (anti-H-2) private antibodies fail to form or are weak in recipients bearing an unfavorable *Ir-1* allele.

In view of all these pitfalls and of ethical considerations, it is desirable that animal immunization be rapidly substituted. The difficulties are well known. Xenogeneic recipients respond primarily to species differences and may not distinguish the subtle differences presented by the HLA alloantigens. Nevertheless, good anti-HLA antibodies are now produced for some specificities using animals made tolerant to human species antigens prior to immunization with alloantigens, or by injecting with purified antigens an animal that closely resembles man (Metzgar and Miller, 1973; Sanderson and Welsh, 1973).

## B. Serological Techniques

The techniques used to detect these antibodies have been progressively refined. They almost all use the intervention of complement.

### 1. *Leukoagglutination*

The first technique described was that of leukoagglutination performed in the presence of complement from the leukocyte donor's own serum (Dausset, 1954). The leukoagglutination reaction using defibrinated blood should be contrasted to the reaction using blood collected into an anticoagulant (usually Sequestrene) in which the complement is inhibited by neutralization of the Ca ions.

The first reaction is probably an *active* phenomenon, similar to immunoadherence (Melief *et al.*, 1967). Rosettes surrounding granulocytes have been observed. The second reaction is probably a *passive* phenomenon. Neither reaction is easily reproducible.

In spite of its apparent simplicity, leukoagglutination has practically been abandoned in favor of lymphocytotoxicity. Attempts to rehabilitate it by introducing a microtechnique were unsuccessful.

### 2. *Lymphocytotoxicity*

In this reaction the presence of a specific antibody is evidenced by the lytic action of complement on target cells. These are exclusively lymphocytes, since granulocytes have practically been eliminated. Cellular death is seen by changes in the permeability of the membrane (penetration of dyes such as trypan blue or eosin), or changes in the vital staining by fluorochrome.

Lymphocytotoxicity in the presence of human complement tends to be weak. Only some sera are active under these conditions. Rabbit complement, on the other hand, potentiates the reaction to a remarkable degree. It is probable that this potentiation is due to the synergic action of anti-human xenoantibodies present in rabbit serum. It follows that the lytic action of an antibody studied *in vitro* may not exist *in vivo*. Certain antibodies may not have a lytic effect in the organism and therefore not really be complement-fixing antibodies proper.

Many variations of the lymphocytotoxic technique have been described. Usually, all the elements used in the reaction are added at once (one-stage reaction; Kissmeyer-Nielsen and Kjerbye, 1967). The two-stage reaction (Terasaki and McClelland, 1964), in which the complement is added after the antibody has been fixed on the cells, is more sensitive. This may be advantageous when a test serum is being studied in detail, but disadvantageous when the classic tissue groups have to be determined by a specific antibody.

These techniques can be rendered more sensitive by two methods: (1) Washing the cells between the first and second stages of the two-stage reaction can be used to reduce the anticomplementary activity of the sera (Amos *et al.*, 1969). (2) The addition of human anti-globulin to the reaction activates the complement even more than does the allo-antibody alone (Johnson *et al.*, 1972). Lymphocytotoxicity is now used for routing tissue typing. Nevertheless the degree of standardization is not yet satisfactory, primarily because of variations in rabbit complement.

### 3. *Complement Fixation*

The third technique, rarely used routinely, is the platelet, or, less commonly, lymphocyte complement-fixation reaction. Its advantage over lymphocytotoxicity is that the results are more quantitative and hence more precise. Because of its rigorous standardization (Colombani *et al.*, 1971), it is possible to measure the number of complement units fixed with great exactness. Additionally, platelets can be stored for several months (at least 6 months) at 4°C without loss of antigenicity. Accordingly, it is possible to have a permanent, complete panel of phenotyped or even genotyped platelets ready to be used for absorption or elution tests. However, the platelet complement-fixation reaction is approximately ten times less sensitive than two-stage lymphocytotoxicity.

Only test sera possessing a lymphocytotoxicity higher than 1:5 can be used, and these are relatively rare. However, this disadvantage is often compensated by the great specificity. Finally, it must be emphasized that although in the vast majority of specificities currently known there is complete parallelism between lymphocytes and platelets, there are nevertheless some specificities, such as B12 and B8, which are not completely expressed on the platelets of certain individuals.

Many other techniques are also used to demonstrate the existence of anti-HLA antibodies. Some are immunofluorescence methods, which have become very popular, especially in the study of antigen redistribution under the influence of antibodies. Others are mixed agglutination using anti-globulins and antibody-coated erythrocytes as revealers, immunocytoadherence, and serotonin liberation by platelets.

### C. Characteristics of Anti-HLA Antibodies

The vast majority of anti-HLA antibodies are IgG immunoglobulins, but small traces of IgM are often present (Arhons and Glavind-Kristensen, 1971). The allotypes and idiotypes of anti-HLA antibodies have not as yet been studied, and it is not known whether different classes of immunoglobulins are involved.

We have emphasized complement-fixing activity since most usual techniques are based on complement activation. However it must be borne in mind that some antibodies are not complement fixing. Thus, an IgM and several IgG antibodies capable of blocking complement fixation have been reported (Colombani *et al.*, 1973). It is becoming more and more apparent that both types of antibody coexist in varying proportions in many sera.

Planned parent–child immunizations permit the appearance of anti-HLA antibodies, their development during antigenic injections, and their progressive disappearance after the termination of injections to be followed precisely.

One such planned immunization will serve to illustrate many characteristics of HLA serology. A father, DEG, was immunized by his daughter who only differed by a single specificity, B5. Additionally, the father possessed a specificity, B18, which has some similarities to B5. It might be expected that any response would be relatively simple. This did not prove to be the case (Legrand and Dausset, 1974). The first antibody that appeared (Fig. 9.3) was directed against the specificity B5; however, from the second leukocyte injection onward the anti-B5 antibody was accompanied by a second antibody that defined a more inclusive or, in *H-2* terminology, a *public* specificity, present not only on cells bearing

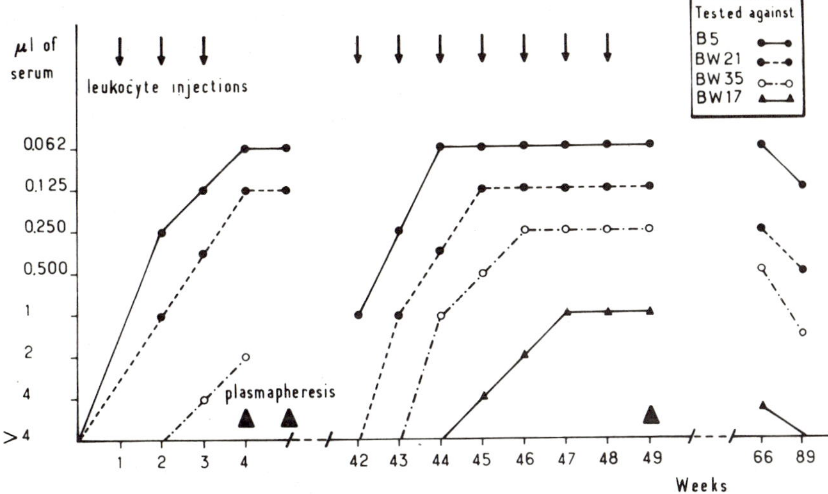


FIG. 9.3. Sequential development and titers of four different antibody populations by immunization of an Aw24, B18/A2, B12 father by his daughter whose maternal haplotype was Aw24, B5. Note that the donor and recipient differ by B5 only and that B18 and B5 are known cross-reacting specificities. The father received two series of leukocyte injections, separated by an interval of 38 weeks. The reactions against B5 and Bw21 cells appeared practically simultaneously; the reactions against Bw35 was much weaker and did not appear until the second injection. Only the reaction against B5 remained between the two series of injections. The other two antibody populations reappeared rapidly, followed, after the third injection, by a fourth, against Bw17. This was the first to disappear.

the donor's known B5 specificity but also cells bearing Bw21. This fact is of great theoretical and practical importance in the comprehension of the serology and genetics of transplantation antigens. Continuing the immunization, a third antibody population was seen to develop, once again apparently directed against a specificity absent from the donor (Bw35).

Injections were discontinued for 38 weeks. The antibody titers diminished, and finally disappeared except the first one directed against B5. A second series of leukocyte injections led to their rapid reappearance at varying titers. A fourth antibody population developed, apparently directed yet again against a specificity not found in the donor (Bw17). This last antibody remained weak.

The existence of several distinct antibody populations is indicated by their sequential appearance in steps and also by their physical separation by means of absorption-elution on cells of the appropriate group. The details of the antibody specificities developed during this experiment will be discussed later. Here we wish to emphasize a unique serological phenomenon that is one of the most striking characteristics of HLA and *H-2* serology: the ability of certain cells to absorb an antibody although no visible reaction occurs (Van Rood and Van Leeuwen, 1965). This is referred to as "agglutination-negative–absorption-positive" (ANAP). It also occurs with lymphocytotoxicity, and is then called "cytotoxicity-negative–absorption-positive" (CYNAP).

During the voluntary immunization taken as an example, this phenomenon was strikingly evident. The second antibody to appear was absorbed by but did not react with certain cells possessing the specificity Bw35. The third antibody was absorbed without reaction on certain cells possessing the specificity Bw17. Finally, the third population was absorbed without reaction on Bw15 (Fig. 9.4).

Another common phenomenon in HLA serology is illustrated in Fig. 9.4 namely, the *inclusion* of the reactivity of an antibody in that of a second antibody appearing later in the course of the immunization. Thus the reactivity of the first antibody, anti-B5, is included in that of the second antibody, which reacts with W21 cells, and so on. The frequency with which this "Russian doll" phenomenon is seen suggests a deep biological and genetic significance, but what this may be is presently unknown.

This example of father–daughter immunization provides a good example of the complexity of HLA serology. It illustrates (1) the possibility of an immunization against a specificity other than the known specificity of the donor's cells; (2) the possibility of completely or partially absorbing an antibody without provoking a reaction (CYNAP) on those cells that will, nonetheless, react directly with the next antibody to appear; (3) the systematic inclusion of the reactivities of the antibodies that appeared first in the reactivities of the antibodies that appeared last; and (4) the *progressive and sequential appearance of several antibody populations* that react with an ever increasing number of cells taken at random from the population. One interpretation of the multiplicity of antibodies is the occurrence of *cross-reactions* between the HLA specificities.

### *1. Cross-Reactions*

The term cross-reaction is used here in its broadest serological sense; no particular interpretation of the results is implied. The observed fact is the possibility of complete or partial absorption of certain antibodies by a cell bearing another determinant in the same allelic series. In 1970 Colombani *et al.* put forward the conception of cross-reacting groups (CREG) or "families" of specificities. The most obvious CREG's are

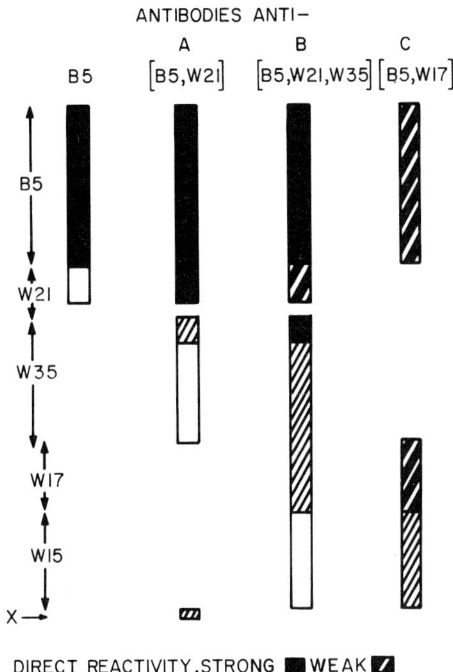


FIG. 9.4. Schematic representation of the serological reactions obtained with the four antibody populations isolated from serum DEG. These antibodies appeared in order from left to right. The antibody against the B5 specificity which was present on the immunising cell appeared first, then the other antibodies. These antibodies reacted with cells in the population which did not contain B5 but another private specificity at the same locus (Bw21, Bw35, Bw17, or Bw15). The anti-B5 reacted with all B5 cells tested and was partially absorbed by all except two Bw21 cells. The anti-A reacted with the above-mentioned B5 and Bw21 cells and was more or less completely absorbed by Bw35 cells. The anti-B reacted with the preceding cells and was absorbed by some Bw35 cells and very weakly by Bw15 cells. The anti-C reacted with B5 and Bw17 cells and very weakly by Bw15 cells. The anti-C reacted with B5 and Bw17 cells and was completely absorbed by Bw15 cells. If the immunization had been pursued, it is possible that the antibody would also have reacted with the Bw35 cells.

at the first or A locus: A1–A3–A11, A2–A28, and to a lessor degree A9–Aw29–Aw30–Aw31–Aw32–Aw33. At the second or B locus: B5–Bw35–Bw15–Bw21, B7–Bw40–B27–Bw22, and B8–B14.

These CREG's are not separate from one another. There are interactions between groups so that there are networks of cross-reactions between a number of allelic products at each of the two main loci. There

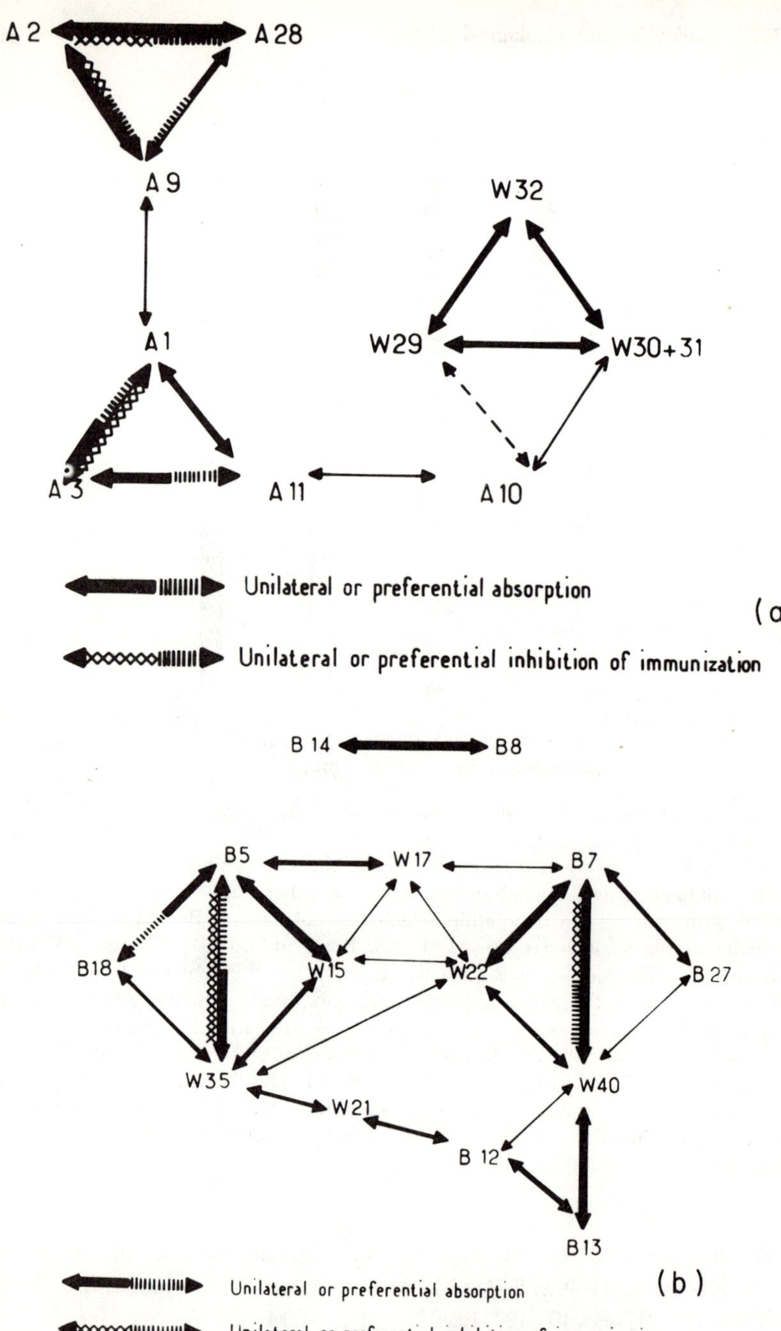


FIG. 9.5. Cross-reactions between alleles of the HLA-A locus (a) and the HLA-B locus (b). A solid line indicates a strong and symmetrical absorption by one of the

are three ways of studying cross-reactions: (1) The oldest and most obvious is *absorption–elution* on cells which do *not* possess the antigen used for the immunization. (2) They can also be demonstrated by *co-occurrence* in the same test serum of antibodies reactive with the products of two alleles, even though they were induced by a single allelic product. (3) Finally, they can be studied by the *inhibition of immunization* when the recipient possesses structures similar to those on the donor's molecules. These three methods have given remarkably consistent results. A graphic representation of the multiple links between specificities is given in Fig. 9.5.

One of the most interesting characteristics of cross-reactions is their frequent *asymmetry*. Some cross-reactions are completely or predominantly unilateral. These asymmetries, again, can be studied by absorption elution or by the frequency of immunization in a given combination. Mittal and Terasaki (1972) described several asymmetries. Anti-A11 is clearly absorbed by A3 cells, but the converse is partial and inconstant. Other asymmetrical pairs are anti-A1 and A3, anti-B7 and Bw40, anti-B5 and Bw35, and anti-B5 and B18.

Asymmetry in reciprocal immunization is especially clear between A2 and A9. A9 individuals are infrequently immunized against A2. The converse situation gives normal immunization. Other immunization asymmetries are less obvious. Thus A2 recipients seldom produce anti-A28 antibodies, but the converse is more common; A3 recipients rarely become immunized against A11. B7 recipients seldom form anti-Bw40 antibodies. The causes of asymmetric absorption may be different from those of asymmetric immunization, e.g., absorption between A2 and A9 is reciprocal, but immunization between these two specificities is distinctly asymmetric.

As previously stated, the CYNAP phenomenon is one of the most striking characteristics of HLA serology. Several degrees of CYNAP are

---

specificities of an antibody directed against the other specificity. A broken line means that the absorption is asymmetrical, weak, or negative for the specificity situated on the side of the arrow. For example, anti-A28 is not, or is weakly, absorbed on A9, though anti-A9 is strongly absorbed on A28. A line of crosses means that symmetrical inhibition of immunization occurs, where the line is complete. Where it is incomplete it means that the inhibition is not symmetrical. For example, A9 individuals rarely produce an anti-A2, although in the reverse direction antibody production is strong. The thickness of the line is in proportion to the intensity of cross-absorption. A weak or dubious cross-reaction is indicated by a dotted line. Based on Colombani *et al.* (1974), Mittal and Terasaki (1972, 1974), Albert *et al.* (1973b), Cullen and Pickles (1972), Morris and Dumble (1973), Degos and Colombani (1973), Staub-Nielsen and Svejgaard (1972), and Staub-Nielsen *et al.* (1973).

possible. Absorption, without lysis, can be [for the normal quantity of platelets used for absorption ($3 \times 10^9$ platelets or $300 \times 10^6$ lymphocytes per ml)] *total* or *partial.* In extreme cases the absorption may be so weak that it cannot be demonstrated by a decrease in the titer of the absorbed serum, but only through the elution of the antibody.

Antibodies reacting in CYNAP are less firmly fixed on their substratum than directly lytic antibodies. They can often be detached simply by washing. Additionally, acid elution is possible at relatively high pH levels (Dorf *et al.*, 1972). They have, therefore, the appearance of imperfectly specific antibodies. They may be considered to be antibodies having cross-reactions with structures that are poorly adapted to their antibody sites. Nevertheless it is not yet understood why complement is not activated. Excessive distance between sites is not a satisfactory explanation, since complement is bound and the cell killed by interaction with directly lytic antibodies directed against the determinants of the same molecule.

### 2. *Possible Interpretations*

At least two nonmutually exclusive interpretations can be given for cross-reactions and the CYNAP phenomenon. The first and simplest is that there are similarities in the structure of the private specificities of the two allelic series that lead to a classic cross-reaction. The same antibody population is capable of being fixed with more or less avidity on products whose amino acid composition and spatial structure are similar but not identical. It is known that antibodies developed late in an immunization schedule show both increased avidity and an increased tendency to cross-react (Gershon and Konko, 1972; Unterdown and Eisen, 1971). This fact in itself could explain a number of properties of the inclusion system. The first interpretation corresponds to Hirschfeld's complex–simple model (1965), in which the antibody is complex but the antigen is simple.

Another interpretation, conversely, concerns the intervention of several antibody populations, at least one of which is directed against a public specificity common to two allelic products. In this case, it is the antigen that is complex, since it possesses an antigenic site or sites in addition to the main or private specificity site of each segregant series. This is Hirschfeld's simple–complex model, in which the antigen is complex and the antibodies are non-cross-reacting.

A third possibility is a combination of the two previous models. The antigen is complex, but the test serum itself also contains several antibody populations, some of which are specific for a single specificity while the others cross react with distinct but related specificities (complex–complex model).

Arguments in favor of the complex–complex hypothesis were found during the study of serum DEG, which has already been discussed in connection with the kinetics of immunization. It was found possible (1) to isolate several antibody populations, monospecific according to the usual criteria, which nevertheless react with several allelic forms at the same locus; (2) to find some privileged cells that possess the private specificity but nevertheless do not possess the public specificity frequently associated to the private in the population, thus illustrating the individuality of each site; (3) to demonstrate that the blocking of one specificity by its specific antibody does not prevent the later fixation of a second antibody on the same cell, again showing that the two specificities are *distinct* and sufficiently far from one another not to lead to steric inhibition; (4) to demonstrate that capping the molecule bearing the first specificity leads to the redistribution of the second, proving that both are on the same molecule (Legrand and Dausset, 1974).

There is one other lesson of possible theoretical importance that can be drawn from serum DEG. Anti-B5 did not react with but was very weakly absorbed (CYNAP) by the Bw21 cells that reacted directly with the second antibody. This, in turn, was absorbed with no reaction on some Bw40 cells, with which the third antibody reacted with no CYNAP (Fig. 9.4).

Thus, it appears that each antibody imperfectly recognizes the specificity against which the antibody appearing next will react directly. These facts suggest the existence of cross-reactions between the various specificities in question, in a certain sequence, as though each specificity depended on the preceding one.

Thus, far from being mutually exclusive, the two theoretical interpretations complement one another. A complex–complex model is necessary to explain the complexity of HLA serology.

### 3. *Differential Immunogenicity of HLA Antigens*

Although several studies have been devoted to this subject, it has not been possible to establish a hierarchy of immunogenicity within each of the two main series. It would appear that each private specificity possesses the same capacity of inducing the formation of circulating antibodies. Naturally the calculation must take into consideration the chances of an immunizer possessing this antigen encountering a recipient who does not possess it.

## III. Immunogenetics of the HLA System

### A. Specificities

#### 1. Definition

The definition of an allelic series in an immunogenetic system is dependent on the monospecificity of the reagents used. Proof of monospecificity is never complete, but can be approximated by the following steps.

A test serum is absorbed on to a certain number of cell varieties that react positively. All absorbates are then retested on the same varieties. If there is only one antibody population in the test serum, all the positive cells will have absorbed the antibody, and consequently all the absorbates will give negative reactions with all the cells. Certainty that the serum in question is monospecific increases as more and more cell varieties are tested, but it is never absolute. In practice, it has been agreed that for a reactivity found in from 10–90% of the population, complete absorption by 30 varieties of positive cells establishes the serum as *operationally monospecific*.

This test is simplified if the test serum is obtained by immunization against a single individual and if cells from the immunizer are available. By definition, these cells contain all the antigens against which an antibody could have been developed and in consequence all absorbates on positive cells should, if monospecific, be negative against them.

In the early days of HLA serology, the definition of a specificity was based mainly on the comparison of sera with similar reactions. The infrequent similar sera stood out from the mass and were accepted as a guide.

Later, comparisons were made by the $\chi^2$ method (Colombani, 1963) and automated by the use of the computer (Van Rood, 1962). The result is even more accurate if the $\chi^2$ is corrected by the number of comparisons. The *correlation coefficient*, $r = (\chi^2/N)^{1/2}$, where $N$ is the number of cells tested with the two sera under comparison, can have a positive or negative value according to whether the association is based on similar or dissimilar reactions. A positive association is interpreted to mean simply that the two sera under comparison show more similar features than the laws of chance allow. On the other hand, a negative association means that the two sera tested tend to react with different cells.

The first HLA specificities were defined by two or more sera reacting in an approximately identical fashion. This left some ambiguity, and the authenticity of specificities was proved only by the genetic relationships that appeared between them in population and family studies.

Genetics came to the help of serology. Although the definition is still somewhat arbitrary, specificities can now be considered as entities and are assigned to the cells of subjects in a given population sample under study.

### 2. *Relationship between Specificities*

The statistics ($\chi^2$ and $r$) that are used to define specificities can also be used to study the relationship between them. Application to even very heterogeneous human populations can yield important inferences.

Positive associations can have several different interpretations. The two specificities studied may be governed by genes that are independent but have a functional association (e.g., ABO and secretor); they may be linked on the same chromosome, as is the case in the HLA system, where one specificity belongs to the first locus and the other to the second; or they may be due to cross-reactions either in the same system or in different systems. The third type of relationship is extremely common within the HLA system when comparing a specificity A included in another specificity B. This situation is found each time a broad (public) specificity is compared with a narrow (private) one.

Conversely, a negative association almost certainly indicates an allelism or pseudoallelism, but in the HLA system the number of alleles is such that negative associations can be very weak or even not occur at all.

A simple population study can furnish valuable clues. Three allelic specificities cannot be present at the same time in the same individual, who, by definition, cannot possess more than two alleles on each homologous chromosome. The search for the "absence of triplets" is accordingly a method used where allelism is suspected. However, only family studies can, in fact, enable allelism to be definitely established.

### 3. *Family Studies*

Family studies have played a major role in illuminating the complexity of serological reactions. Even when they are mixtures of several anti-HLA antibodies, as is most often the case, anti-leukocyte sera divide the children of any one family into categories, the number of which, except in the rare instances where recombination has occurred, does not exceed four. Four types of reactivity are observed, indicating that the corresponding genes are situated on homologous chromosomes that are transmitted to the child in one of four combinations. This simple discovery proved that the vast majority of antibodies then known were directed against the products of a single system but did not reveal the complexity of this system.

## B. The Two Main Allelic Series

### 1. *How Allelic Series Are Established*

Above all, however, family studies enabled the allelism (or pseudoallelism) of a certain number of specificities to be proved by the double-backcross method. Families in which one of the parents possesses two specificities (whether or not these are linked by a negative association in the population), both of which the other parent lacks, may be informative. If it is proved that each child receives one, and only one, of the two specificities possessed by a given parent, it may be suspected that the two specificities studied are allelic. This result, however, may be due to chance. In order to prove the allelism of these specificities, a sufficient number of informative families all giving the same result is necessary. The number of families needed depends on the number of children. An allelic series is thus established step by step. A1 and A2 were first of all shown to behave like alleles, then A1 and A3, and A2 and A3, etc. The same was true for the second allelic series, as shown in Table 9.5.

### 2. *The First Allelic Series (Locus A)*

By means of leukoagglutination with defibrinated blood, Payne *et al.* (1964) demonstrated the first two HLA specificities LA1 and LA2

TABLE 9.5
Probability of Allelism between Several Specificities Belonging to an Allelic Series Determined by Double-Backcross Mating[a]

| Specificities borne by one heterozygous parent | Number of families | Number of children with the First | Second | Both | Neither | Probability (in the absence of linkage) |
|---|---|---|---|---|---|---|
| B12 and 5 | 3 | 9 | 4 | 0 | 0 | $\leq 10^{-3}$ |
| B12 and 8 | 1 | 4 | 2 | 0 | 0 | 0.0313 |
| B5 and 8 | 5 | 12 | 12 | 0 | 0 | $\leq 10^{-5}$ |
| B12 and 7 | 3 | 3 | 8 | 0 | 0 | 0.004 |
| B5 and 7 | 1 | 3 | 2 | 0 | 0 | 0.06 |

[a] Probability is calculated using Morton's method (1955). Allelism is extremely probable for the two pairs of specificities B12 B5 and B5 B8. From these observations the allelism of B12 and B8 can be deduced in spite of the insufficient number of children observed. The same is true, in this example, for the specificity B7 (Dausset *et al.*, 1968). A greater number of informative families was studied later on, and the allelism of the four specificities was confirmed.

(LA2 is equivalent to Mac or, in revised nomenclature, A2) which, on the basis of both population and family studies, fulfilled the criteria of allelism. Since LA1 was present in 25% of the population and LA2 in 51%, many individuals in the population possessed neither LA1 nor LA2. The existence of at least one other allele could be predicted. In 1966 this prediction was fulfilled by the description of LA3 that had a frequency of 35% (Bodmer *et al.*, 1966). The original LA3 probably corresponds to the specificities A3 + A11, known to possess strong cross-reactions with one another. A9, a fourth specificity in the first series, was described by Terasaki *et al.* (1965), but its allelism was not proved until some years later.

A further step in HLA analysis was taken when it was agreed that new specificities may be defined by *difference* between two specificities, one of which is included in the other. Cells that possessed the wider specificity but not the shorter were regarded as possessing a specificity, although at that time there was no antiserum specific for these cells. The first example was that of cells that possessed Da2 but were negative for Da1. The cells reacting with anti-Da1 and anti-Da2 were called $Da1^A$ (A2). The cells reacting with anti-Da2 only were called $Da1^B$ (A28) (Dausset *et al.*, 1967).

This method was also followed by Svejgaard and Kissmeyer-Nielsen (1968) who described Ba* (A28) as the part of Ba (A2 + A28) that did not correspond to A2. Sera specific for A28 were later found which behaved as previously described (Section III,A) in connection with the definition of specificities.

It was soon noticed that the specificities defined under A9 and A10 could both be divided into two distinct allelic specificities. Thus A9 covers two allelic specificities with strong similarities between them; these are the specificities Aw23 and Aw24. In the same way, A10 covers two allelic specificities, Aw25 and Aw26. The public specificity Aw19 was also subdivided into five private specificities, A29, Aw30, Aw31, Aw32, and Aw33.

It is practically impossible, except in exceptional cases, to attribute the discovery of an antigen to one team or to another. Very often, the same specificity was discovered simultaneously and independently by several laboratories (Tables 9.1–9.4).

At the beginning of 1975, 14 specificities of the first allelic series were recognized in Caucasoids. All are well defined serologically and show Mendelian inheritance. Transmission is autosomal, monofactorial, and dominant.

There are also alleles for which no specificity is yet known. These "blank" genes have a cumulative gene frequency of 4.9% (Table 9.6).

TABLE 9.6

ANTIGEN AND GENE FREQUENCY FOR HLA-A, B, C, AND D LOCI IN CAUCASOIDS (FRENCH)

| A locus | | | B locus | | |
|---|---|---|---|---|---|
| Antigens | Antigen frequency (%) | Gene frequency (%) | Antigens | Antigen frequency (%) | Gene frequency (%) |
| A1 | 25.1 | 13.4 | B5 | 15.2 | 7.9 |
| A2 | 44.8 | 25.7 | B7 | 18.2 | 9.5 |
| A3 | 22.6 | 12.0 | B8 | 16.7 | 8.7 |
| Aw23 } A9 | 4.3 | 2.2 | B12 | 32.5 | 17.8 |
| Aw24 } A9 | 18.2 | 9.5 | B13 | 5.4 | 2.7 |
| Aw25 } A10 | 3.9 | 1.9 | B14 | 8.8 | 4.5 |
| Aw26 } A10 | 8.3 | 4.2 | B18 | 11.3 | 5.8 |
| A11 | 11.8 | 6.0 | B27 | 7.8 | 4.0 |
| A28 | 9.8 | 5.0 | Bw35 (W5) | 15.2 | 7.9 |
| A29 | 10.3 | 5.3 | Bw40 (W10) | 13.7 | 7.1 |
| Aw30 | 2.4 | 1.2 | Bw15 | 12.3 | 6.3 |
| Aw31 | 6.8 | 3.5 | Bw39 } Bw16 | 0.9 | 0.4 |
| Aw32 | 9.8 | 5.0 | Bw38 } Bw16 | 2.4 | 1.2 |
| Aw33 | 1.9 | 0.9 | Bw17 | 5.9 | 3.0 |
| Blank | | 4.9 | Bw21 | 4.9 | 2.4 |
| | | | Bw22 | 7.1 | 3.7 |
| | | | Bw37 | 2.9 | 1.4 |
| | | | Bw41 | 4.9 | 2.4 |
| | | | Blank[a] | | 4.4 |

| C locus | | | D locus | | |
|---|---|---|---|---|---|
| Antigens | Antigen frequency (%) | Gene frequency (%) | Antigens | Antigen frequency (%) | Gene frequency (%) |
| Cw1 | 10.0 | 5.0 | Dw1 | 19.3 | 10.2 |
| Cw2 | 14.9 | 8.0 | Dw2 | 15.2 | 7.8 |
| Cw3 | 26.0 | 14.6 | Dw3 | 16.4 | 8.5 |
| Cw4 | 19.7 | 11.1 | Dw4 | 15.6 | 8.2 |
| Cw5 | 14.0 | 7.4 | Dw5 | 14.6 | 7.5 |
| Blank | | 53.9 | Dw6 | 10.5 | 5.4 |
| | | | Blank | | 52.4 |

[a] Other B antigens in Caucasoids: HR (gene frequency = <1); KSO* (JA) (gene frequency = <1); 407* (gene frequency = <1); TT* (gene frequency = <1).

The product of these genes is possibly nonimmunogenic or nonreactive in our present tests. More probably, an antibody or antibodies recognizing the gene product or products will be discovered in the future.

The somewhat arbitrary nature of the existing classification should be emphasized. If only the specificities with a wide distribution are considered, it is possible to describe this allelic series differently. This is, in fact, what happened in the past. Such an allelic series can have only six specificities, A1, A2 + A28, A3 + A11, A9, A10, and Aw19. Undoubtedly the process of fission of specificities is still unfinished. Many of the specificities currently recognized will be further divided. Hence some symbols are, prudently, still treated as provisional.

### 3. *The Second Allelic Series* (*Series B*)

Some of the antigens detected by Van Rood, using leukoagglutination, had antithetical distributions, which suggested the existence of additional allelic series. Thus the two widely distributed specificities 4a and 4b appeared to be allelic, although too many individuals were heterozygous (Van Rood, 1962). Narrower antigens were discovered after the introduction of the lymphocytotoxicity test. Most of these are totally included in either 4a or 4b.

The first indication of allelism between private specificities detected by lymphocytotoxicity was the observation that the three specificities B5, B8, and B12 were never found together in the same individual (Dausset *et al.*, 1965). If specificities belong to the same series, triplets cannot exist. The allelism of these three specificities was confirmed by joint family studies during the Third Workshop (Ceppellini *et al.*, 1967). But the conception that these might be part of a second HLA series could not be established until the allelic relationships between these and other specificities was proved by extended family studies.

Since 1967, new antigens have been detected rapidly, often, as with the first series, simultaneously and independently by various laboratories (Tables 9.1–9.4). At present, the number of private specificities at the B locus can be estimated as more than 20, but the exact figure varies according to the subdivisions that are included.

In Caucasoids, certainly no fewer than 19 specificities all showing monofactorial codominant inheritance, make up the B allelic series. Alleles of this series must exist for which no reaction has been identified. The gene frequency corresponding to these blank reactions is 4.49 (Table 9.6).

As in the A series, the boundary of individual specificities may be arbitrary. Some specificities that are now considered clearly defined will doubtless undergo a process of dichotomy as antibodies are discovered which recognize narrower and narrower specificities.

After 12 years of study the place of 4a and 4b in the HLA system is still uncertain. The specificities at the second locus, which are currently recognized by lymphocytotoxicity and platelet complement fixation, can now be grouped on the basis of cross-reactions into two large families. The first group is made up of B5, B12, B13, B14, B18, Bw15, Bw21, and Bw35 and the second of B7, B8, B27, Bw22, and Bw40. With some exceptions the first group is linked by the common specificity 4a, the second by the common specificity 4b. According to d'Amaro (1975), 4a includes B5, 13, Bw27, Bw17, and part of B12, and 4b includes B7, 8, 14, Bw15, Bw22, Bw35, Bw40, and part of B12. Thus they have a sharply contrasting distribution in the Caucasoid population.

The exact definition of 4a and 4b is difficult because the antisera that recognize them are not homogeneous. Their monospecificity has not been definitely established; in many cases, they seem to contain mixtures of antibodies that are active against the various specificities in each of the two large "families." Nevertheless, in some rare cases a monospecificity or at any rate an operational monospecificity is thought to have been found. In these respects, the serological properties of 4a and 4b resemble those of some long public H-2 specificities (Chapter 6, Section V,B).

### 4. *The Relationship between the A and B Series*

As the alleles in the two series became better known, it grew obvious that the private specificities often segregated in families in groups of two (Dausset *et al.*, 1966). Each child in the four categories previously mentioned received two specificities from each parent, one belonging to the first allelic series, and the other to the second. This suggested that the specificities were governed by genes closely linked on the same chromosome. The genes on one chromosome were referred to as an HLA haplotype, i.e., half an HLA genotype.

Each individual, therefore, possesses two HLA haplotypes (father: a and b; mother: c and d). The four types of children possess the haplotypes ac, ad, bc, and bd, respectively. Inasmuch as each haplotype contains at least two genes, each individual possesses four HLA genes that, except in the case of homozygotes, determine four different antigens.

In the vast majority of families, segregation of the parental haplotypes occurs *en bloc* with no recombination between the first and second locus. However, approximately 1 gamete in 100 (0.80%) shows recombination, leading to the appearance of a new haplotype. An example of a family where paternal recombination has taken place is given in Table

9.7. Crossing-over in this system, as is usually the case, is more frequent in women than in men (0.99 versus 0.61). There is a tendency for recombinations to occur in the second half of the sibship. The average age of the parents does not appear to have an influence.

One unusual feature of HLA genetics is the occurrence of preferential gametic associations between genes at the A and B loci. Thus the genes A1 and B8, belonging to A and B series, respectively, are often associated in the Caucasoid population. The same applies to A3 and B7. There is thus a linkage disequilibrium, which can be measured by the difference between observed and expected haplotype frequencies ($\Delta$). $\Delta$ may be calculated from the phenotype of individuals (Bodmer *et al.*, 1969; Mattiuz *et al.*, 1970) according to the formula

$$\Delta = (\theta 4)^{1/2} - [(\theta 2 + \theta 4)(\theta 3 + \theta 4)]^{1/2}$$

in which $\theta 2$ is the frequency of individuals possessing the first specificity only, $\theta 3$ frequency of individuals possessing the second specificity only

TABLE 9.7
CROSSING-OVER BETWEEN A AND B AND BETWEEN B AND D LOCI IN ONE FAMILY (KA)[a]

| | Haplotype formula | Specificities and D types |
|---|---|---|
| Father | aw/bx | A2,B8,w/A11,Bw35,x |
| Mother | cy/dz | A3,B7,y/A1,B8,z |
| Child | | |
| 1 | bx/cy | A11,Bw35,x/A3,B7,y |
| 2 | bx/cy | A11,Bw35,x/A3,B7y |
| 3 | bx/*dy* | A11,Bw35,x/A1,*B8,y* |
| 4 | bx/dz | A11,Bw35,x/A1,B8,z |
| 5 | bx/dz | A11,Bw35,x/A1,B8,z |
| 6 | aw/dz | A2,B8,w/A1,B8,z |
| 7 | aw/dz | A2,B8,w/A1,B8,z |
| 8 | aw/cy | A2,B8,w/A3,B7,y |
| 9 | aw/cy | A2,B8,w/A3,B7,y |
| 10 | *abx*/cy | *A2,Bw35*,x/A3,B7,y |

[a] The HLA haplotypes are designated by a, b, c, and d and the D (MLR) type by w, x, y, and z. Crossovers are indicated in italics. Note the paternal crossing over between A and B loci in child number 10 and the maternal crossing over between B and D loci in child number 3. MLR was positive between children numbers 3 and 4, but negative between numbers 3 and 1 and numbers 3 and 10. (From Eijsvoogel *et al.*, 1972.)

and $\theta 4$ frequency of individuals possessing neither specificity, $\theta 1$ being the frequency of individuals possessing both specificities.

Thus in a sample of 247 individuals tested for A1 and B8, where $\theta 1$ is 18/169, $\theta 2$ is 22/169, $\theta 3$ is 8/169, and $\theta 4$ is 121/169, the $\Delta$ will be 0.042.

If the gene frequency of A1 is $p1 = 0.134$ and that of B8 is $p2 = 0.087$, the expected theoretical haplotype frequency of A1, B8 is $p1p2 = 0.011$. In fact, the A1,B8 haplotype frequency is $\Delta + p1p2 = 0.042 + 0.011 = 0.053$.

Table 9.8 shows the significant Caucasoid haplotype frequencies and $\Delta$'s.

## 5. *HLA Polymorphism*

The polymorphism of the HLA system is extraordinary. Even if no complexities other than those of the two allelic series are taken into account, there are already $15 \times 20 = 300$ possible haplotypes, 20,246 phenotypes, and 45,245 genotypes. If the other series are included in the calculations, the number of combinations exceeds several million. The HLA system is, therefore, the most polymorphic human group system yet discovered. In addition, it is the closest linkage so far demonstrated in man for which recombinations can be studied. It is these characteristics that make the HLA system the most powerful genetic marker and an invaluable tool in population genetics.

TABLE 9.8
Significant Linkage Disequilibria ($p < 0.001$)
(in Caucasoids)[a]

| Between A and B | | | Between B and C | | |
|---|---|---|---|---|---|
| $\Delta$ ($\times 10^3$) | Haplotype | Frequency ($\times 10^3$) | $\Delta$ ($\times 10^3$) | Haplotype | Frequency ($\times 10^3$) |
| 42 | A1, B8 | 53 | 51 | Bw35, Cw4 | 66 |
| 41 | A3, B7 | 56 | 46 | Bw15, Cw8 | 46 |
| 34 | A29, B12 | 45 | 14 | Bw22*, Cw3 | 24 |
| 19 | A1, Bw17 | 23 | 19 | Bw40, Cw2 | 15 |
| 8 | Aw31, B13 | 9 | 15 | B12, Cw5 | 21 |
| 8 | Aw32, Bw37 | 9 | 6 | Da30, Cw1 | 6 |
| 8 | Aw26, Bw41 | 9 | | | |
| 6 | Aw33, B14 | 6 | | | |

[a] For most haplotypes, haplotype frequencies are the product of the gene frequencies of the two specificities. Some haplotypes, however, differ significantly from the expected frequency, e.g., the haplotype A1, B8 should have a frequency of 0.011, but the observed frequency is 0.056. Such differences are expressed by $\Delta$ (see text). The $\Delta$ between the B and C loci are those given by Pierres *et al.* (1975).

### 6. *The Third Allelic Series* (*Series C*)

A serum with an odd reactivity attracted the attention of the Scandinavian workers in 1969 (Sandberg *et al.*, 1970; Kissmeyer-Nielsen *et al.*, 1971). This serum, AJ, reacted only with a few B5, Bw15, Bw22, and B27 individuals, and was not associated with other antigens. This phenomenon may be called a partial inclusion phenomenon. Additionally, in each family where the AJ characteristic was associated with one of these B series specificities, the two were transmitted together.

It was not until some years later that sera with reactions that were allelic with those of the first serum were discovered by Svejgaard *et al.* (1973). Like AJ, each of these sera reacted with only a certain percentage of individuals possessing a given second locus specificity. The sera reacting in this way were 170, UPS, and 315.

Mayr *et al.* (1973) took up this study using new sera. They confirmed that AJ, 170, UPS, and 315 (Cw1 to Cw4 in new terminology) identify an allelic series. They added two new alleles, Cw5 and T6. By studying many families, the frequent association of Cw1 with B5, Bw15, Bw22, and B27; of Cw2 with B27 and Bw40; of Cw3 with Bw40, Bw15, and Bw22; and Cw4 with Bw35 were confirmed. The last-named association is so strong that the respective sera can be and have been mistaken for one another. Some Cw4, however, are associated with B12 and Bw15. Finally, Cw5 is associated with B12 and sometimes with Bw18, and T6 with B8.

The strongest linkage disequilibria are given in Table 9.8. The linkage between the second locus and this third locus is very close, so close that up to the present time only one convincing example of recombination between the two loci has been found (Low *et al.*, 1974). This recombination places the third locus between the A and B loci, very close to the B (Fig. 9.6).

Capping experiments (Chapter 11) done independently by three different teams with specific antibodies seem to show that the aggregation of a C locus specificity at one pole of a cell does not block the cytotoxic action of an antibody directed against a B locus specificity. Similarly, the fixation of a fluorescent anti-globulin of one color onto antibodies directed against a B locus specificity whose aggregation at one pole of a cell has been provoked does not prevent a fluorescent antibody of another color directed against a specificity of the C series being fixed on the entire cell surface.

If each individual does indeed possess three HLA genes on each chromosome, everyone except homozygotes should have six specificities on his lymphocyte surfaces. This suggests a polymorphism so extensive as

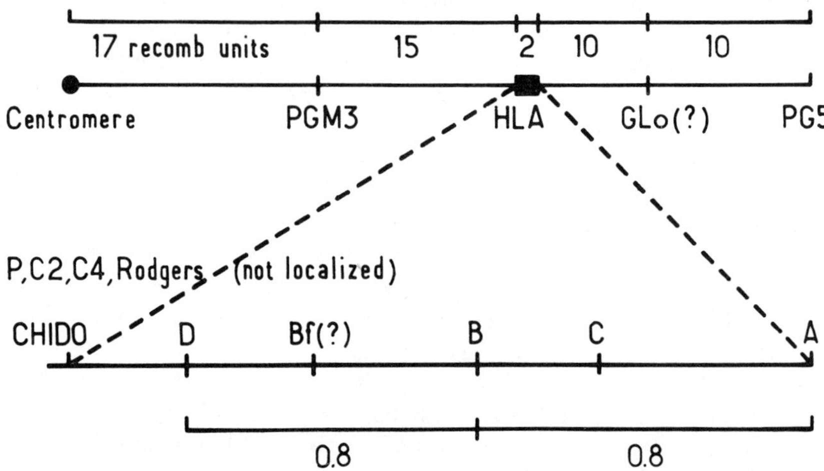


FIG. 9.6. Schematic representation of the human chromosome 6 with an enlargement of the HLA complex. The site of the centromere is not definitely established and is given only by analogy with the mouse. The HLA linkage group comprises the following genes: the red cell blood groups P, CHIDO, and Rodgers; the enzymes phosphoglucomutase 3 (PGM3), cytoplasmic malic enzyme (ME-1), indophenol tetrameric oxidase (IPO-B or SOD-2); the urinary pepsinogen 5 (PG5); and glyoxalase 1 (GLo). It also comprises structural or regulatory genes involved in C3 activation: the C3 proactivator (factor B of the properdin system, Bf), genes controlling the second (C2) and fourth (C4) component of the complement. Probably close to the D locus are the genes coding for the human Ia analogue (locus Ly-Li, Legrand and Dausset 1975b; locus Ag, Van Rood *et al.*, 1975a, 1976).

to ensure an extraordinary degree of HLA individuality. Already, with only six alleles detected at the C locus there are 1800 possible haplotypes, 323,936 phenotypes, and 1,620,900 genotypes.

## C. Distribution of HLA Specificities in Other Populations

### *1. Gene Frequencies*

Because of the extraordinary polymorphism and geographic variation, HLA specificities are uniquely powerful markers for anthropological studies. Better than any others, they enable the genetic distances between different populations to be appreciated, and they give valuable hints for the construction of phylogenic trees and for attacking the problem of selection and homogenization by gene drift or founder effect.

The HLA system has an advantage over other systems in that it contains at least two loci that, although they are closely linked, are subject to recombination. One consequence of this situation is the development of anthropologically informative disequilibria following migration, selection or gene drift.

A few anthropological studies, mainly done before 1972, had already shown great variations in gene frequency in different populations. But it was the Fifth Workshop that first brought together data from all over the world.

It has been found that a high level of A1, 3, B7, 8, 12, and possibly A29 is a Caucasoid characteristic. *Negroids* have a high frequency of A9(Aw23), A10(Aw26), Aw30, and Bw17 and possess genes Aw36, Aw43, and Bw42 that are extremely rare in Caucasoids. *Mongoloids* have A9(Aw24), Bw40, Bw15, Bw22, and a gene provisionally known as Malay (Aw33). It is necessary to distinguish the American Indians from other Mongoloid populations, since, although they have a distinctly Mongoloid HLA profile, they lack some of the usual alleles [A10 (Aw25 and Aw26), A11, B13, Bw22]. The number of HLA specificities in American Indian tribes is remarkably limited. At the A locus they possess A2, A9(Aw24), A28, Aw31, and Aw33 and at the B locus, B5, B27, Bw35, Bw40, Bw15, Bw16, and KSO*. It is odd that W21, a Mediterranean specificity, should be found in certain tribes. A28 and Aw31 are found in Asia only among the former inhabitants of Japan, the Ainus. Moreover, Bw15 and Aw31 are found mainly in South America and not in North America.

An *Australoid* characteristic is the frequency of A10 and Bw22, although the latter gene occurs relatively infrequently in Asia (Table 9.9).

Midway between the Mongoloids of the Asian continent and the Australoids come the inhabitants of the Pacific, especially the Polynesians. Their main characteristic is a high rate of Bw22 and the presence of KSO.*

The study of gametic association or Δ in these various populations was especially instructive. In Caucasoids, the frequent association between A1 and B8 is very striking. Not all Caucasoid populations possess this characteristic. It is absent from Indian populations and increases progressively to reach a peak in Northern Europe.

Similarly, the gametic association of A3 and B7 is a Caucasoid characteristic, but is only obvious in northern Europe (Scandinavia). Other significant associations are also known in Europe, e.g., A2, B12 (especially in the North), A29, B12 and Aw33, Bw14 (especially in the South), and finally Aw30, B18 in Basques and Sardinians.

TABLE 9.9
WORLD DISTRIBUTION OF HLA GENES ACCORDING TO THE RESULTS OF THE FIFTH WORKSHOP[a]

| | Caucasoids | | | Mongoloids | | | Negroids | |
|---|---|---|---|---|---|---|---|---|
| Gene | Europe (average) | Middle East (average) | India (average) | Mongoloids (average) | Australia (average) | American Indian (average) | Negroids (average) | Hottentots |
| A1 | 17 | 13 | 12 | *2* | *0* | *1* | 4 | 5 |
| A2 | 28 | 20 | 15 | 18 | 11 | 48 | 17 | 12 |
| A3 | 15 | 10 | 7 | *1* | *0* | *1* | 8 | 8 |
| Aw23 } A9 | 2 } 9 | 6 } 19 | 2 } 14 | *2* } 41 | *6* } 28 | *0* } 25 | **8** } 13 | **7** } 13 |
| Aw24 | 7 | 13 | 12 | **39** | **22** | **25** | 5 | 6 |
| Aw25 } A10 | 2 } 6 | 1 } 5 | 1 } 7 | 2 } 7 | 15 } 25 | 0 } 0 | 1 } 8 | 1 } 24 |
| Aw26 | 4 | 4 | 6 | 5 | 10 | 0 | **7** | **23** |
| A11 | 6 | 6 | 18 | 13 | 6 | 1 | *1* | *0* |
| A28 | 4 | 6 | 6 | 2 | 0 | 9 | 9 | 10 |
| A29 | 4 | 1 | 1 | *1* | *1* | *0* | 5 | 9 |
| Aw30 | 2 | 4 | 1 | 2 | 2 | 1 | **16** | **8** |
| Aw31 | 1 | 2 | 1 | 0 | 0 | 9 | 2 | 3 |
| Aw32 | 4 | 4 | 3 | *0* | *0* | *0* | 4 | 3 |
| Aw33 | 2 | 5 | 7 | **7** | **20** | 4 | 7 | 5 |
| Blank | 2 | 5 | 8 | 6[c] | **7** | 1 | 6[f] | 0 |
| B5 | 6 | 15 | 19 | 9 | 0 | 10 | 8 | 6 |
| B7 | 13 | 3 | 5 | *2* | *0* | *1* | 12 | 13 |
| B8 | 11 | 3 | 8 | *1* | *0* | *0* | 4 | 2 |
| B12 | 16 | 9 | 10 | *3* | *0* | *1* | 12 | 14 |
| B13 | 2 | 3 | 2 | 4 | 11 | 0 | 1 | 1 |
| Bw35 (W5) | 10 | 13 | 12 | 6 | 0 | 24 | 6 | 8 |
| Bw40 (W10) | 6 | 4 | 6 | **24** | **32** | **15** | 7 | 7 |
| B14 | 4 | 4 | 0 | *0* | *0* | *1* | 3 | 8 |
| Bw15 | 6 | 1 | 8 | **16** | **15** | **14** | 4 | 5 |
| Bw16 | 4 | 6 | 1 | 4 | 1 | 12 | 1 | 2 |
| Bw17 | 4 | 5 | 8 | 2 | 0 | 1 | **21** | **14** |
| B18 | 5 | 5 | 2 | 1 | 0 | 1 | 3 | 6 |
| Bw21 | 2 | 9 | 1 | 0 | 0 | 4 | 1 | 0 |
| Bw22 | 3 | 3 | 3 | **13** | **37** | 0 | *1* | *1* |
| B27 | 4 | 2 | 2 | 3 | 0 | 3 | *1* | *3* |
| Blank | 4[b] | 15 | 13 | 12[d] | 4 | 13[e] | 15[g] | 10 |

[a] World distribution of HLA genes according to the results of the Fifth Workshop (see Dausset and Colombani, 1973). The gene frequencies, which are diminished in comparison with Caucasoids are printed in *italics*, and those which are increased are printed in **bold type**.

[b] Contains Bw41 (gene frequency: 2) and Bw37 (gene frequency: 1).

[c] Contains Aw34 (gene frequency: 11 in Malaysia).

[d] Contains Hs (SIN-2) in Orientals.

[e] Contains KSO* (JA) (gene frequency: 10 in Eskimos).

[f] Contains Aw 36 (Mo*) and Aw43 (BK) in Negroids.

[g] Contains Bw 42 (MWA) in Negroids.

In other population groups, the $\Delta$ are less striking since associations of specificities are infrequent. Nevertheless, the association of A2 and Bw40, A9 and Bw35 in Mongoloids, of A9 and Bw17 in Negroids, and of A11 and Bw40 in Australoids should be noted.

Some of the populations studied for the HLA system are true *isolates*. These populations are small and their isolation virtually complete, either because of geographical distance (Easter Island) or because of moral, social (Twaregs), or religious (Moslem Arabs in Israel) taboos. The degree of consanguinuity is sometimes difficult to establish and sometimes well known, when genealogies are available.

In true isolates, an unusual frequency of certain genes due to gene drift or the founder effect, can be observed. This is the case for Bw35 (91% of the population) in the American Indians of San Juan la Laguma in Guatemala (Cann *et al.*, 1973). Some haplotypes are particularly frequent in isolates. This linkage disequilibrium does not have the same meaning as in panmictic populations. The two haplotypes A11, Bw21 and A28, B7, for example, are especially common in Twaregs.

Other isolates are relatively large, for example, the Greenland Eskimos. Physical isolation of the Eskimos has existed for many millenia. Founder effect and gene drift have led to characteristics similar to those of small isolates, i.e., homogeneity in their HLA genes. These people are Mongoloid, as shown by the preponderance of Aw24, Bw40, and Bw15.

The American Indians are also a virtual isolate, since they have been practically cut off from the rest of the world for at least 50,000 years. A great homogeneity of HLA genes is observed within individual tribes, a situation not usually seen in other group systems. Similarly, the Papua of New Guinea are remarkably homogeneous for the HLA system. Only four genes at the A locus and six at the B have been found.

### 2. *Genetic Distance and Phylogenetic Trees*

Using the material obtained during the Fifth Workshop, one team tried to represent *genetic distances* in the form of a graph based on observed gene frequencies. In spite of some limitations in the methods employed, the dispersion of racial groups, as measured by gene distances calculated from the gene frequencies of the alleles at the A and B loci, shows a close resemblance to geographic dispersion (Degos and Dausset, 1974).

Other attempts have been made to use these distances to trace *phylogenetic trees* (Piazza *et al.*, 1975). The results are probably very crude since the differences in gene frequency have diverse origins (migration, selection, drift, etc.). Also these trees only take fission into consideration (a parental population giving rise to two or more populations) and do not consider possible later fusion. Nevertheless, the trees obtained correlate well with other historical and geographical evidence.

## D. The HLA Linkage Group

Up to the present we have considered only the loci of the HLA system. Because of the excellence of HLA genes as markers, it has been possible to identify other neighboring and even relatively distant genes on the same chromosome. This group of genes may be called the HLA linkage group (Fig. 9.6).

Basically, there are two methods of analyzing such a linkage group. The first, the classic genetic method, uses the probability of a certain characteristic segregating with an HLA haplotype in a family. It is known that this technique is not powerful and cannot cover a distance of more than 25 crossover units. A characteristic calculated in this way with a negative result (more than 25 units) must be regarded as independent, although a remote location on the same chromosome is not ruled out. The more recent cell hybridation method partly corrects this insufficiency. The principle is as follows: a hybrid cell (e.g., man/mouse or man/hamster) progressively loses human chromosomes at random during successive passages. When two well-defined characteristics are lost at the same time on many occasions, it can be inferred that they are on the same chromosome. The two characteristics are said to be *syntenic.*

### 1. *Classic Familial Method: Linkage*

The classic genetic method has been used to demonstrate a linkage between HLA and the erythrocyte isoenzyme phosphoglucomutase 3 ($PGM_3$). Recombination frequency was 0.14 in men and 0.27 in women, i.e., at the very limits of the method. This conforms to the usual rule that, in mammals, recombination frequency is higher in females than in males. In a study in which both HLA loci were followed, the $PGM_3$ gene accompanied the second locus. Similarly the Bf locus which governs proactivation of C3 was found to be closely linked to the HLA system (Allen, 1974). Families with a deficit of C2 and of C4 indicate that C2 and C4 are governed or regulated by genes close to HLA (Fu *et al.*, 1974; Rittner *et al.*, 1975). This correlates with the fact that a gene governing the amount of complement in mice has been localized in the *Ss* region of the *H-2* complex (Démant, 1973). *Ss* has been tied to C4 (T. Meo, personal communication). A linkage of HLA with the erythrocyte groups Chido (Middleton *et al.*, 1974) and Rodgers has been suggested. A linkage has also been suggested with the erythrocyte isoenzyme glyoxalase I (GLO) (Bender and Grzeschik, 1976) and urinary pepsinogen 5 (Weitkamp *et al.*, 1975) (Fig. 9.6).

### 2. *Cell Hybridation Method: Synteny*

One exceptional family with 14 children indicated a possible association of HLA with the *P* system. The cell hybridation method confirmed this. The loss of the HLA chromosome was always accompanied by the loss of the P antigens from man/mouse hybrid cells (Fellous *et al.*, 1973).

Cell hybridation studies indicate that the HLA complex is situated on chromosome 6. The $PGM_3$, $ME_1$ (malic cytoplasmic enzyme), and IPO-B (indophenol tetrameric oxidase) genes are syntenic. Similarly HLA is syntenic with these three markers. As the $ME_1$ gene has been localized on chromosome 6, it is logical to think that the linkage group $PGM_3$–IPO-B–$ME_1$–HLA is on this chromosome. It is currently impossible to state the distance between these genes and their order on the chromosome (see Edwards *et al.*, 1973). However if the second or B locus is analogous to the *H-2K* locus because of its greater influence on graft survival, mixed lymphocyte reaction (MLR) intensity and graft versus host (GVH), it is tempting to place the centromere on the B side, for *H-2K* is closer to the *T* locus, which is itself next to the centromere. However since the relative positions of the A, B, C, and D loci (see Section VI) appear to be different in man and in mice, it seems quite likely that an inversion has occurred which may or may not have changed the order of these loci in relation to the centromere.

## IV. General Conception and Evolution of the HLA System

Before discussing other genes in the HLA complex, it may be useful to set down some speculations concerning the structure and evolution of the HLA antigens. We believe that these help to unify a great mass of experimental data. In view of the apparent homology of the major histocompatibility systems of mammals and possibly other vertebrates, they should be applicable to major histocompatibility systems in general.

### A. Speculations Concerning the Structure of the HLA Antigens

#### 1. *Number of HLA Molecules*

In 1965, Dausset and Iványi wrote: "The Hu-1 system is a complex system, composed of many antigenic factors" (Dausset *et al.*, 1965). Today this statement is supported by a large number of related facts that, taken together, permit a general, although still provisional, interpretation of the HLA system. This interpretation will probably be modified and certainly be filled out as more discoveries are made.

In man as in the mouse (Chapter 6, Section VIII) there are doubtless many loci within the small chromosome area that comprises the major histocompatibility complex (MHC). Three of these are serologically defined loci, each of which determines a distinct series of allelic specificities. The two loci determining the two major series are at the ends of the system, about 0.8 recombination units apart.

Biochemical and cell surface redistribution (capping) tests indicate that there are at least three distinct entities (or molecules). Each of these biochemical entities possesses or determines one of the private specificities of one of the three allelic series. None determines specificities in more than one series. The conclusion can therefore be drawn that the three molecules are each governed by a different cistron and that there are at least three HLA cistrons. Each of these molecules is itself complex. They bear the private specificities that make up the three allelic series, and they most likely bear several other public specificities as well.

### 2. *Number of HLA Antigenic Sites*

The number of amino acids that make up the HLA molecule is more than sufficient to allow several antigenic sites to exist on its surface. Voluntary immunization experiments seem to indicate, according to the immunization and detection techniques used, that the number of antigenic sites capable of provoking an antibody is relatively limited (three to five per molecule) (Legrand and Dausset, 1974). There must, therefore, be many pairs of nucleotides whose product seems at the present time to be immunologically "silent."

In a given population, certain public specificities are frequently associated with a single private specificity. Let us take as an example a Caucasoid A1 molecule, which almost always contains the public specificities A and B (Fig. 9.7). Public specificity A is shared with the molecules A3 and A11; public specificity B with A11 only. The anti-B antibody will react with both HLA-A1 and HLA-A11 cells, giving the appearance of cross-reactions between these two products. Another specificity, C, is not present on the A1 molecule, but is shared by the A3 and A11 molecules. Anti-C antibodies will give the appearance of a cross-reaction between A3 and A11.

Sometimes a specificity, e.g., D is almost always present on the A1 molecule in a given population. A test serum containing anti-A1 and anti-D would appear monospecific since both specificities exist on most A1 cells used for absorption. However if one of the rare cells not possessing D happens to be used, the anti-D will not be absorbed but will remain in the supernatant, demonstrating that the serum is polyspecific.

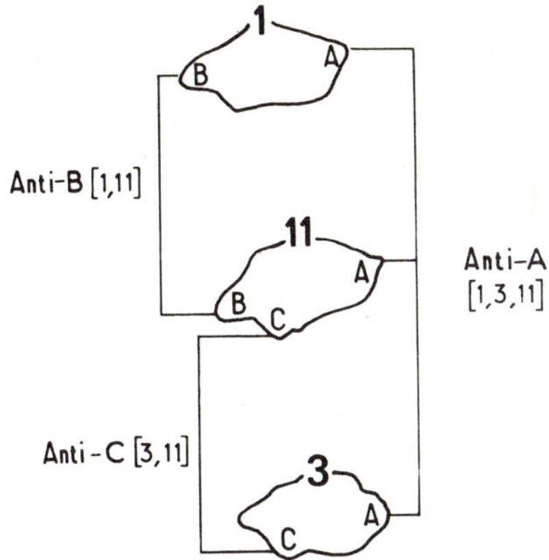


FIG. 9.7. Schematic representation of the product of the A1, A3, and A11 alleles of the first HLA locus. The private specificities A1, A3 and A11 characterize each of these products. Nevertheless, they also possess public specificities common to several products: A is common to all three molecules; B is shared by A1 and A11; C by A3 and A11; and D, in the population studied, is almost always associated with A1.

In another population, the probability of finding a cell without D is greater since the association between A1 and D may be less strong.

This general description of the HLA system as presented here only differs from descriptions published by other authors in small details. The existence of antigenic sites on the same molecule which are physically distinct from one another is possibly the most debated point. Batchelor and Sanderson (1970) as well as Walford (1970) consider that on the surface of the HLA molecule there are no distinct sites but a *continuum* of structures that can all be antigenic. Batchelor and Sanderson postulate antigenic sites a, b, c, d, and e against which anti-ab, anti-bcd, or anti-abcde antibodies could develop. They attribute the broadening of the antibody specificity observed during immunization to the appearance of antibodies with a broader and broader spectrum. For example an anti-abcde antibody could react with an abcdef antigenic site. The illusion that the sites are distinct stems from the recipients' inability to become immunized against the sites they already possess. For example, an nmcdop recipient in the presence of an abcde donor could produce anti-ab and anti-e antibodies, but not anti-cd, since he possesses cd himself.

It is also necessary to take tertiary structures, as well as primary and secondary, into consideration. A tertiary configuration could lead to the appearance of immunogenic structures that would not exist in another tertiary combination of the same primary chain.

Thus, although there is a general consensus as to the complexity of the HLA gene products, many people still consider the existence of multiple sites to be merely an abstract concept. It is true that specific test sera against public specificities have not yet been studied precisely and exchanged between laboratories, but this research will probably make up the next serological and genetic stage in our knowledge of the HLA system.

### 3. *Specificities Common to A and B Molecules: Interlocus Specificities*

Other arguments should also be put forward concerning the existence of antigenic sites common to various HLA molecules. It is known that in mice some public specificities are found on both *K* and *D* gene products (Shreffler *et al.*, 1966; Démant *et al.*, 1971; Snell and Cherry, 1974; Snell *et al.*, 1971, 1974). The same phenomenon was found in man by the study of a serum that was striking in that it contained an anti-A9 (A series) with an anti-B12 and anti-B27 (B series). This serum is operationally monospecific but reacts with and is equally well absorbed by cells differing from the serum donor by a single specificity at either the A (A9) or the B (B27) locus. Capping one or other of these molecules leads to the elimination of the reaction with this serum. Moreover a distinct antigenic site does seem to exist, as indicated by absorption inhibition tests (Legrand and Dausset, 1974).

## B. Speculations Concerning the Evolution of the HLA Antigens

Our conception of the HLA system leads us to formulate a hypothesis concerning the formation of the HLA complex during the evolution of man. It has been seen (Fig. 9.4) that the reactivities of the antibodies that appeared during the course of an immunization became broader and broader, and that the narrowest was completely included in the broadest. We also showed that each antibody could be absorbed, without visible reaction (CYNAP), but the cells reacted directly with the next antibody to appear as though they contained cascading structures similar to those indicated by cross-reactions. This situation suggests that there are very great similarities between the current antigenic sites present on one HLA molecule which could all, consequentially, have been formed by successive duplications of a common ancestral gene. The oldest gene would be the one that is the most widespread in the population. It would, however, also be *the least immunogenic since it would be the least modified in comparison with the ancestral gene.* According to this hypothesis, therefore, there should be repeated motifs in the HLA molecule, or briefly, the equivalent of immunoglobulin *domains.*

Accordingly, it was expected that several domains would be found in the human HLA molecule. In each of these domains there would be an antigenic site formed by duplication and mutation of a gene governing another older site. These sites, derived one from the other, would have structures that were so similar that there would frequently be cross-reactions between them.

From the point of view of phylogenic evolution, one cannot help but be struck by the great similarity between the MHC in the different vertebrate species studied up to the present time.

It would seem that in each species there is a single *main system* whose importance dominates that of all other systems. Moreover this main system, in many species, including humans, mice, chimpanzees, rhesus monkeys, and probably dogs, is made up of at least two closely linked loci, each determinant a complex series of alleles. It can be imagined that these two loci arose by duplication of a common ancestral locus at a remote time in evolution, before the differentiation of the different vertebrate species.

Moreover it is striking that, in spite of its extreme polymorphism, the human histocompatibility system does have certain structural similarities with the analogous systems found in all mammals studied.

In the light of our combined serological, genetic, and biochemical knowledge of the vertebrate MHC, it is clear that any hypothesis concerning MHC evolution must, on the one hand, account for its extreme complexity both at the species and the individual level and, on the other, account for its remarkable persistance with no fundamental modification during phylogenic diversification.

## V. The Natural History of HLA Antigens

### Distribution in the Organism

The HLA gene products are found on the membrane of almost all the nucleated cells in the organism. This ubiquitous distribution very probably indicates that they have an important role in biology, but the nature of this role is as yet unknown. In attempts to solve this mystery, numerous studies have been carried out on the situation, number, and turnover of the MHC gene products and their relationship with the other elements of the cell membrane.

HLA molecules exist mainly on the *external* cell membrane. This has been shown by labeling studies as well as by classic serological tests. HLA antigens may be identified on the cell surface by using labeled anti-HLA antibodies, which can be seen with a visual (fluorescent label) or electron (antibodies labeled with viruses) microscope. Sometimes the so-called sandwich technique, with labeled anti-human globulins, has been profitably used.

These techniques, used systematically, have proved very informative and have led not only to an approximation of the number of HLA sites but also to important ideas about their reconstruction after destruction or physical elimination, in other words, their natural history.

*1. On Blood Elements*

The *lymphocyte* is the main point of reference, since it is in daily use for the determination of individual HLA types. It also has an exceptionally high content of HLA antigens. The most precise studies were done using this cell.

Microscopic techniques have established that there are approximately $10^3$ HLA sites per specificity on a lymphocyte membrane. This figure has been corroborated by biochemical studies that have yielded an estimate of approximately 7000 HLA molecules per specificity (Sanderson and Welsh, 1974) or 28,500 for four specificities. These figures should be regarded as no more than rough approximations. The HLA molecules make up approximately 1% of the proteins on the lymphocyte surface.

No precise study has been made comparing the number of HLA sites on human B and T lymphocytes. It would seem that whatever their origin (blood, lymph nodes, thoracic duct), lymphocytes react identically to HLA antibodies (Patel, 1971). Chronic lymphocytic leukemia lymphocytes, which are mainly B cells, seem to possess a high HLA content. In mice, B lymphocytes absorb anti-H-2 antibodies more efficiently than T lymphocytes (Shevach *et al.*, 1973).

The number of HLA sites on the internal membrane is still unknown, but appears to be low and perhaps zero (Dausset, 1965; Wilson and Amos, 1972). The number of sites on white blood cells other than lymphocytes has not yet been studied in detail. However, it is known that granulocytes, monocytes, platelets, and reticulocytes all possess HLA molecules. They also exist on erythrocytes, but only in very small quantities.

The presence of transplantation antigens on *granulocytes* was proved by the presence of these cells in agglutinates provoked by anti-leukocyte antibodies. All three categories of polymorphonuclear cells—neutrophils, eosinophils, and basophils—are observed. Indeed, it has been proved that granulocytes are indispensable to the formation of these agglutinates. Pathological granulocytes from myeloid leukemia patients are also strongly agglutinated by leukocytic antibodies and may be used for absorptions (Bialek *et al.*, 1966; Thorsby, 1969).

*Monocytes*, too, have been shown to possess HLA antigens (Kourilsky *et al.*, 1971). *Platelets*, next to lymphocytes, are the best-studied blood elements. They are in daily use for tissue typing and systematic absorptions. As a general rule, platelets are rich in HLA antigens. Although a platelet has a much smaller surface area than a lymphocyte, the same absorption can be done if ten (Dausset *et al.*, 1960) or twenty (Bialek *et al.*, 1966) platelets per lymphocyte are used. Although present on platelets, the expression of the antigen may be modified. Thus B12 is sometimes expressed exactly as it is on lymphocytes, and sometimes B12 is scarcely expressed at all (Dausset *et al.*, 1970). In this last case, only very sensitive absorption tests were able to show that a small quantity of B12 was in fact present. The antigens B8 and Bw40 are subject to the same phenomenon and other specificities may show it also.

It is interesting to note that the ability of platelets to react to specific antibodies increases with storage. When fresh, platelets scarcely fix any antibodies, but after 4 or (better still) 8 days of storage at +4°C, reaction is at a maximum. The mechanics of this phenomenon is still unclear; it could be due to the presence of a plasma-derived film (platelet "atmosphere") which physical or enzymatic treatments could eliminate, making the platelets usable in serological tests on the very day of collection.

The presence of H-2 antigens on mouse *erythrocytes* and the apparent absence of HLA antigens on human red blood cells was at one time regarded as a major distinction between the two systems. Proof that HLA sites exist on *reticulocytes* was the first step in closing the gap. This was established not only from serological tests on reticulocyte-rich pathological blood (Harris and Zervas, 1969) but also from labeled visualization tests (Silvestre *et al.*, 1970).

The existence of HLA sites on mature erythrocytes could be proved only by extremely sensitive techniques, such as bromeline agglutination used with the autoanalyzer. The antigens $Bg^a$, $Bg^b$, and $Bg^c$ were defined in this way. At first these were thought to be new erythrocyte groups (Morton *et al.*, 1969, 1971; Doughty *et al.*, 1973), and it was not until 1969 that a comparison with HLA antigens led to the proof that each has an HLA equivalent ($Bg^a$ = A7; $Bg^b$ = B17; $Bg^c$ = A28) (Tables 9.1–9.4). It is notable that some HLA specificities are detected on erythrocytes more easily than others, and it is to be hoped that manipulations, such as those used for platelets, will lead to easier methods of demonstrating all specificities on these cells, since this would enormously simplify tissue typing.

### 2. *On Fibroblasts*

Skin fibroblasts isolated by treatment with trypsin have been found to be susceptible to lysis by anti-leukocyte antibodies. Fibroblasts in culture possess HLA antigens that can be detected by various techniques, including complement fixation (Fellous *et al.*, 1973).

The expression of HLA antigens on hybrid cells (e.g., man/mouse) can be demonstrated during the whole time the chromosome or chromosomes bearing the HLA genes remain in the hybrid.

Tissue typing on amniotic cells obtained by amniocentesis is probably possible, and could have practical consequences in the elimination of abnormal genes linked to the HLA loci.

### 3. *On Spermatozoa*

Spermatozoa definitely possess HLA antigens (Fellous, 1969; Piazza *et al.*, 1969; Fellous and Dausset, 1970; Kerek and Afzelius, 1972; Halim *et al.*, 1974). They are apparently assembled on the postchromosomal band. Of major interest is the question whether their expression on a given spermatozoon is haploid or diploid, in other words, whether a spermatozoon only expresses the antigens governed by the autosome it contains or whether antigens governed by both chromosomes persist on its surface. Fellous and Dausset's experiments (1970) are strongly in favor of a haploid expression, since no more than 50% of the spermatozoa are killed by an antibody directed against a specificity for which the subject is heterozygous. On the other hand, 80% are killed when the specificity is doubly present in a homozygote. Moreover, when two specificities on the same autosome (cis position) are attacked simultaneously by the corresponding antibodies, no more than 50% of the spermatozoa are killed, whereas if the antibodies are directed against two specificities on different autosomes (trans or allelic position), approximately 80% are killed. This experiment, although strongly indicative of haploid expression, is inconclusive because the failure to observe 100% lysis cannot easily be explained, and the difference between 50 and 80% is so small that it could be due to technical difficulties. However, direct visualization of two distinct spermatozoal populations labeled by fluorescent antibodies has recently been performed successfully (Halim *et al.*, 1974). Similiar tests with *H-2* in mice have not given a definite answer, but there is evidence that the *T* locus antigen in mice shows haploid expression (Chapter 5, Section II,C).

While the possibility remains that HLA antigens from the spermatogonia are carried over to the surface of the spermatozoon, this hypothesis seems unlikely in view of the relative times necessary for two successive meioses and the renewal of HLA antigens.

It is unnecessary to emphasize the significance that haploid expression would have. From a theoretical point of view, it would demonstrate that the genome of male germinal cells is indeed active. Practically, it would be possible to eliminate spermatozoa bearing an HLA-linked defect by means of anti-HLA antibodies.

It has recently been observed that H-2 and HLA antigens are apparently absent from the spermatogonia of impuberal mice or men, although the T antigen is present. The same is true of H-2 in the embryonic cells of teratomas (Artzt and Jacob, 1974).

### 4. *On Tissues*

The *placenta* was the first organ to be used as a source of HLA antigens for absorption and solubilization (Bruning *et al.*, 1964). The placenta is rich in HLA antigens, but is difficult to study because it is of both maternal and fetal origin. Whether *trophoblasts* possess HLA antigens is still uncertain. Preliminary studies seem to have established that they are not expressed, at any rate not in a detectable form (Loke *et al.*, 1971); yet the trophoblast genome is thought to be able to express them in a different environment, since tumors of trophoblastic origin, such as chorioepitheliomas, do possess them.

To our knowledge, the relative density of HLA antigens on the various human organs has only once been investigated (Berah *et al.*, 1970). The deficiencies in this kind of comparison should be emphasized, especially the failure to use methods that would permit the study of different categories of cells. In spite of these imperfections, it is apparent that, as in mice, the organ with the most HLA antigens is the spleen, followed by the lung, the liver, the intestines, the kidney, and the heart in that order. Although the nervous system is known to possess H-2 antigens in mice (see Table 5.4), the human brain was found to be incapable of absorbing anti-leukocyte antibodies that were specific to the organ donor's antigens.

It would be unwise to draw any conclusions from these data as to the relative "transplantability" of different organs. Antibody absorption depends not only on the presence but also on the presentation and accessibility of the antigens. For example, *in vitro* absorption on fresh platelets is weak, but HLA incompatible platelets are rapidly destroyed by sensitized recipients.

### 5. *In Body Fluids*

By concentrating normal plasma, it is possible partially or totally to inhibit an antibody corresponding to one of the plasma donor's antigens (Van Rood *et al.*, 1970; Miyakawa *et al.*, 1973). The form of these HLA antigens in plasma is unknown. The entire HLA molecule or only a haptenic determinant may be present or the antigen may be linked to lipoproteins (Schultz and Schreffler, 1972; Aster *et al.*, 1973). In any case, the presence of HLA determinants in plasma is certainly relevant to the conceptions of turnover and shedding of HLA antigens discussed in Chapter 11.

HLA antigens have also been found in urines during pathological kidney conditions, such as tubulopathies (Robert *et al.*, 1974). This is doubtless the consequence of the presence of HLA antigens in plasma. HLA antigens, moreover, are excreted in milk (Dawson *et al.*, 1974).

### 6. *On Abnormal or Pathological Elements*

The behavior of HLA antigens in abnormal situations, such as cells in culture, tumor, or other pathological cells, has yet to be considered. A distinction should be made between those cells that are still liable to the phenomenon of aging (normal fibroblasts in culture) and those which can reproduce indefinitely (lymphoid cells in culture, cancer cells).

It is known that normal fibroblasts in culture do not usually survive longer than approximately 40 successive generations. HLA antigens under these conditions were studied by three teams with contradictory results. Sasportes *et al.* (1971) found that HLA antigens were only weakly detectable after the thirtieth generation, and that during the few remaining generations prior to the extinction of the line, first the B locus antigens and then all HLA antigens disappeared. Goldstein and Singal (1972) confirmed the disappearance of antigens during the last few generations, especially those at the B locus. Brautbar *et al.* (1973), on the other hand, working on cultures *en masse*, did not find any modification. It is possible that cultures *en masse* do not enable clonal modifications to be distinguished.

The interest of this study is mainly centered on the possible role of HLA antigens in intercellular relationships. Are surface antigens indispensable to survival? It is known that they are absent from progeria syndrome fibroblasts (Singal and Goldstein, 1973). It is also known that man/mouse hybrid cells can survive without HLA antigens. However, these cells do possess H-2 antigens that could be sufficient for survival.

In established lymphoid cell lines, HLA antigens appear to be stable. Lymphoid cells in culture are a frequent source of soluble HLA antigens; hence the presence and persistance of HLA structures are certain. Nevertheless, the membrane may be modified to such an extent that detection methods perfected on peripheral lymphocytes are too sensitive when applied to lymphocytes in culture. A quantitative study has shown that the density of detected antigens is ten times greater on cultured cells than it is on lymphocytes from the peripheral blood of the same donor.

It is possible that it is merely the presentation of the antigenic sites which is modified, rather than their expression itself. A. R. Sanderson (personal communication) considers that these cells carry seven times as many HLA sites as the corresponding lymphocytes.

Cells in culture may show abnormal reactions, due to antibodies directed against specificities that are known to cross-react with a specificity on the cultured cell. Thus, according to H. M. Dick (personal communication), an A1 cell may react with anti-A3 or anti-A11 sera, or an A2 cell may react with an anti-A28 and then an anti-A9. In other words, cross-reacting specificities appear during culture. Some aberrational reactions, however, cannot be classified. They could be reactions directed against viral antigens, although preliminary study seems to have eliminated Epstein-Barr viral antigens. It is more likely that they are the human homologue of Ia specificities (Chapter 6, Section VIII,B).

Cell lines from solid tumors fully express HLA antigens, and this expression appears to persist indefinitely. However, few systematic comparisons have been made with the patients' lymphocytes. HLA antigens are also expressed normally on indigenous tumors. Tests of Burkitt tumors, for example, and peripheral lymphocytes have revealed no significant differences (Dausset *et al.*, 1974).

Thus, as a general rule, the antigens of the main hisotocompatibility system are expressed on almost all nucleated cells. The antigens are, therefore, ubiquitous and are not differentiation antigens. They do not disappear from cells in continuous culture nor from tumor cells. They are, therefore, a permanent part of cell membranes.

## VI. The Genes Governing the Mixed Lymphocyte Reaction (D Series)

It has been observed that when two allogeneic lymphocyte populations are cultivated in contact with one another, the lymphocytes undergo substantial morphological alterations: the nucleus increases in volume, mitoses occur, and large intranuclear nucleoli appear; the cytoplasm enlarges and takes on an aspect that gives the cells all the characteristics of immature blast cells.

It was Bain and Lowenstein (1964) followed by Bach and Hirschhorn (1964) who introduced this test into human biology. The *mixed lymphocyte reaction* (MLR) rapidly came to play an important role in transplantation (reviewed by Sørensen, 1972). The reaction was first set up so that the two populations responded to each other (bilateral reaction); it was later adapted so that only one of the populations could respond (unilateral reaction). If one of the cell populations is treated with agents such as mitomycin or X-rays, it remains alive but is incapable of synthesizing DNA and therefore of dividing and multiplying. The introduction of the unilateral reaction enabled the genetics of the reaction to be studied efficiently.

### A. Genetics of the D Series Products

An early study of the relationship between MLR and HLA incompatibilities had suggested a correlation between major incompatibilities at HLA and a positive MLR (Dausset *et al.*, 1965; Iványi *et al.*, 1967). But it was Bach and Amos (1967) who showed that MLR is governed by the same chromosomal region as the HLA system. Studying MLR's between members of many families, they observed that the reaction is negative between 25% of the brothers and sisters in the same family, and that these are the brothers and sisters who inherited identical HLA haplotypes. They did observe one exception to this rule.

At first there was a tendency to liken lymphocyte transformations observed *in vitro* in the presence of another lymphocyte population to the allogeneic immune response, especially the response to incompatibilities involving the HLA antigens. The MLR was interpreted as the *in vitro* equivalent of graft rejection *in vivo*. However, it soon became obvious that a number of characteristics of this reaction were different from those of the classic immune response. (1) No apparent preimmunization is necessary to produce a reaction between two allogeneic cells. (2) The stimulating cell has to be living, and a plasma factor is indispensable. (3) The intensity of the reaction does not significantly increase during immunization; similarly there is only minor modification of the MLR if it is repeated after a skin or kidney graft. Accordingly, it was stated that no secondary or anamnestic response occurs. In fact, recent studies have shown that a secondary response is indicated, not by an increase in intensity, but by an earlier reaction (Bondevik and Thorsby, 1973; Fradelizi and Dausset, 1975). (4) The MLR is stronger where the two partners in the reaction are close on the phylogenic scale, and the MLR is particularly strong between two members of the same species. (5) Although platelets contain HLA antigens, they are incapable of stimulating allogeneic lymphocytes. This is also true for fibroblasts. Nevertheless, it appears that epithelial cells and spermatozoa can stimulate.

Once again the way was shown by the murine model. In 1970 Rychlíková *et al.* observed that allogeneic blast transformation in mice was mainly associated with the *K* end of the *H-2* complex. An incompatibility at the *D* locus led to weak blast transformation only. Several teams, using families with recombinants between the HLA-A and B loci, made similar observations in connection with man (reviewed by Dausset *et al.*, 1973). It was noted that only differences at the B locus lead to an appreciable stimulation. The MLR, therefore, was governed either by the B locus or by a gene closely linked to it.

### 1. *The Main Locus Governing the MLR (D Series)*

It was now evident that the genetic control of MLR was not directly tied to HLA antigens. Guided by the exception to the rule, reported by Bach and Amos (1967) that MLR can be positive between two HLA identical sibs, Yunis and Amos (1971) studying an appropriate family suggested that the MLR is governed by an independent gene. Similarly, other families showed positive reactions between HLA identical sibs and negative reactions between HLA semi-identical sibs. The results were interpreted to mean that there is an MLR locus separate from and outside of the two main HLA loci (Fig. 9.8). The locus was designated D. From the number of mutually stimulating HLA identical sibs, it is estimated that the distance between B and D is approximately 1 recombination unit. The order is probably D, B, C, A (Fig. 9.6).

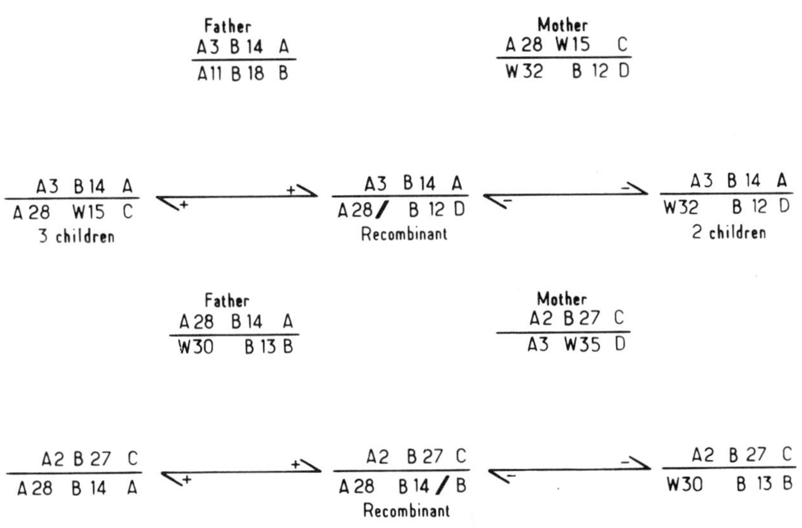


FIG. 9.8. MLC reactivity in families with a recombination between the two A and B loci (above) or between the B and D loci (below). The former indicates that the locus governing the MLR is situated next to the B locus. The latter shows that the MLR locus is distinct from the B locus since it can be separated from it by recombination. The distances between the A and B loci and the B and D loci are approximately the same (1 recombination unit). The results of reciprocal MLR's between two individuals joined by an arrow are indicated at the end of the arrow adjacent to the stimulating cell.

Our knowledge of the genetics of the D series is still rudimentary. How polymorphic is it? Is it a single, very polymorphic gene or a series of less polymorphic genes that can be combined in a great diversity of ways? Either hypothesis is compatible with the fact that negative reactions are rare (1/10,000) between unrelated individuals. These negative reactions, however, are more frequent between individuals of HLA identical phenotype, whether or not they are related. In fact, approximately 10% of the reactions between individuals of phenotype A1, B8, A3, B7, i.e., individuals who probably possess the two most frequent haplotypes (A1, B8 and A3, B7) are negative.

A similar observation was made in studies of MLR's between HLA phenotypically identical parents and children. This situation is found where the two parents possess the same HLA haplotype. In these cases, the percentage of negative reactions is distinctly higher (30%) than when the two individuals tested are unrelated. But this figure is certainly biased, for these cases are isolated and have been reported without data as to the number of families studied. Here again the common haplotype is very often A1, B8.

It follows from the above that some specificities at the B locus are preferentially associated with certain alleles at the D locus. This linkage disequilibrium ($\Delta$) is best established for A1, B8 and A3, B7 (Albert *et al.*, 1973a). In any case, in these haplotypes at least three genes are strongly associated with one another in spite of the relatively large distance between them. It will later be shown that yet more genes are suspected of being associated in disequilibrium with these same two haplotypes, especially a gene present in patients suffering from multiple sclerosis and juvenile diabetes (Chapter 12, Section II).

### 2. *Do Other MLR-Governing Genes Exist?*

Family studies soon indicated that, in fact, the system must be even more complicated since not all MLR's could be explained by possible combinations of D genes. Lebrun *et al.* (1973) noticed that when both A and B loci differences were present, the reaction was greater than when the B locus alone was mismatched. From this they deduced that the A locus region played a part in MLR. Eijsvoogel *et al.* (1972) observed weak MLR's in certain combinations differing at the A locus only, and likewise concluded that there is a gene linked to the A locus which governs a weak MLR. The existence of this locus was also suggested by two families with recombinations studied by Dupont *et al.* (1974). Additionally, Mempel *et al.* (1973a) noted that the average intensity of MLR reactions in the presence of a single A locus incompatibility differs from the average between unrelated serologically identical individuals. The existence of an MLR effect linked to the A locus is, therefore, probable.

There is evidence for possibly other MLR loci. A difference in reactivity between two HLA identical brothers was noted in an informative family in which there was a probable recombination between the B and D loci. The results can be explained by the existence of a third MLR gene situated not far from the B locus, but whose internal or external situation in relation to the A–B interval cannot be definitely established (Sasportes *et al.*, 1973). Thorsby *et al.* (1973b) have come to similar conclusions from studies on another family. It should be emphasized that fuller confirmation of the existence of these other MLR genes is necessary.

However, the murine model shows that MLR can be activated by several regions in the *H-2* complex. The strongest reaction is produced by a difference at the *I* region situated between the left or *K* extremity and the *Ss* locus, but detectable reactions result from differences apparently at *H-2K* and *H-2D* themselves and at a region including or to the right of *Ss* (Chapter 8, Section I,A; Festenstein and Démant, 1973).

It seems therefore that the MHC of man is unlike that of mice in that his main MLR locus is situated outside the two main A and B loci, but similar in that he possesses other supplementary loci along the length of the complex.

Another considerable difference is the apparent absence in man of a locus similar to the *Mls* locus (Festenstein, 1966; Chapter 8, Section I,B). This locus is independent of *H-2* and is unusual in that it does not induce the development of effector cells capable of lysis, as do the MLR loci of the major histocompatibility complexes in both men and mice.

The discovery of MLR genes provides at most a partial explanation of poorly understood complex phenomena. An unexplained aspect of these phenomena is the *asymmetric reactions* that are positive in one direction and negative in the other. The most simple and logical situation is that which exists between individuals who are, respectively, heterozygous and homozygous for the main D series gene. This has been observed in those special families in which both parents possess the same D gene in one of their HLA complexes. Such pairs were found by the systematic examination of families in which the two parents shared an HLA haplotype. Confirmation that both parents possess the same D gene is given by the negative reaction obtained between the parents and their phenotypically identical children. In these families, some children are homozygous for the haplotype common to both parents and thus for D (Fig. 9.9).

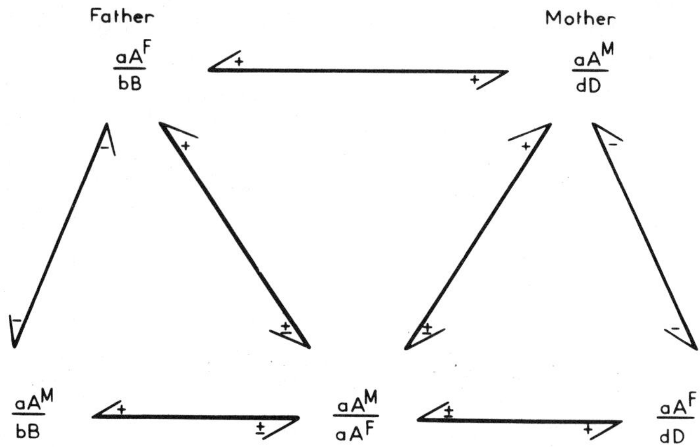


FIG. 9.9. MLR in families with shared HLA haplotypes and principle of D typing. a, b, and d are the HLA haplotypes and A, B and D the corresponding D locus products. Identity of $A^F$ and $A^M$ can be demonstrated by the negative two-way MLR between the sibs who are phenotypically identical to their parents and the asymmetric reaction against the homozygous cell. The homozygous cell may be used as a stimulating cell for D typing. A heterozygous A cell will react in the same way as the father's or heterozygous sibs' cells. Arrows have the same meaning as in Fig. 9.8.

According to the classic compatibility rules, the homozygote's reaction to the heterozygote should be positive (which has indeed been observed), and the heterozygote's reaction to the homozygote should be negative. In fact, the latter reaction is not completely negative. The weakly positive reaction is paradoxical, but is possibly due to mitogenic factors emitted by the homozygous cells, which, in spite of mitomycin, are capable of a faint reaction against the heterozygous cells. Although not entirely negative in one direction, these reactions between homozygotes and heterozygotes may be considered true asymmetric reactions.

Asymmetric reactions have also been observed in genetic situations other than the relatively clear one described above. The exact mechanisms of these are not understood. The reactions observed in families where an asymmetric reaction occurs cannot always be interpreted as due to the presence of a D homozygote. As in serology, therefore, the idea of *inclusion* was suggested; one of the cells could possess a certain series of MLR D-stimulating products, and the other a second series completely included in the first (Eisjvoogel *et al.*, 1972; Dupont *et al.*, 1973a). This implies that there is an entire region of D genes, possibly formed by duplication followed by mutation of an ancestral gene, a concept which is similar to that presented in this chapter concerning serologically defined genes. However speculative this may be, it provides one possible explanation of the puzzling results sometimes obtained from intrafamily studies.

### B. Determining D Types

The polymorphism of D genes is confirmed by the very wide occurrence of positive MLR's between unrelated individuals. The products of the D genes are not known. Are there membrane structures similar to those governed by the A,B,C genes, or a diffusible metabolic product?

One cannot help but be struck by the difficulty of proving the existence of this product by classic serological tests. Since the inception of studies of antibodies that fix complement to human lymphocytes, no antibodies have been found whose action can strictly be associated with MLR. This does not, of course, exclude the existence of anti-D antibodies. Moreover, antibodies directed against the products of genes situated in the same region of the *H-2* complex as that governing MLR have been detected in mice. These anti-Ia antibodies are able to block MLR-stimulating cells (Chapter 8, Section I,D,1), but there is as yet no formal proof that these are antibodies against the mouse homologue of D gene products.

#### 1. *Direct MLR Typing*

Because no anti-D antibodies were available, research was done into methods of typing using MLR itself. One of the first methods consisted of using cells from unrelated HLA phenotypically identical individuals. Such individuals are most common in the phenotype A1, A3, B8, B7. Testing 19 of these individuals in all possible combinations, Mempel *et al.* (1973a) found two pairs and one group of five individuals who were incapable of mutual stimulation in either direction. MLR was positive between the individuals making up the two pairs and the group of five. Similarly, testing 14 individuals whose HLA phenotype was A1, B8, A2, B7, they observed a group of five mutually nonreacting individuals. Moreover a non-reacting trio was found in a group of 11 A1, B8, A2, B12 individuals. These first, very encouraging results indicate that D polymorphism is limited and now amenable to our methods of investigation.

A second procedure (Mempel *et al.*, 1973b) consisted of using known D homozygous cells for typing. These cells are found in those families in which the parents possess the same HLA haplotype. When MLR is negative in both directions between one parent and at least one phenotypically identical child, it can be agreed that the children in this family who received the haplotypes bearing the D gene common to both parents are indeed homozygous at the D locus (Fig. 9.9). Their cells can accordingly be used as reagents (i.e., in the same way as a test serum). In the presence of an unrelated cell that is homozygous for the same D locus, MLR is negative in both directions. In the presence of a heterozygous cell containing the same D allele, an asymmetrical reaction will be obtained. The heterozygote's reaction to the homozygote will be practically negative (ignoring the paradoxal reaction noted above). The homozygote's reaction to the heterozygote will be equivalent in intensity to that obtained where only a single D difference exists (one haplotype difference).

This method has proved extremely fruitful. Mempel *et al.* (1973b) studied the reactions of two A3, B7 homozygous cell types found in two families in which the parents both possessed the haplotype A3, B7. The D allele, named Pi, possessed by the two cells was the same, since the MLR between them was negative. Pi was found in six out of 48 individuals tested, giving a phenotype frequency of 14%. But Pi was more frequently observed in individuals possessing A7, where it was found in 33% of the individuals tested. There is, therefore, a linkage disequilibrium between A7 and Pi ($\Delta = 0.039$), a disequilibrium that is similar to the one that exists between A3 and B7 ($\Delta = 0.05$). It would, therefore, appear that the group of genes making up the haplotype A3, B7, Pi have preferential gametic associations.

The Scandinavian team took a similar approach to the problem of D typing (Jørgensen *et al.*, 1973; Dupont *et al.*, 1973b), also using homozygous A3, B7 cells found in special families. The homozygous D allele was called 7a (Dw2). It was found in 10% of unrelated subjects, 56% of subjects possessing A7, 7% of subjects not possessing A7, and, very interestingly, in 70% of multiple sclerosis patients. The Dw2 gene segregated with HLA genes in three families. It has now been proved that Dw2 and Pi are identical.

Another source of D homozygous cells is from those rare families in which the two parents are first cousins and have inherited the same haplotype from their common ancestors. Unless a recombination between B and D loci has taken place, it is certain that the D genes are identical. The children who are homozygous for this haplotype are homozygous for D and for all the other D genes in the region.

Jørgensen *et al.* (1973) used a homozygous A2, B27 cell of this kind to determine the frequency of the associated D gene, called j, in the Danish population (0.14). This cell was shown to detect a D specificity (Dw2) identical to the Pi previously described by Mempel *et al.* (1973b). Another D product was independently discovered by several teams, this time associated with B8 (Dw3).

Van den Twell *et al.*, (1973) used six cell types from marriages between first cousins, tested among themselves and against eight unrelated cells (selected for their negative reactions with other phenotypically identical cells) to define provisionally five sets of mutually nonreacting cells. Later, 22 homozygous cells were used and several different D determinants were recognized. An attempt to correlate the D types obtained by this direct method and the indirect methods (see below) has been made. At present eight D products are internationally recognized by direct MLR typing (Table 9.6) (Thomsen *et al.*, 1975).

Still further possibilities exist in connection with the direct determination of D types. The use of secondary response of cells primed *in vitro* against one D product seems promising (Fradelizi and Dausset, 1975; Bach *et al.*, 1975).

### 2. *Typing by MLR Inhibition*

MLR is inhibited by certain sera (Ceppellini *et al.*, 1971; Thorsby *et al.*, 1973a) possessing anti-HLA antibodies directed against either the stimulating cell or the responding cell (in the second case the inhibition is stronger), and also sometimes by sera that do not appear to contain anti-HLA antibodies, at any rate antibodies detectable by usual techniques (Gatti *et al.*, 1973; Robert *et al.*, 1973).

MLR inhibition is very frequently encountered in the presence of plasma from patients immunized by transfusion, even where cytotoxic antibodies appear to be absent (Wernet and Kunkel, 1973). Sengar *et al.* (1973) found that there was a virtually direct ratio between the number of transfusions and MLR blocking. Similarly, the plasmas of pregnant women with no cytotoxic antibodies suppress 23% of MLR's, whereas normal plasmas only suppress 2.8%.

D typing by means of MLR inhibition can only be attempted with specific anti-D sera. In theory, the best test sera should be obtained from immunizations between HLA identical sibs who differ at the D locus or loci. Van Leeuwen *et al.* (1973) used a slightly different approach. In this approach, the reactive cell is HLA identical to the one used to immunize the serum donor. In this way, the possibility of responding to HLA antigens is theoretically eliminated, although differences at the C locus or the antigenic factors of all three loci could still exist. The mechanism and dynamics of inhibition are still too uncertain to enable firm genetic conclusions to be drawn.

### 3. *Typing by Classic Serological Methods*

Typing for MLR with sera studied by immunofluorescence, whether or not these block MLR, is perhaps more promising. If the sera are

IgG, it should be possible to visualize their fixation by immunofluorescence on leukocyte surfaces. Some parallelism was noted between MLR typing and positive immunofluorescence, and four D types were provisionally defined (Van Leeuwen *et al.*, 1973).

Efforts made by several teams to use a direct cytotoxic test turned out to detect cellular structures specific for B lymphocytes, which seem to be governed by genes close to, but distinct from, the D locus. The antibodies thus detected are probably the equivalent of the murine Ia antibodies.

## C. B Lymphocyte Specificities

Beside the classical anti-HLA antibodies, many sera contain other antibodies that are probably responsible for a number of unexpected reactions. They have been ignored for a long time because their reaction was apparently weak and poorly reproducible. This was probably due to the fact that they reacted only against a small proportion of the peripheral blood lymphocytes, the B subpopulation.

To detect these antibodies, special procedures were devised. In order to eliminate the HLA antibodies they were looked for (1) in sera developed by volunteer immunization between HLA phenotype identical, MLR positive individuals (Legrand and Dausset, 1975b; Solheim *et al.*, 1975), (2) in sera from multiparous women in which no anti-HLA antibodies were detected (Ferrone, personal communication), and (3) in sera absorbed on platelets (Terasaki *et al.*, 1975). Sera proved to inhibit the MLR were also selected (Van Rood *et al.*, 1975a,b). Screening for positive sera was performed on monoclonal B cells from chronic lymphocytic leukemia blood or from cell lines (Winchester *et al.*, 1975a,b; Bodmer *et al.*, 1975). One cell line (from a Burkitt patient) called Daudi apparently devoid of HLA antigens was especially useful (Fellous *et al.*, 1975).

The techniques used to define the B specificities were either direct using immunofluorescence or a modified lymphocytotoxicity test or indirect using absorption. The test serum was first absorbed on the lymphocytes to be typed and subsequently tested on a panel of B cell lines or of B chronic lymphocytic leukemia cells. Thanks to these various methods most of the teams reached the conclusion that it is possible to detect in many human sera antibodies reacting against normal B lymphocytes.

The first step was the observation of "abnormal" reactions of some sera on chronic lymphocytic leukemia cells. Walford *et al.* (1975) took advantage of these reactions to define a lymphocyte system called Merrit. The possibility that these reactions were directed against leukemic antigens was eliminated by the demonstration of the specificities on normal lymphocytes (Gossett *et al.*, 1975).

An interesting point is that most of the B specificities are governed by a gene (or genes) that is closely linked to the HLA complex. In families they segregate with an HLA haplotype (Legrand and Dausset, 1975b). Ly-Li1 and Ly-Li2 (Chapter 10, Table 10.3) are two specificities in this category. The gene Ly-Li is close to HLA-D. In population studies, two sera were found which strictly follow Dw3 and could be true anti-HLA-D antibodies. Three other sera seem to detect three alleles of a new locus (Ag) very close to, but distinct from, HLA-D (Van Rood *et al.*, 1975a, 1976). As in the HLA system, some specificities seem to be "included" in others (Legrand and Dausset 1975b). The corresponding determinants are absent from erythrocytes, platelets, and T lymphocytes but are present on monocytes, epithelial cells, and spermatozoa (Fellous *et al.*, 1975) as are the Ia antigens in the mouse. They are not linked to $\beta_2$-microglobulin (Fellous *et al.*, 1975; Solheim *et al.*, 1975).

New information will be accumulated very rapidly. Although the importance of these B specificities is yet to be established, it could be considerable not only in our understanding of the B–T cell interraction but also from a practical point of view. They seem governed by a gene or genes so close to the HLA-D locus that they can serve as markers for HLA-D typing before organ or bone marrow transplantation and they could be very closely associated with some diseases.

## REFERENCES


Ahrons, S. 1971. Leukocyte antibodies: Occurrence in primigravidae. *Tissue Antigens* **1**:178–183.

Ahrons, S., and S. Glavind-Kristensen. 1971. Cytotoxic HL-A antibodies: Immunoglobulin classification. *Tissue Antigens* **1**:129–136.

Albert, E. D., W. Mempel, and H. Grosse-Wilde. 1973a. Linkage disequilibrium between *HL-A7* and the *MLC* specificity Pi. *Transplant Proc* **5**:1551–1554.

Albert, E. D., M. R. Mickey, and P. I. Terasaki. 1973b. A new approach to cross-reactivity in the HL-A system. *Symp Ser Immunobiol Stand* **18**:156–164.

Allen, F. H. 1974. Linkage of *HL-A* and *GBG*. *Vox Sang* **27**:382–384.

Amos, D. B. 1953. The agglutination of mouse leucocytes by iso-immune sera. *Br J Exp Pathol* 34:464–470.

Amos, D. B., and F. H. Bach. 1968. Phenotypic expressions of the major histocompatibility locus in man (*HL-A*): Leukocyte antigens and mixed leucocyte culture reactivity. *J Exp Med* **128**:623–637.

Amos, D. B., H. Bashir, W. Boyle, M. MacQueen, and A. Tiilikainen. 1969. A simple micro-cytotoxicity test. *Transplantation* **7**:220–222.

Artzt, K., and F. Jacob. 1974. Absence of serologically detectable H-2 on primitive teratocarcinoma cells in culture. *Transplantation* **17**:632–634.

Aster, R. H., B. H. Miskovich, and G. E. Rodey. 1973. Histocompatibility antigens of human plasma. *Transplantation* **16**:205–210.

Bach, F. H., and D. B. Amos. 1967. *Hu-1:* Major histocompatibility locus in man. *Science* **156**:1506–1508.

Bach, F. H., and K. Hirschhorn. 1964. Lymphocyte interaction: A potential histocompatibility test *in vitro*. *Science* **143**:813–814.

Bach, F. H., P. M. Sondel, M. J. Sheehy, R. Wank, B. J. Alter, and M. L. Bach, 1975. The complexity of the HLA LD System: A PLT analysis. Pages 576–580 *in* F. Kissmeyer–Nielsen, ed. Histocompatibility Testing 1975. Munksgaard, Copenhagen.

Bain, B., and L. Lowenstein. 1964. Genetic studies on the mixed leukocyte reaction. *Science* **145**:1315–1316.

Balner, H., F. J. Cleton, and J. G. Eernisse, eds. 1965. Histocompatibility Testing 1965. Munksgaard, Copenhagen.

Batchelor, J. R., and A. R. Sanderson. 1970. Implications of cross-reactivity in the HL-A system. *Transplant Proc* **2**:133–143.

Bender, K., and K. H. Grzeschik. 1976. Possible assignment of the gluoxalase I (GLo) gene to chromosome 6 using man–mouse somatic cell hybrids. *Humangenetik* in press.

Berah, M., J. Hors, and J. Dausset. 1970. A study of HL-A antigens in human organs. *Transplantation* **9**:185–192.

Bialek, J. W., W. F. Bodmer, J. G. Bodmer, and R. Payne. 1966. Distribution and quantity of leukocyte antigens in the formed elements of the blood. *Transfusion* **6**:193–205.

Bodmer, W. F., and R. Payne. 1965. Theoretical consideration of leukocyte grouping using multispecific sera. Pages 141–149 *in* H. Balner, F. L. Cleton, and J. G. Eernisse, eds. Histocompatibility Testing 1965. Munksgaard, Copenhagen.

Bodmer, W. F., J. G. Bodmer, S. Adler, R. Payne, and J. Bialek. 1966. Genetics of "4" and "LA" human leucocyte groups. *Ann NY Acad Sci* **129**:473–489.

Bodmer, W. F., J. G. Bodmer, D. Ihde, and S. Adler. 1969. Genetic and serological association analysis of the HL-A leukocyte system. Pages 117–126 *in* N. E. Morton, ed. Computer applications in genetics. University of Hawaii Press, Honolulu.

Bodmer, W. F., E. A. Jones, D. Young, P. N. Goodfellow, J. C. Bodmer, H. M. Dick, and C. M. Steel. Serology of human Ia type antigens detected on lymphoid lines. Pages 677–684 *in* F. Kissmeyer–Nielsen, ed. Histocompatibility Testing 1975. Munksgaard, Copenhagen.

Bondevick, H., and E. Thorsby. 1973. The response of alloimmune human lymphocytes in mixed lymphocyte culture tests. *Transplant Proc* **4**:1477–1480.

Brautbar, C., E. J. Stanbridge, M. A. Pellegrino, S. Ferrone, R. A. Reisfeld, R. Payne, and L. Hayflick. 1973. Expression of HL-A antigens on cultured human fibroblasts infected with mycoplasma. *J. Immunol* **111**:1783–1789.

Bruning, J. W., A. Van Leeuwen, and J. J. Van Rood. 1964. Purification of leucocyte group substances from human placental tissue. *Transplantation* **2**:649–653.

Cann, H. M., J. G. Bodmer, and W. F. Bodmer. 1973. The HL-A polymorphism in Mayan Indians of San Juan La Laguna, Guatemala. Pages 367–376 *in* J. Dausset and J. Colombani, eds. Histocompatibility Testing 1972. Munksgaard, Copenhagen.

Ceppellini, R., and J. J. Van Rood. 1974. The HL-A system. I. Genetics and molecular biology. *Semin Hematol* **11**:233–251.

Ceppellini, R., E. S. Curtoni, P. L. Mattiuz, V. Miggiano, G. Scudeller, and A. Serrs. 1967. Genetics of leukocyte antigens: A family study of segregation and linkage. Pages 149–187 *in* E. S. Curtoni, P. L. Mattiuz, and R. M. Tosi, eds. Histocompatibility Testing 1967. Munksgaard, Copenhagen.

Ceppellini, R., G. D. Bonnard, F. Coppo, V. C. Miggiano, M. Pospisil, E. S. Curtoni, and M. Pellegrino. 1971. Mixed leukocyte cultures and HL-A antigens. I. Reactivity of young fetuses, newborns and mothers at delivery. *Transplant Proc* 3:58–70.

Collins, Z. V., P. F. Arnold, F. Peetoom, G. S. Smith, and R. L. Walford. 1973. A naturally occurring monospecific anti-HL-A8 isoantibody. *Tissue Antigens* 3:358–363.

Colombani, J. 1963. Leukocyte agglutination. Page 56 *in* C. Steffen, ed. Methods of immunohaematologic research. Karger, Basel.

Colombani, J., M. Colombani, and J. Dausset. 1970. Cross-reactions in the HL-A system with special reference to Da6 cross-reacting group. Pages 79–82 *in* P. I. Terasaki, ed. Histocompatibility Testing 1972. Munksgaard, Copenhagen.

Colombani, J., J. D'Amaro, B. Gabb, G. Smith, and A. Svejgaard. 1971. International agreement on a microtechnique of platelet complement fixation (Pl C Fix). *Transplant Proc* 3:121–126.

Colombani, J., M. Colombani, and J. Dausset. 1973. Non-complement-fixing IgM antibodies with anti-HL-A2 specificity and blocking activity. *Transplantation* **16**:257–260.

Colombani, J., M. Colombani, L. Degos, E. Terrier, Y. Gaudy, and H. Dastot. 1974. Effect of cross-reactions on HL-A antigen immunogenicity. *Tissue Antigens* **4**:136–145.

Cullen, P. R., and M. M. Pickles. 1972. *HL-A2* and *HL-A9*. A possible relationship. *Tissue Antigens* **2**:341–343.

Curtoni, E. S., P. L. Mattiuz, and R. M. Tosi, eds. 1967. Histocompatibility Testing 1967. Munksgaard, Copenhagen.

D'Amaro, J. 1975. W4 (4a) and W6 (4b) in diverse human populations. *Tissue Antigens* **5**:386–394.

Dausset, J. 1954. Leuco-agglutinins. IV. Leuco-agglutinins and blood transfusion. *Vox Sang* **4**:190–198.

Dausset, J. 1956. Immuno-hématologie biologique et clinique. Flammarion, Paris.

Dausset, J. 1958. Iso-leuco-anticorps. *Acta Haematol (Basel)* **20**:156–166.

Dausset, J. 1965. Auto-antileukocyte ribosomal fraction in leukoneutropenia. *Ann NY Acad Sci* **124**:550–562.

Dausset, J., and J. Colombani, eds. 1973. Histocompatibility Testing 1972. Munksgaard, Copenhagen.

Dausset, J., and A. Nenna. 1952. Présence d'une leuco-agglutinine dans le sérum d'un cas d'agranulocytose chronique. *C R Soc Biol (Paris)* **146**:1539–1541.

Dausset, J., M. Colin, and J. Colombani. 1960. Immune platelet iso-antibodies. *Vox Sang* **5**:4–31.

Dausset, J., P. Iványi, and D. Iványi. 1965. Tissue alloantigens in humans: Identification of a complex system (*Hu-1*). Pages 51–62 *in* H. Balner, F. L. Cleton, and J. G. Eernisse, eds. Histocompatibility Testing 1965. Munksgaard, Copenhagen.

Dausset, J., P. Iványi, and N. Feingold. 1966. Tissue alloantigens present in human leucocytes. *Ann NY Acad Sci* **129**:386–407.

Dausset, J., P. Iványi, J. Colombani, N. Feingold, and L. Legrand. 1967. The *Hu-1* system. Pages 189–292 *in* E. S. Curtoni, P. L. Mattiuz, and R. M. Tosi, eds. Histocompatibility Testing 1967. Munksgaard, Copenhagen.

Dausset, J., J. Colombani, L. Legrand, and N. Feingold. 1968. Le deuxième sub-locus du systéme HL-A. *Nouv Rev Fr Hematol* **8**:841–846.

Dausset, J., J. Colombani, L. Legrand, and M. Fellous. 1970. Genetics of the *HL-A* system: Deduction of 480 haplotypes. Pages 53–77 *in* P. Terasaki, ed. Histocompatibility Testing 1970. Munksgaard, Copenhagen.

Dausset, J., M. Sasportes, and A. Lebrun. 1973. Mixed lymphocyte cultures (MLC) between serologically HL-A identical parent and child and between HL-A homozygous and heterozygous individuals. *Transplant Proc* **5**:1511–1515.

Dausset, J., S. Singh, J. L. Gourand, L. Degos, C. Solal, and G. Klein. 1974. HL-A and Burkitt's disease. *Tissue Antigens* **5**:48–51.

Dawson, J. R., S. S. Shasby, and D. B. Amos. 1974. The serologic detection of HL-A antigens in human milk. *Tissue Antigens* **4**:76–82.

Degos, L., and J. Colombani. 1973. Quantification of cross-reactions between HLA antigens by Bayes' method. Pages 479–483 *in* J. Dausset and J. Colombani, eds. Histocompatibility Testing 1972. Munksgaard, Copenhagen.

Degos, L., and J. Dausset. 1975. Comparison of genetic (factorial correspondence analysis) and geographical distances. *Tissue Antigens* **5**:464–466.

Démant, P. 1973. *H-2* gene complex and its role in alloimmune reactions. *Transplant Rev* **15**:162–200.

Démant, P., G. D. Snell, and M. Cherry. 1971. Hemagglutinating and cytotoxic studies of *H-2*. III. A family of 3-like specificities not in the *C* cross-over region. *Transplantation* **11**:242–259.

Dorf, M. E., J. Y. Eguro, J. Dawson, E. J. Rauckman, and D. B. Amos. 1972. Cross-reactions of HL-A antibodies. II. Continuous pH gradient elution. *J Immunol* **109**:681–685.

Doughty, R. W., S. R. Goodier, and K. Gelsthorpe. 1973. Further evidence for HL-A antigens present on adult peripheral red blood cells. *Tissue Antigens* 3:189–194.

Dupont, B., C. Jersild, G. S. Hansen, L. Staub-Nielsen, M. Thomsen, and A. Svejgaard. 1973a. Multiple MLC (LD) determinants on the same *HL-A* halotype. *Transplant Proc* **5**:1481–1487.

Dupont, B., C. Jersild, G. S. Hansen, L. Staub-Nielsen, M. Thomsen, and A. Svejgaard. 1973b. Typing for MLC determinants by means of LD-homozygous and LD-heterozygous test cells. *Transplant Proc* **5**:1543–1549.

Dupont, B., R. A. Good, G. S. Hansen, C. Jersild, L. Staub-Nielsen, B. H. Park, A. Svejgaard, M. Thomsen, and E. J. Yunis. 1974. Two separate genes controlling stimulation in mixed lymphocyte reaction in man. *Proc Natl Acad Sci* USA **71**:52–56.

Edwards, J. H., F. H. Allen, K. P. Glenn, L. U. Lamm, and E. B. Robson. 1973. The linkage relationships of HL-A. Pages 745–751 *in* J. Dausset and J. Colombani, eds. Histocompatibility Testing 1972. Munksgaard, Copenhagen.

Eijsvoogel, V. P., J. J. Van Rood, E. D. du Toit, and P. T. A. Schellekens. 1972. Position of a locus determining mixed lymphocyte reaction distinct from the known *HL-A* loci. *Eur J Immunol* **2**:413–418.

Fellous, M. 1969. Mise en évidences des antigènes de transplantation sur les spermatozoïdes et leur expression probablement haploïde. Thesis, Univ. Paris.

Fellous, M., and J. Dausset. 1970. Probable haploid expression of HL-A antigens on human spermatozoon. *Nature (Lond)* **225**:191–193.

Fellous, M., P. Couillin, Neauport-Sautès, C. Billardon, and J. Dausset. 1973. Study of expression of human alloantigens in man × mouse hybrid cell. *Eur J Immunol* 3:543–548.

Fellous, M., F. Mortchelewicz, M. Kamoun, and J. Dausset. 1975. The use of a lymphoid cell line to define new B lymphocyte specificities, probably controlled by the MHC region. Pages 708–712 *in* F. Kissmeyer-Nielsen, ed. Histocompatibility Testing 1975. Munksgaard, Copenhagen.

Festenstein, H. 1966. Antigenic strength investigated by mixed cultures of allogeneic mouse spleen cells. *Ann NY Acad Sci* **129**:567–572.

Festenstein, H., and P. Démant. 1973. Workshop summary on genetic determinants of cell-mediated immune reactions in the mouse. *Transplant Proc* **5**:1321–1327.

Fradelizi, D., and J. Dausset. 1975. Mixed lymphocyte reactivity of human lymphocytes primed *in vitro*. I. Secondary response to allogenic lymphocytes. *Eur J Immunol* **5**:295–301.

Fu, S. M., H. G. Kunkel, H. P. Brusman, F. H. Allen, and M. Fotino. 1974. Evidence for linkage between *HL-A* histocompatibility genes and those involved in the synthesis of second component of complement. *J Exp Med* **140**:1108–1111.

Gatti, R. A., E. J. Yunis, and R. A. Good. 1973. Characterization of a serum inhibitor of MLC reactions. *Clin Exp Immunol* **13**:427–437.

Gershon, R. K., and K. Kondo. 1972. Degeneracy of the immune response to sheep red cells. *Immunology* **23**:321–324.

Goldstein, S., and D. P. Singal. 1972. Loss of reactivity of HL-A antigens in clonal population of cultured human fibroblasts during aging *in vitro*. *Exp Cell Res* **75**:278–282.

Gossett, T., R. L. Walford, G. S. Smith, A. Robins, and G. B. Ferrara. 1975. The *Merrit* alloantigen system of humans lymphocytes. Pages 687–691 *in* F. Kissmeyer-Nielsen, ed. Histocompatibility Testing 1975. Munksgaard, Copenhagen.

Halim, A., K. Abbasi, and H. Festenstein. 1974. The expression of the HL-A antigens on human spermatozoa. *Tissue Antigens* **4**:1–6.

Harris, R., and J. D. Zervas. 1969. Reticulocyte HL-A antigens. *Nature (Lond)* **221**:1062–1063.

Hirschfeld, J. 1965. Serologic codes: Interpretation of immunogenetic systems. *Science* **148**:968–971.

Iványi, P., and J. Dausset. 1966. Alloantigens and antigenic factors of human leucocytes. *Vox Sang* **11**:326–331.

Iványi, D., M. Rychlíková, M. Sasportes, P. Iványi, and J. Dausset. 1967. Leukocyte antigens and the mixed lymphocyte culture reaction. *Vox Sang* **12**:186–198.

Jensen, K. G. 1962. Leucocyte antibodies in serums of pregnant women. Serology and clinic. *Vox Sang* **7**:454–469.

Jensen, K. G. 1966. Leucocyte antibodies and pregnancy. A survey. Munksgaard, Copenhagen.

Johnson, A. H., R. D. Rossen, and W. T. Butler. 1972. Detection of alloantibodies using a sensitive antiglobulin microcytotoxicity test. *Tissue Antigens* **2**:215–226.

Jørgensen, F., L. U. Lamm, and F. Kissmeyer-Nielsen. 1973. Mixed lymphocyte culture with inbred individuals: An approach to MLC typing. *Tissue Antigens* **3**:323–339.

Kerek, G., and B. A. Afzelius. 1972. The HL-A antigens on human spermatozoa. *Int J Fertil* **17**:120–126.

Kissmeyer-Nielsen, F. 1975. Histocompatibility Testing 1975. Munksgaard, Copenhagen.

Kissmeyer-Nielsen, F., and K. E. Kjerbye. 1967. Lymphocytotoxic microtechnique. Purification of lymphocytes by flotation. Pages 381–383 *in* E. S. Curtoni, P. L. Mattiuz, and R. M. Tosi, eds. Histocompatibility Testing 1967. Munksgaard, Copenhagen.

Kissmeyer-Nielsen, F., and E. Thorsby. 1970. Human transplantation antigens. *Transplant Rev* **4**:1–176.

Kissmeyer-Nielsen, F., A. Svejgaard, and M. Hauge. 1968. Genetics of the human *HL-A* transplantation system. *Nature (Lond)* **219**:1116–1119.

Kissmeyer-Nielsen, F., A. Svejgaard, and E. Thorsby. 1971. Human transplantation antigens. The *HL-A* system. *Bibl Haematol* **38**:276–281.

Kourilsky, F. M., D. Silvestre, J. P. Levy, J. Dausset, M. G. Niccolai, and A. Senik. 1971. Immunoferritin study of the distribution of HL-A antigens on human blood cells. *J Immunol* **106**:454–466.

Lebrun, A., M. Sasportes, and J. Dausset. 1973. La culture mixed lymphocytaire. Rôle possible de la région du premier locus *HL-A*. *C R Acad Sci (Paris)* **276**: 1763–1765.

Legrand, L., and J. Dausset. 1974. The complexity of the *HL-A* gene product. I. Study of a serum produced against HL-A5 in an HL-A semi-identical situation. *Tissue Antigens* **4**:329–345.

Legrand, L., and J. Dausset. 1975a. The complexity of the *HL-A* gene product. II. Possible evidence for a "public" determinant common to the 1st and 2nd *HL-A* series. *Transplantation* **19**:177–180.

Legrand, L., and J. Dausset. 1975b. A second lymphocyte system (Ly-Li). Pages 665–668 *in* F. Kissmeyer-Nielsen, ed. Histocompatibility Testing 1975. Munksgaard, Copenhagen.

Loke, Y. W., V. C. Josey, and R. Borland. 1971. HL-A antigens on human trophoblast cells. *Nature (Lond)* **232**:403–405.

Low, B., L. Messeter, S. Mansson, and T. Lindholm. 1974. Crossing-over between the $SD_2$ (*FOUR*) and $SD_3$ (*AJ*) loci of the human major histocompatibility chromosomal region. *Tissue Antigens* **4**:405.

Marchal, G., J. Dausset, J. Colombani, G. Bilski-Pasquier, B. Jaulmes, H. Brecy, J. Evelin. 1958. Immunisation anti-leucocytaire provoquée par l'injection répétée du même sang. *Sang* **29**:549–560.

Mattiuz, P. L., D. Ihde, A. Piazza, R. Ceppellini, and W. F. Bodmer. 1970. New approaches to the population. Genetic and segregation analysis of the HL-A system. Pages 193–205 *in* P. I. Terasaki, ed. Histocompatibility Testing 1970. Munksgaard, Copenhagen.

Mayr, W. R., D. Bernoco, M. de Marchi, and R. Ceppellini. 1973. Genetic analysis and biological properties of products of the third *SD* (*AJ*) locus of the *HL-A* region. *Transplant Proc* **5**:1581–1593.

Melief, C. J. M., M. Van der Hart, C. P. Engelfriet, and J. J. Van Loghem. 1967. Immune adherence of leucocytes and fibroblasts derived from skin, sensitized by cytotoxic leucocyte iso-antibodies and complement, to the surface of indicator cells. *Vox Sang* **12**:374–389.

Mempel, W., H. Grosse-Wilde, E. Albert, and S. Thierfelder. 1973a. Atypical MLC reactions in HL-A typed related and unrelated pairs. *Transplant Proc* **5**:401–408.

Mempel, W., H. Grosse-Wilde, P. Baumann, B. Netzel, I. Steinbauer-Rosenthal, S. Scholz, J. Bertrams, and E. S. Albert. 1973b. Population genetics of the MLC response: Typing for MLC determinants using homozygous and heterozygous reference cells. *Transplant Proc* **5**:1529–1534.

Metzgar, R. S., and J. L. Miller. 1973. Production of precipitating primate antibodies to human membrane antigen(s) with HL-A activity by immunisation with soluble HL-A antigens. *J Immunol* **110**:1097–1107.

Middleton, J., M. C. Crookston, J. A. Falk, E. B. Robson, P. J. C. Cook, J. R. Batchelor, J. Bodmer, G. V. Ferrara, H. Festenstein, R. Harris, F. Kissmeyer-Nielsen, S. D. Lawler, J. A. Sachs, and I. Wolf. 1974. Linkage of *chido* and *HL-A*. *Tissue Antigens* **4**:366–373.

Miescher, P., and M. Fauconnet. 1954. Mise en évidence de différents groupes leucocytaires chez l'homme. *Schweiz Med Wochenschr* **84**:597.

Mittal, K. K., and P. I. Terasaki. 1972. Cross-reactivity in the *HL-A* system. *Tissue Antigens* **2**:94–104.

Mittal, K. K., and P. I. Terasaki. 1974. Serological cross-reactivity in the *HL-A* system. *Tissue Antigens* **4**:146–156.

Miyakawa, Y., N. Tanigaki, V. P. Kreiter, G. E. Moore, and D. Pressman. 1973. Characterization of soluble substances in the plasma carrying HL-A alloantigenic activity and HL-A common antigenic activity. *Transplantation* **15**:312–319.

Moeschlin, S., and R. Wagner. 1952. Agranulocytosis due to the occurrence of leucocyte agglutinins (pyramidon and cold agglutinins). *Acta Haematol* **8**:29–41.

Morris, P. J., and L. Dumble. 1973. The capacity to form anti-HL-A2 cytotoxins. *Symp Ser Immunobiol Stand* **18**:179–181.

Morton, N. E. 1955. Sequential tests for the detection of linkage. *Am J Hum Genet* **7**:277.

Morton, J. A., M. M. Pickles, and L. Sutton. 1969. The correlation of the $Bg^a$ blood group with the HL-A7 leucocyte group. Demonstration of antigenic sites on red cells and leucocytes. *Vox Sang* **17**:536–547.

Morton, J. A., M. M. Pickles, L. Sutton, and S. Skov. 1971. Identification of further antigens or red cells and genetic evidence confirming the localization of Sutter in the Kell blood lymphocytes. Association of $Bg^b$ with W17 (Te 57) and $Bg^c$ with W18 (Da15, Ba*) *Vox Sang* **21**:141–153.

Nymand, G. 1974. Complement-fixing and lymphocytotoxic antibodies in serum of pregnant women at delivery. *Vox Sang* **27**:322–337.

Opelz, G., M. R. Mickey, and P. I. Terasaki. 1973. Blood transfusions and unresponsiveness to HL-A. *Transplantation* **16**:649–654.

Overweg, J., and C. P. Engelfriet. 1969. Cytotoxic leucocyte iso-antibodies formed during the first pregnancy. *Vox Sang* **16**:97–104.

Patel, R. 1971. Cytotoxic reactions of lymphocytes of blood, lymph node and thoracic duct origin with monospecific anti-HL-A antisera. *Transplantation* **11**:348–351.

Payne, R. 1957. The association of febrile transfusion reactions with leukoagglutinins. *Vox Sang* **2**:233–241.

Payne, R. 1964. Neonatal neutropenia and leukoagglutinins. *Pediatrics* **33**:193–204.

Payne, R. 1962. The development and persistence of leukoagglutinins in parous women. *Blood* **19**:411–424.

Payne, R., and M. R. Rolfs. 1958. Fetomaternal leukocyte incompatibility. *J Clin Invest* **37**:1756–1763.

Payne, R., M. Tripp, J. Weigle, W. F. Bodmer, and J. Bodmer. 1964. A new leukocyte iso-antigen system in man. *Cold Spring Harbor Symp Quant Biol* **29**:285–295.

Piazza, A., P. L. Mattiuz, and R. Ceppellini. 1969. Assortimento per gli aplotipi del sisteme *HL-A* come possible meccanismo de selezione gametica o zigotica. *Haematologica* **54**:703–720.

Piazza, A., L. Sgaramella-Zonta, P. Gluckman, and L. L. Cavalli-Sforza. 1975. The fifth histocompatibility workshop gene frequency data. A phylogenetic analysis. *Tissue Antigens* **5**:445–463.

Pierres, M., D. Fradelizi, C. Neauport-Sautès, and J. Dausset. 1975. Third *HL-A* segregant series: Genetic analysis and molecular independence on the lymphocyte surface. *Tissue Antigens* **5**:266–279.

Rittner, C., G. Hauptmann, H. Grosse-Wilde, E. Grosshans, M. M. Tongio, and S. Mayer. 1975. Linkage between *HL-A* (major histocompatibility complex) and genes controlling the synthesis of the fourth component of complement. Pages 945–954 *in* F. Kissmeyer-Nielsen, ed. Histocompatibility Testing 1975. Munksgaard, Copenhagen.

Robert, M., H. Betuel, and J. P. Revillard. 1973. Inhibition of the mixed lymphocyte reaction by sera from multipares. *Tissue Antigens* **3**:39–56.

Robert, M., C. Vincent, and J. P. Revillard. 1974. Antigène HL-A et beta-2-microglobuline dans l'urine. *C R Acad Sci (Paris)* **278**:2237–2240.

Russell, P. S., H. J. Winn, and D. B. Amos, eds. 1965. Histocompatibility Testing. Natl. Acad. Sci., Washington, D.C.

Rychlíková, M., P. Démant, and P. Iványi. 1970. The predominant role of the *K* end of the *H-2* locus in lymphocyte transformation in mixed cultures. *Folia Biol (Praha)* **16**:218–221.

Salmon, C., and D. Schwartz. 1960. Analyse statistique d'une série de 639 malades polytransfusés: Essai d'une interprétation des conditions d'iso-immunisation. *Rev Hematol* **15**:162–173.

Sandberg, L., E. Thorsby, F. Kissmeyer-Nielsen, and A. Lindholm. 1970. Evidence of a third sublocus within the *HL-A* chromosomal region. Pages 165–169 *in* P. I. Terasaki, ed. Histocompatibility Testing 1970. Munksgaard, Copenhagen.

Sanderson, A. R., and K. I. Welsh. 1973. HL-A reagents from primates. I. Antigen preparation, immunization and preliminary analysis of sera. *Transplantation* **16**:304–312.

Sanderson, A. R., and K. I. Welsh. 1974. Properties of histocompatibility (HL-A) determinants. I. Site density of antigens of the two HL-A segregant series on peripheral human lymphocytes. *Transplantation* **17**:281–289.

Sasportes, M., C. Dehay, and M. Fellous. 1971. Variations of the expression of HL-A antigens on human diploid fibroblasts in vitro. *Nature (Lond)* **233**:332–334.

Sasportes, M., C. Mawas, A. Bernard, Y. Christen, and J. Dausset. 1973. MLR in families with an *HL-A* haplotype shared by parents: Recombination between $SD_2$ and $LD_2$ and possible evidence for an $LD_3$ locus. *Transplant Proc* **5**:1517–1522.

Schultz, J. S., and D. C. Schreffler. 1972. Studies on the serum fraction containing soluble inhibitors of anti-HL-A sera. *Transplantation* **13**:186–188.

Sengar, D. P. S., G. Opelz, and P. I. Terasaki. 1973. Suppression of mixed leukocyte response by plasma from hemodialysis patients. *Tissue Antigens* **3**:22–29.

Shevach, E. M., D. L. Rosenstreich, and I. Green. 1973. The distribution of histocompatibility antigens on T and B cells in the guinea pig. *Transplantation* **16**:126–133.

Shreffler, D. C., D. B. Amos, and R. Mark. 1966. Serological analysis of a recombination in the *H-2* region of the mouse. *Transplantation* **4**:300–322.

Shulman, N. R., V. J. Marder, M. C. Hiller, and E. M. Collier. 1964. Platelet and leukocyte isoantigens and their antibodies: Serologic, physiologic and clinical studies. *Progr Hematol* **4**:222–304.

Silvestre, D., F. M. Kourilsky, M. G. Nicolai, and J. P. Levy. 1970. Presence of HL-A antigens on human reticulocytes as demonstrated by electron microscopy. *Nature (Lond)* **228**:67–68.

Singal, D. P., and S. Goldstein. 1973. Absence of detectable HL-A antigens on cultured fibroblasts in progeria. *J Clin Invest* **52**:2259–2263.

Singal, D. P., M. R. Mickey, K. K. Mittal, and P. I. Terasaki. 1968. Serotyping for homotransplantation. XVII. Preliminary studies of *HL-A* subunits and alleles. *Transplantation* **6**:904–912.

Snell, G. D., and M. Cherry. 1974. Hemagglutination and cytotoxic studies of *H-2*. IV. Evidence that there are 3-like antigenic sites determined by both the *K* and the *D* cross-over regions. *Folia Biol (Praha)* **20**:81–100.

Snell, G. D., P. Démant, and M. Cherry. 1971. Hemagglutinating and cytotoxic studies of *H-2*. I. *H-2.1* and related specificities in the *EK* crossover region. *Transplantation* **11**:210–237.

Snell, G. D., P. Démant, and M. Cherry. 1974. Hemagglutination and cytotoxic studies of *H-2*. V. The anti-27, 28, 29 family of antibodies. *Folia Biol (Praha)* **20**:145–160.

Solheim, B. G., A. Bratlie, N. Winther, and E. Thorsby. 1975. LD antisera prepared by planned immunizations. Pages 713–718 *in* F. Kissmeyer-Nielsen, ed. Histocompatibility Testing 1975. Munksgaard, Copenhagen.

Sørensen, S. F. 1972. The mixed lymphocyte culture interaction. Techniques and immunogenetics. *Acta Pathol Microbiol Scand* **230**:1–82.

Staub-Nielsen, L., and A. Svejgaard. 1972. HL-A immunisation and HL-A types in pregnancy. *Tissue Antigens* **2**:316–327.

Staub-Nielsen, L., L. Ryder, and A. Svejgaard. 1973. HL-A immunisation in pregnancy. *Symp Ser Immunobiol Stand* **18**:182–192.

Svejgaard, A. 1969. Iso-antigenic systems of human blood platelets. A survey. *Ser Haematol* **11**:3.

Svejgaard, A., and F. Kissmeyer-Nielsen. 1968. Cross-reactive human HL-A isoantibodies. *Nature (Lond)* **219**:868–869.

Svejgaard, A., L. Staub-Nielsen, L. Ryder, F. Kissmeyer-Nielsen, L. Sandberg, A. Lindholm, and E. Thorsby. 1973. Subdivision of HL-A antigens. Evidence of a new segregant series. Pages 465–474 *in* J. Dausset and J. Colombani, eds. Histocompatibility Testing 1972. Munksgaard, Copenhagen.

Terasaki, P. I. 1970. Histocompatibility Testing 1970. Munksgaard, Copenhagen.

Terasaki, P. I., and J. D. McClelland. 1964. Microdroplet assay of human serum cytotoxins. *Nature (Lond)* **204**:998–1000.

Terasaki, P. I., M. R. Mickey, D. L. Vredevoe, and D. R. Goyette. 1965. Serotyping for homotransplantation. IV. Grouping and evaluation of lymphotoxic sera. *Vox Sang* **11**:350–376.

Terasaki, P. I., G. Opelz, M. Park, and M. R. Mickey. 1975. B-lymphocyte specificities. Pages 657–664 *in* F. Kissmeyer-Nielsen, ed. Histocompatibility Testing 1975. Munksgaard, Copenhagen.

Thomsen, M., B. Jacobsen, P. Platz, L. P. Ryder, L. Staub-Nielsen, and A. Svejgaard. 1975 LD typing, polymorphism of MLC determinants. Pages 509–518 *in* F. Kissmeyer-Nielsen, ed. Histocompatibility Testing 1975. Munksgaard, Copenhagen.

Thorsby, E. 1969. HL-A antigens on human granulocytes studied with cytotoxic isoantisera obtained by skin grafting. *Scand J Haematol* **6**:119–127.

Thorsby, E., H. Bondevick, and G. B. Solheim. 1973a. The inhibition effect of HL-A antibodies on lymphocyte transformation in vitro. *Transplant Proc* **5**:343–348.

Thorsby, E., H. Hirschberg, and A. Helgesen. 1973b. A second locus determining human MLC response: Separate lymphocyte populations recognize the products of each different *MLC* locus allele in allogeneic combination. *Transplant Proc* **5**:1523–1528.

Unterdown, B. J., and H. N. Eisen. 1971. Cross-reactions between 2,4-dinitrophenyl and 5-acethracil groups. *J Immunol* **106**:1431–1440.

Van den Twell, J. G., A Blussé van Oud Ablas, J. J. Keuning, E. Goulmy, A. Termijtelen, M. L. Bach, and J. J. Van Rood. 1973. Typing for MLC (LD). I. Lymphocytes from cousin-marriage offspring as typing cells. *Transplant Proc* **5**:1535–1538.

Van Leeuwen, A., R. Schuit, and J. J. Van Rood. 1973. Typing for MLC (LD). II. The selection of non-stimulator cells by MLC inhibition test using SD identical stimulator cells (MISIS) and fluorescent antibody studies. *Transplant Proc* **5**:1539–1542.

Van Rood, J. J. 1962. Leucocyte grouping. A method and its application. Thesis, Leiden.

Van Rood, J. J., and A. Van Leeuwen. 1963. Leukocyte grouping. A method and its applications. *J Clin Invest* **42**:1382–1390.

Van Rood, J. J., and A. Van Leeuwen. 1965. Defined leukocyte antigenic groups in men. Pages 21–36 *in* P. S. Russell, H. J. Winn, and D. B. Amos, eds. Histocompatibility Testing. Natl. Acad. Sci., Washington, D.C.

Van Rood, J. J., J. G. Eernisse, and A. Van Leeuwen. 1958. Leucocyte antibodies in sera from pregnant women. *Nature (Lond)* **181**:1735–1736.

Van Rood, J. J., A. Van Leeuwen, H. M. J. Schippers, W. H. Vooys, E. Frederiks, H. Balner, and J. G. Eernisse. 1965. Leukocyte groups, the normal lymphocyte transfer test and homograft sensitivity. Pages 37–50 *in* H. Balner, F. L. Cleton, and J. G. Eernisse, eds. Histocompatibility Testing 1965. Munksgaard, Copenhagen.

Van Rood, J. J., A. Van Leeuwen, and M. C. F. Van Santen. 1970. Anti-HL-A2 inhibitor in normal human serum. *Nature (Lond)* **226**:366–367.

Van Rood, J. J., A. Van Leeuwen, J. J. Keuning, and A. Blussé van Oud Alblas. 1975a. The serological recognition of the human *MLC* determinants using a modified cytotoxicity technique. *Tissue Antigens* **5**:73–79.

Van Rood, J. J., Van Leeuwen, J. J. Keuning, and A. Termijtelen. 1975b. Serotyping for MLC. III. Family and population studies with an MLC inhibiting serum Pl. *Transplant Proc* **7**:31–34.

Van Rood, J. J., A. Van Leeuwen, A. Termijtelen, and J. J. Keuning. 1976. The genetics of the major histocompatibility complex in man, HLA. *In* D. H. Katz and B. Benacerraf, eds. The role of the products of the histocompatibility gene complex in immune responses. Academic Press, New York.

Vredovoe, M. R., M. R. Mickey, D. R. Goyette, N. S. Magnuson, and P. I. Terasaki. 1966. Serotyping for homotransplantation. VIII. Grouping of antisera from various laboratories into five groups. *Ann NY Acad Sci* **129**:521–528.

Walford, R. L. 1960. Leukocyte antigens and antibodies. Grune & Stratton, New York.

Walford, R. L. 1969. The isoantigenic systems of human leukocytes; medical and biological significance. *Ser Haematol* 2(2):16.

Walford, R. L. 1970. Antibody diversity, histocompatibility systems, disease states and ageing. *Lancet* **2**:1226–1229.

Walford, R. L., G. S. Smith, E. Zeller, and J. Wilkinson. 1975. A new alloantigenic system on human lymphocytes. *Tissue Antigens* **5**:196–204.

Weitkamp, L. R., J. J. Van Rood, E. Thorsby, W. Bias, M. Fotino, S. D. Lawler, J. Dausset, W. R. Mayr, J. Bodmer, F. E. Ward, J. Seignalet, R. Payne, F. Kissmeyer-Nielsen, R. A. Gatti, J A. Sachs, and L. U. Lamm. 1973. The relation of parental sex and age to recombination in the *HL-A* system. *Hum Hered* **23**:197–205.

Weitkamp, L. R., P. L. Townes, and A. Johnston. 1975. Linkage data on urinary pepsinogen and Kell blood group. Pages 281–282 *in* D. Bergsma ed. Human gene mapping 2. Karger, Basel.

Wernet, P., and H. G. Kunkel. 1973. Antibodies to a specific surface antigen of T cells in human sera inhibiting mixed leukocyte culture reactions. *J Exp Med* **138**:1021–1026.

Wilson, L. A., and D. B. Amos. 1972. Subcellular location of HL-A antigens. *Tissue Antigens* **2**:105–111.

Winchester, R. J., S. M. Fu, P. Wernet, H. G. Kunkel, B. Dupont, and C. Jeersild. 1975a. Recognition by pregnancy serums of non-HL-A alloantigens selectively expressed on B lymphocytes. *J Exp Med* **141**:924–929.

Winchester, R. J., B. Dupont, P. Wernet, S. M. Fu, J. Hansen, N. Laursen, and H. G. Kunkel. 1975b. Studies on the correlation between LD determinants and HL-B, a non HL-A alloantigen system selectively expressed on B lymphocytes. Pages 651–656 *in* F. Kissmeyer-Nielsen, ed. Histocompatibility Testing 1975. Munksgaard, Copenhagen.

Yunis, F. J., and D. B. Amos. 1971. Three closely-linked genetic systems relevant to transplantation. *Proc Natl Acad Sci USA* **68**:3031–3035.

CHAPTER 10

# THE HLA COMPLEX: PRACTICAL IMPLICATIONS



## I. Organ Transplantation

The best known and most spectacular practical implication of HLA immunogenetics is without doubt transplantation. Kidney transplantation has become a daily therapy. Bone marrow grafts are still in the experimental stage. However, clarity of the experimental data still stands in sharp contrast to the persistent difficulties at the medical level.

### A. Experimental Data: Skin Grafts

The average survival of random skin grafts between unrelated donors was established as 10.5 days. The survival of grafts from different individuals placed on a recipient previously immunized by a first graft is variable, a finding that suggested the possibility of human tissue groups (Rapaport *et al.*, 1960).

### *1. Influence of the HLA Complex*

A correlation between leukocyte antigens and skin graft survival was made simultaneously in Paris (Dausset *et al.*, 1965) and in Leiden (Van Rood *et al.*, 1965) using the preimmunization technique perfected in monkeys (Balner and Dersjant, 1965). Volunteers were preimmunized by the injection of leukocyte suspensions from a donor possessing at least one incompatible HLA antigen. At that time only a few antigens had been clearly defined. The antigens A2, B7, Bw4, and Bw6 were used. Fifteen days after the immunization, skin grafts from other donors, whether or not these had the antigen against which the volunteers had been preimmunized, were performed. All donors were ABO compatible. The results showed unequivocally that it was possible to predict the destiny of skin grafts by the presence or absence of the antigen against which preimmunization had occurred. This was the first demonstration of the role of the genes at the HLA complex.

As a second step, intrafamily skin grafts were done. One important fact clearly emerged. The survival of skin grafts between HLA identical sibs is particularly long (20–25 days) when compared to that of those between HLA semiidentical (14 days) and different (11–12) sibs. It should be noted that there is only a small difference between the last two survival times, but that graft survival where the influence of the HLA complex has been eliminated is quite clearly lengthened (Amos *et al.*, 1967; Ceppellini, 1968).

These figures show the extreme importance of the HLA complex in transplantation. They also indicate, no less clearly, since grafts between HLA identical sibs are also rejected that there are other genetic controls in man; in other words, there are histocompatibility systems other than the main system.

In order to study the role of the HLA antigens themselves more precisely, skin grafts from several children in the same sibship were placed on their father's arm. Graft survival was compared with the degree of match or mismatch of the father's genotype with the haplotype that the child had inherited from the mother. Analysis of 143 grafts showed a statistical correlation ($p < 0.001$) between the number of incompatibilities and the length of survival (Table 10.1). When the most obvious cross-reactions were taken into consideration, the correlation became even more clear-cut; an incompatibility between two antigens in the same cross-reaction group seems to be intermediate between an identity

TABLE 10.1
143 SKIN GRAFTS (CHILDREN TO FATHERS) IN HLA SEMI-IDENTICAL SITUATIONS[a]

| | Without cross-reactions | | | With cross-reactions[b] | | |
|---|---|---|---|---|---|---|
| | Number of grafts | Survival (days) | | Number of grafts | Survival (days) | |
| 0 Mismatches | 4 | 14.75 | 14.17 | 13 | 14.31 | 13.71 |
| 1 Mismatch | | | | | | |
| 1st locus only | 9 | 13.44 | | 16 | 14.06 | |
| 2nd locus only | 22 | 14.36 | | 30 | 13.27 | |
| 2 Mismatches | 108 | 11.85[c] | | 84 | 11.51[d] | |

[a] Data from Dausset *et al.*, 1970. In all cases, compatibility for both *A* and *B* loci could be established. (There were no unknown relationships due to "blank" antigens or possible homozygosity.)

[b] Cross-reactions considered: CREG B5, Bw35, Bw15, Bw21; CREG B7, Bw40, Bw22, B27.

[c] $p$ values between 11.85, 14.36, and 14.17 are, respectively, 0.01 and 0.007.

[d] $p$ values between 11.51, 13.27, and 13.71 are, respectively, 0.01 and 0.001.

and an incompatibility (Dausset *et al.*, 1970). Other teams came to similar conclusions concerning the influence of the HLA system on skin grafts (Ceppellini *et al.*, 1969b; Amos *et al.*, 1969).

### 2. INFLUENCE OF THE ABO AND P SYSTEMS

During these studies, ABO matching was consistently practiced, and, oddly enough, it was not until later that the influence of ABO incompatibility was systematically studied, first by preimmunization (Rapaport *et al.*, 1968) and then without immunization (Ceppellini *et al.*, 1969a).

Group O volunteers were preimmunized using group A erythrocytes almost completely separated from leukocytes or using A substances from a pig's stomach. Fifteen days later, the volunteers were grafted with skin from group O or A donors; HLA compatibility was not taken into consideration. Most of the ABO incompatible grafts did not even become vascularized but were immediately rejected as "white" grafts. If vascularization did begin, it was rapidly followed by accelerated rejection (Table 10.2).

The influence of ABO without preimmunization is less explosive but nevertheless very significant (Ceppellini *et al.*, 1969a). Grafts were performed between unrelated individuals, without taking incompatibilities at the HLA system into account. Compatible grafts (O → O and O → A, etc.) were rejected after an average of 12.2 days, and incompatible

TABLE 10.2
DEMONSTRATION OF THE ROLE OF A AND B ANTIGENS IN TRANSPLANTATION[a]

| Blood group O recipients preimmunized by | Mean survival time (days) of skin grafts from donors of blood groups | | | |
|---|---|---|---|---|
| | O | $A_1$ | $A_2$ | B |
| Erythrocytes $A_1$ | 10.5 | 4.0 | | |
| Erythrocytes $A_2B$ | 7.5 | W.G.[b] | 4.5 | |
| Erythrocytes B | 11 | | | 4.5 |
| Soluble substance A | 12.5 | W.G. | | |
| Soluble substance B | | | | W.G. |

[a] Data from Dausset and Rapaport (1968).
[b] W.G., white graft.

grafts (A → O, B → O) after 9.1 days. An interesting phenomenon was observed in the case of grafts from $A_2$ individuals. These grafts behaved almost as though they were group O when placed on group O individuals (rejection time 11.6 days).

Studies with other immunogenetic systems did not reveal a significant influence. The P system, where Ceppellini *et al.* (1966) found that compatible grafts survived for 12.4 days compared to 10.8 days for incompatible ones, is a possible exception.

## B. Kidney Transplantation

The first organ to be grafted was the kidney, an organ that is easy to transplant and which, because of the effective substitutional therapy available from the artificial kidney, permits a relatively long waiting period for a compatible donor. Kidney transplantation has become a routine procedure, and more than 15,000 have been performed throughout the world. National and regional organizations have been created to promote organ exchange.

The HLA types of all potential recipients are determined using batteries of specific antisera against all possible HLA specificities. Microlymphocytotoxicity is the most widely used technique. Some laboratories use microcomplement fixation on platelets in parallel. The donors are preferably typed with the same reagents. The most compatible recipient is chosen from the waiting list of patients. The graft is then performed provided that no circulating antibodies are detectable against the donor's lymphocytes using the most sensitive techniques (negative *cross match*).

### 1. Acute Rejection Associated with a Positive Cross Match

From the first attempts it appeared that disparities in the leukocyte antigen pattern of the donor and the recipient, detected by reactions obtained from several leukoagglutinins of unknown specificity, very often led to a rapid cessation of the function of the grafted kidney (Dausset and Colombani, 1962). The patients, all polytransfused, were strongly preimmunized, as shown by actual tests for antibodies. The role of these preformed antibodies on the immediate fate of the graft was clearly established later on—they can lead to hyperacute rejection of the graft on the operating table (Kissmeyer-Nielsen *et al.*, 1966; Starlz *et al.*, 1968). But there are also reports of hyperacute rejection in cases where no antibodies can be proved, even by the most sensitive techniques. Everyone is agreed on the importance of pretransplantation cross matching. No transplantation should be done if there is the smallest doubt as to its negativity.

When the recipient has not been preimmunized against one or more of the donor's antigens, immunization occurs after the graft. In patients who have received immunosuppressive treatment, rejection symptoms are delayed and often lessened, or even absent. "Rejection crises," shown by a fall in creatinine clearance, are a manifestation of incompatibility. Statistics concerning the early occurrence, intensity, and number of rejection crises illustrate the influence of compatibility at the HLA complex.

### 2. Correlation with HLA Incompatibilities

In weighing the significance of correlations between HLA incompatibility and graft failure, it should be remembered that failures are not all due to immunological causes. Infection, or the original disease recurring in the graft, are added to and intermingle with immunological rejection reactions. Because it was impossible to distinguish the different influences, it seemed more sensible to analyze the global results, making no exceptions. The only criterion of failure was the inability of a grafted kidney to keep a patient alive without the help of extrarenal hemodialysis. An immune reaction was assumed, for the purposes of the study, to be responsible for all failures, even technical ones.

1. The preponderant role of the HLA complex in organ transplantation was established beyond doubt when a sufficient number of grafts had been done between sibs. The best results were obtained when the donor was an HLA identical sib (Van Rood *et al.*, 1967; Dausset *et al.*, 1969; Singal *et al.*, 1969). Failures of these cases were very rare. It was, however, necessary to wait several years before a significant statistical com-

parison could be made between this privileged category and that made up of grafts from non-HLA-identical sibs (mostly haploidentical) (Hors *et al.*, 1971). It appeared that in the well-defined genetic situation provided by grafts between sibs and with the accompaniment of immunosuppression, the HLA chromosomal area governs the fate of kidney grafts almost alone.

2. When the donor is one of the parents, the survival curve is very similar to those from HLA haploidentical sibs. In both cases, donor and recipient differ genetically by a single HLA complex.

3. When the donor and recipient differ at both HLA complexes, as is the case for almost all grafts from unrelated donors, the survival curve is less favorable. The comparison of the actuarial curves obtained where neither, one, or both HLA complexes differ is given in Fig. 10.1. These early studies served to demonstrate the obvious influence of the HLA complex as a whole in kidney transplantation.

In order to establish the role of the HLA system itself, it was necessary to find a significant correlation between the number of incompatible

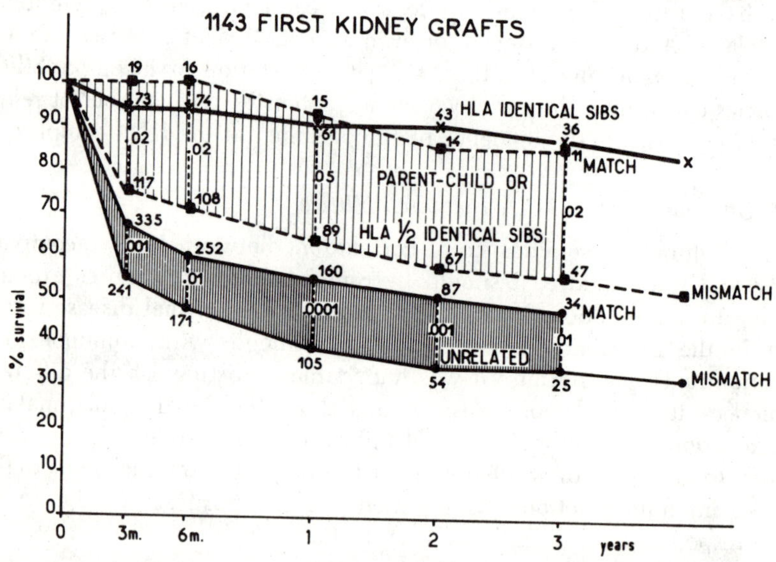


Fig. 10.1. Actuarial graft survival according to the donors relationship with the recipient (1143 first transplants). *HLA identical* siblings share both HLA complexes with the donor. *Parent–child* pairs as well as *HLA semi-identical* siblings, share only one HLA haplotype. The figures next to the graphs indicate the number of patients under observation for each consecutive interval. The "matched" semi-identical donors are phenotypically identical with the recipients. The "matched" unrelated donors have zero or one incompatibility with the recipients. The "mismatched" in both categories possess more incompatibilities than the "matched."

antigens and the length of graft survival. This was a long and difficult task, since our knowledge of the HLA antigens was still fragmentary and the materials were heterogeneous. An analysis that did not take into account the many serologically undefined "blank" antigens could only lead to false conclusions. The introduction of a method of calculating the probability of incompatibility of the "blank" antigens (due to untested or homozygous antigens) was an important advance (Hors *et al.*, 1971). Later, the number of "full house" grafts, i.e., those where all the donor's antigens are known, became large enough almost to eliminate this problem.

The effect of HLA incompatibilities is mainly long term. For this reason it was necessary to wait until a relatively large number of cases, performed under relatively uniform conditions, had been accumulated and a sufficient time had elapsed to evaluate the outcome for each level of incompatibility. It was from 918 cadaver kidney grafts performed within the France Transplant Group (533) and London Transplant Group (385) networks (Dausset *et al.*, 1974) that for the first time the correlation, expected in theory, was found to be significant. A regular increase in the percentage of survival at 2 years was observed depending on the number of identities, starting with none or one, passing through two, then three and ending up with four (Fig. 10.2). It was observed that there was 35% survival at 2 years where there was only one, or no identities, and over 70% when the donor and recipient are serologically indistinguishable at the two major HLA loci. The chances of graft survival are, therefore, doubled when the risk of immunization against the main antigens of the HLA system is eliminated.

An even more stringent analysis was made possible by the use of only those grafts for which all four of the donor's antigens had been serologically determined (full house donor), i.e., those where there was no uncertainty because of a possible homozygosity of one or both of the donor's antigens. The expected correlation was also found (Dausset *et al.*, 1974).

As available material increases, the analysis of HLA incompatibilities may be extended further. One of the first questions is the respective influence of imcompatibilities at the first and second loci.

It is known that in mice the *D* locus appears to be less immunogenic than the *K* locus. Incompatibilities at *D* lead to slower graft rejection, weaker MLR's and less violent GVH's (Chapter 6, Section IX). They are more sensitive to the action of anti-lymphocyte sera. The human homologue of the *D* locus is believed to be the first or A locus. And indeed, analysis has shown that cadaver kidney grafts with an incompatibility at the A locus only have a longer survival time than those with

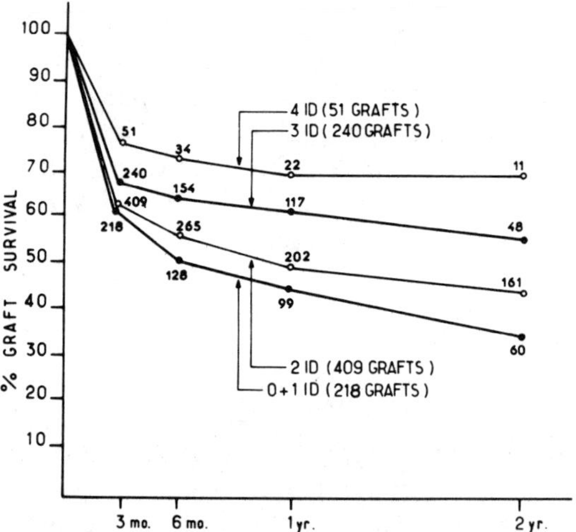


FIG. 10.2. Actuarial graft survival and degree of HLA identity (ID) between donor and recipient (308 first transplants). Figures next to the graphs indicate the number of patients under observation for each consecutive interval. At 3, 6, 12 and 24 months, respectively; 4 ID versus 2, $p < 0.05$, $<0.05$, $<0.05$, not significant; 4 ID versus $1 + 0$, $p < 0.05$, $<0.02$, $<0.001$, $<0.005$; 3 ID versus $1 + 0$, $p$ not significant $<0.01$, $<0.01$, $<0.001$. (From Dausset *et al.*, 1974, reprinted by permission from the *New England Journal of Medicine* **290**, 979–983.

an incompatibility at the B locus only. If this observation is confirmed on a larger scale, it could have important consequences and facilitate the choice of the best donor. Priority should be given to compatibility at the B locus. It is possible that the greater immunogenity of the B locus is only apparent (it is not obvious in humoral immunity) and is in fact due to incompatibilities at the C locus, which are in most cases added to those at the B. If this is indeed the case, HLA typing at the B locus detects incompatibilities at two different loci. It is also known that there is a linkage disequilibrium between the B locus and the main D locus which would also explain the observed difference. As in skin grafts, no one antigen was found, in kidney grafts, to be obviously more immunogenic than another.

Histocompatibility is certainly not the only factor to influence kidney graft fate. There are undoubtedly uncontrollable variations that sometimes mask the influence of histocompatibility in certain statistics. One reason some teams have been unable to find a correlation with the number of incompatibilities is possibly the absence of extremes. Indeed, when the number of patients awaiting transplantation is small but the number of available kidneys relatively large, very incompatible grafts are usually avoided. Very few grafts with four incompatibilities will, therefore, occur. There will also be very few grafts that are very compatible (four identities). The vast majority of grafts will be in the median zone with two or three identities, and therefore the correlation will not appear. Many other factors also partially mask the influence of histocompatibility, the main ones being the heterogeneity of clinical and therapeutic methods and the heterogeneity of serological techniques and criteria. Several other factors are currently under discussion.

The influence of preimmunization (with negative cross match) as defined by the number of pregnancies, transfusions, or previous grafts is evaluated differently. Although the number of pregnancies correlates with appearance of anti-HLA antibodies, it does not seem to influence the fate of the graft. Also, contrary to expectations, it has not been clearly proved that multiple transfusions have a harmful effect. The patient heavily transfused through dialysis is scarcely penalized. It has even been said that graft survival was shortened in a *nontransfused* patient (Opelz *et al.*, 1973). This would tend to indicate that some transfusions, given under appropriate, though still unknown conditions of such variables as number, rhythm, and date in relation to the transplantation operation, may have a beneficial effect. If this were to be confirmed, it would suggest the intervention of enhancing antibodies or the establishment, through transfusion, of a state of cellular unresponsiveness of some kind. This effect has been observed mainly when the graft is compatible.

The influence of preimmunization defined as the presence of antilymphocyte antibodies in the recipient's serum *before* the graft is also variously estimated. Van Hooff *et al.* (1972) consider that the correlation with HLA incompatibility can only be observed in preimmunized patients. Dausset *et al.* (1974), on the other hand, found the same correlation whether or not preformed antibodies existed, but confirmed (1975) that where the preformed antibodies are broadly reactive, interacting with more than 50% of the panel cells, kidney survival is often shortened (Clark *et al.*, 1974). It is also likely that the circulating antibodies to the donor's antigens are mainly active during the first weeks after transplantation, being responsible for the frequent pathological pattern observed at this time, characterized by vascular lesions. Antibodies detectable by the lymphocyte-dependent antibody (LDA) technique could be active at this time (Ting and Terasaki, 1975).

Approximately 30% of chronic dialysis patients develop cytotoxic antibodies. Those patients who do not develop antibodies in spite of many transfusions may be considered as unable to mount, at any rate, easily an immune response. They are commonly referred to as *nonresponders*. Opelz *et al.* (1974) claimed that they were better able to tolerate their grafts, but this has not been found in other studies (Dausset *et al.*, 1974). There are probably several causes of nonresponse: cross-reactions between the donor's and recipient's antigens, production of blocking antibodies which obscure any existing cytotoxic antibodies, and genetic factors that could be aspecific or specific, e.g., the postulated *Ir* genes. These factors must be dissociated before any conclusions can be drawn.

Because it is so easy to show that the HLA complex has a role in kidney graft survival, but so difficult to prove a correlation with the number of incompatible HLA antigens, the question arose whether graft rejection might not in fact be governed by other genes in the complex. Suspicion naturally turned to the D genes governing MLR. Skin grafts between serologically and MLR identical unrelated individuals have been found to have above average survival (15 days), although lower than that of skin grafts between identical sibs (20–25 days). MLR intensity also seems to be connected with skin graft survival—the higher the MLR index, the faster the graft is rejected (Koch *et al.*, 1973). Similarly the studies of Hamburger *et al.* (1971) and Cochrum *et al.* (1973) seem to show that the fate of a kidney graft may be indicated by the intensity of a pregraft MLR between the donor and the recipient.

Another argument in favor of the influence of D factors was sought from the survival of kidneys bearing an HLA haplotype known to have a linkage disequilibrium (Δ) between the D and B loci. There is, for example, a strong Δ between A3, B7, and Dw2, and others are suspected in the haplotypes A1, B8 and A2, B12. The survival of grafts on recipients matched for one of these antigenic patterns and with no preformed antibodies has been found globally improved (Van Hooff *et al.*, 1974). The survival of A1, B8 kidneys in A1, B8 recipients is 71% at 2 years, compared to only 52% in the controls (Dausset *et al.*, 1975).

Observations of the effect of HLA-D identity are in accord with theory, since it is believed that reaction against D incompatibilities occurs before any reaction against A or B locus incompatibilities, although D locus products are not the target for the effector cells (Mawas *et al.*, 1975). Perhaps, as in mice, the ability to produce effector cells is governed by genes of the main histocompatibility system (Festenstein *et al.*, 1974). Should a human equivalent of these genes be situated close to the D locus, the same effect would be observed.

The non-*H-2* systems play an important role in graft rejection in mice (Chapter 3). The existence of comparable systems in man is indicated by, among other evidence, cellular techniques such as CML (Mawas *et al.*, 1973). A B lymphocyte system with a possible influence on skin grafts has been described (Legrand and Dausset, 1975a) (Table 10.3). One other, apparently ubiquitous system, i.e., one whose products like

TABLE 10.3
GENE FREQUENCIES OF LYMPHOCYTE ANTIGENS[a]

| System | Gene | Frequency | Localization |
|---|---|---|---|
| $Ly^D$ | $Ly^{D1}$ | 0.20 | |
| Ly-Co | Ly-Co1 | 0.21 | Probably B lymphocytes |
| Ly-Li | Ly-Li1 | 0.44 | |
| | Ly-Li2 | 0.16 | |

[a] Only 3 anti-$Ly^D$ antibodies have been observed (Shulman *et al.*, 1964), one of which was in a multiparous woman whose children were normal. The Ly-Co system (provisional appelation) was defined by a lymphocytotoxic antibody developed by voluntary immunization between an HLA identical father and daughter. The implications of this system in transplantation have been suggested by skin grafts (Legrand and Dausset, 1975a). A comparison between $Ly^D$ and Ly-Co has not yet been possible. The Ly-Li system (Legrand and Dausset, 1975b), is governed by a gene closely linked to the HLA-D locus (Chapter 9, Section VI,C).

those of the HLA system are found on all the tissues in the organism is the *five* system (Van Leeuwen *et al.*, 1964), with two alleles $5^a$ and $5^b$ (gene frequency 0.326 and 0.964, respectively). The few skin grafts that have been performed with an incompatibility at 5 seem to indicate its irrelevance in transplantation (Van Rood *et al.*, 1965). The existence of differentiation antigens specific for a certain organ, e.g., the kidney, has been suggested. Although this is probable, it does not seem that they play an important role in human transplantation, since this would not account for the almost invariably good results obtained between HLA identical sibs.

ABO compatibility should be respected, as for transfusion (Wilbrandt *et al.*, 1969). It has been claimed that O recipients ($O \rightarrow O$) tolerate their graft longer than non-O ones ($O \rightarrow A$, $A \rightarrow A$, etc.) (Joysey *et al.*, 1973). This difference could be due to anti-$A_1$ antibodies which are sometimes found in the sera of $A_2$ recipients. Another observation is that incompatibilities at the P system have a possibly harmful effect (R. T. D. Oliver, personal communication).

The role of sex has been studied in several analyses. It was feared that because of fetal–maternal interrelations a mother's kidney would be tolerated less well than a father's. No difference was found, however. Nevertheless, a Y-linked antigen has been described in man (Wachtel *et al.*, 1974), and according to Oliver (1974) male cadaver grafts on female recipients survive better than female grafts, which the author explains by an enhancing effect.

### C. Other Organs

Because of the emotional overtones, heart transplants have provoked many well-known objections. In point of fact, the surgical technique has been perfected, but heart transplants suffer from several severe handicaps. The absence of an artificial heart, which can provide a supplement to the failing organ like that offered by the artificial kidney, means that heart transplantation is the last hope and the patient cannot wait long for the most compatible organ. Consequently, the results are almost comparable to those obtained from random kidney transplants (30% survival at 2 years).

Of the other organs, the liver has a special place, at least in current experimentation. The facility with which an allogeneic liver is tolerated in certain pigs has not yet been explained. Is it due to a tolerogenicity peculiar to hepatic antigens, or is it a consequence of the action of hepatic enzymes that modify the immunogenicity of the antigens (Nimelstein *et al.*, 1973)? However, even in pigs this special tolerance does not occur constantly. Encouraging results have been observed in humans, especially children, in spite of the great difficulty of the liver transplant surgical procedure and, here again, the absence of a supplementary apparatus. Some attempts at pancreas transplantation in diabetics have been made. Simultaneous transplantation of pancreas and kidneys is under study. The lung is particularly difficult to transplant because of its many vascular and nervous connections. Some attempts at "heart–lung" transplantation *en bloc* have been made. The intestines and the spleen are also candidates for transplantation, but failure has been the rule. In another field, interstitial corneal transplantation, an everyday procedure, could doubtless benefit if donors were chosen by histocompatibility. It was found that in the presence of marked vascularization of the graft bed, the rate of irreversible graft rejection was significantly influenced by HLA compatibility (Batchelor *et al.*, 1976).

For the treatment of severe burn cases (>60% of the body surface), a selection of skin donors in order to cover the burnt areas for as long as possible has been urged (Chambler and Batchelor, 1969). This is a logical step and the results are as expected. The exact benefits obtained have yet to be established. The creation of a skin bank ought to simplify the logistics of this form of transplantation.

## II. Bone Marrow Grafts

The difficulties and uncertainties which we have just discussed concerning organ transplantation are even more apparent in attempts to graft hematopoietic cells. A major reason for this is the tendency of the immunocompetent cells in the marrow graft to attack the recipient's incompatible alloantigens. The resulting graft-versus-host reaction plus the likelihood of infections in recipients with aplastic anemia leads to an unfavorable prognosis in most such cases.

Nevertheless, since the first attempts in France by Mathé *et al.* (1965), considerable efforts, both clinical and experimental, have been made to overcome these difficulties (reviewed by Bortin, 1970).

Marrow grafts are indicated in all hemopathies that are fatal when usual therapy is given and whose etiology is not a metabolic malfunction or an exterior cause likely to become active on the grafted marrow. This definition could exclude leukemias altogether if their viral origin is accepted, and in fact relapses affecting the grafted marrow have been reported. The best indications are currently immune deficiences, aplastic anemias, Marchiafava–Micheli's syndrome, and possibly hereditary hemoglobulinopathies (see Storb *et al.*, 1974; Dooren *et al.*, 1974).

Two large categories of immune deficiency should be distinguished, depending on whether or not the recipient is able to mount an immune response. When the deficiency is *total,* involving both cellular and humoral response, the same theoretical situation arises as in organ transplants, but it is reversed. Here the recipient cannot reject the graft, but the graft, on the other hand, can attack the recipient; thus, the necessary compatibility is once again unilateral. The recipient merely has to be compatible with the graft.

This clear-cut situation is, however, rarely found, and in most cases the immune deficiency is *partial.* The recipient is still able to mount an immune response against the graft. In this situation, the compatibility has to be good in both directions, and, in fact, identity would be necessary.

## A. The Main Obstacles

Unlike organ transplants bone marrow grafts are still in the experimental stage. Our discussion will be focused on the three main causes of failure: nontake or rejection, graft-versus-host (GVH) reaction, and infection.

### 1. *Nontake or Immunological Rejection*

In the absence of an abortive attempt at take, it is practically impossible to distinguish between nontake and immunological rejection. Failure depends on varying factors: insufficient preparation of the recipient, the number of cells injected, and the existence of preformed antibodies against the donor's cells.

If the recipient has global immune deficiency, only limited or even no preparation is required. However, where the immune system is intact, intensive preparation is needed. Leukemia patients are given total irradiation in the hope of eradicating all the leukemic cells as well, since if they continue to proliferate they could cause a relapse. Aplastic anemia patients are more usually given strong doses of cyclophosphamide (Santos *et al.*, 1972).

One of the most important factors is the number of cells injected. The lowest limit at which a take can be expected has not yet been precisely established in man. In practice as many cells as possible are taken from the donor—adult or child. Experience has shown that graft takes can be obtained with very variable numbers of cells (from $1 \times 10^8$ to $9.4 \times 10^8$ marrow cells per kilogram). It is not known whether a genetic situation exists in man similar to that described by Cudkowicz in mice: nontake due to postulated recessive genes present in the *H-2* complex (*Hh* genes) (Chapter 8, Section II,A).

A role in rejection of a previous immunization by transfusion has been definitely established, primarily by experiments on dogs (Storb *et al.*, 1970). In man, too, a greater number of failures caused by nontake or by rejection has been observed among those patients who had received a large number of transfusions before the graft, even though the cross-match test was negative. Clinicians should thus be forewarned against giving transfusions that are not absolutely vital to patients who may later benefit from a bone marrow graft. It is even advisable to foresee this eventuality on a long-term basis and to avoid using HLA identical sibs as blood donors. It would be better to risk an immunization against antigens that the donor's family do not possess and to keep the chances of sibling graft success high.

### 2. *Graft-versus-Host (GVH) Reaction*

If the preliminary preparatory and compatibility conditions are adequate, signs of graft take, such as a rapid increase of granulocytes, lymphocytes, and then platelets, are observed starting between the fifteenth and thirtieth day.

The major risk is then the appearance of graft-versus-host reaction due to the reaction of donor cells in contact with the recipient's constitutional differences. GVH is unfortunately a very frequent phenomenon, since it is observed in 70% of cases, even when the donor is an HLA identical sib. It causes death in 20% of cases. When it appears early (tenth–twentieth day), this is a sign of gravity. The cutaneous symptoms are constant, occurring in the form of an erythematous eruption, which turns maculopapulous, covering the entire body, especially the extremities (palms, feet, ears). The hepatic attack is manifested by hepatomegaly with an increase of transaminase. Intestinal troubles are often severe. Glandular necroses predominate in the ileum.

Severe and early forms are usually fatal, in spite of the introduction of immunosuppressive therapy. In the forms of only average severity, GVH does not appear until the fifteenth–thirtieth day. The symptoms are milder but involve the same tissues.

Certain heterogeneous complications are sometimes known as *chronic GVH*. It is not certain that these complications are really due to the same mechanism as the graft-versus-host reaction, and they are better referred to as *secondary diseases*. The immunological conflict, however, must be the starting point leading to a state of immune deficiency that takes months to overcome. Although the circulating lymphocytes originate from the healthy donor, they are immunologically incompetent, possibly because of a lack of thymic information since the thymus is destroyed in preparation for the graft. This immune deficit is often the cause of the later death of the patient, especially by virus infection.

The mechanism of GVH is still unknown. There is a tendency to equate MLR and GVH reaction in mice. In man, however, it is obvious that GVH reaction can occur between HLA identical, MLR negative sibs. More probably, differences at other chromosomal areas are capable of leading to the same disorders. In this connection, it should be noted that non-HLA circulating antibodies have been found after GVH reaction between HLA identical sibs (Jeannet *et al.*, 1973; Gluckman, 1974). In one case, the antibodies were active against skin cells.

### B. The Choice of the Donor

Although this may seem paradoxal, a monozygotic twin is not always the ideal donor. If the affliction is genetic in origin, the twin is also liable to be affected, and in cases of malignant hemopathy he is, as has been seen, perhaps the most likely to contract the disease.

In the current state of our knowledge, an HLA identical sib is virtually the only acceptable donor. In some cases, the ABO barrier has been successfully ignored. The chance of a patient having such a sib depends on the number of children in the sibship. In many cases an HLA identical donor does not exist. The search for an HLA identical, MLR negative donor can then be pursued through other members of the family. Among close relatives there is a chance of finding such a donor. If none is found, the last resort is an HLA identical MLR negative unrelated donor, or even one that is only MLR negative. The chance of finding such a donor is about 10% in the most frequent Caucasoid combinations, A1, B8 and A3, B7, in which the B–D locus linkage disequilibrium is strongest. The most rational approach for the future is obviously D typing. At best it can be hoped only to find a situation similar to that of the HLA identical sib, a situation in which there is nevertheless a high percentage of GVH due to unidentified immunogenic differences. Selection by any form of typing will become more and more demanding as the number of known immunogenic systems governing both rejection and GVH increases. In spite of the difficulties, bone marrow grafting is doubtless a therapy of the future.

## III. Implications in Blood Transfusion

Immunization against the antigens of the HLA system occurs very frequently in polytransfused patients. About 50% of patients who have received 30 transfusions possess antibodies that can be detected either by leukoagglutination or by lymphocytotoxicity.

### A. Nonhemolytic Transfusion Reactions

Such immunization by transfusion leads to the appearance of nonhemolytic transfusion reactions—febrile in 80% and with urticarial reactions in 20% of cases. These are often severe and may delay transfusion therapy. For a long time it was thought that mysterious pyrogenic substances in blood were responsible for transfusion shocks. Following the discovery of leukocyte groups, it was realized that most, if not all, transfusion reactions could be the result of the immunological conflict between the recipient's anti-leukocyte antibodies and the injected leukocytes, with the attendant release from damaged leukocytes of pyrogenic substances.

There is no absolute correlation, however, between antibody titers and the intensity of the shock. Doubtless the varied specificity of the antibody or antibodies present in the recipient is responsible for this absence of correlation. Moreover, antibodies are not always demonstrable (see Heinrich *et al.*, 1973; Thulstrup, 1971).

The use of "leukocyte-free" blood from which most of the leukocytes and platelets have been eliminated by mechanical means, effectively prevents most shocks. Blood of this type, in spite of its name, is only partially leukocyte-free, but the number of leukocytes is reduced below the level at which these shocks occur. This level varies from one patient to another. It is somewhere between $5 \times 10^5$ and $10^6$ transfused leukocytes.

## B. Platelet Transfusions

There is a second unfavorable consequence of anti-HLA alloimmunization. Even where there is no transfusion reaction, the survival of platelets and leukocytes is shortened. In a normal state, transfused leukocytes are rapidly sequestered in the lungs, thus making the effect on platelet survival clearer. A sensitive indication of leukoplatelet antibodies can be obtained by measuring the survival time of platelets labeled with radioactive elements. Survival may even be shortened in the absence of antibodies detectable by the usual serological techniques.

The length of survival is related to the number of incompatibilities at the HLA complex. Platelets from an HLA identical sib have a normal length of survival, even in patients who cannot tolerate platelet transfusions from unrelated donors (Yankee *et al.*, 1973). This indicates that immunization against non-HLA antigens, especially the platelet systems Ko and $Pl^A$, at which the individual sibs may differ, are rarely involved. This conclusion is reinforced by the observation that similar survival occurs following transfusion of platelets from HLA phenotypically identical unrelated donors (Lohrmann *et al.*, 1974). Moreover, the efficiency of the platelet contribution increases with the degree of compatibility at the first two loci (Fig. 10.3). A transfusion of identical platelets (A match) gives an increase of 12,500 platelets/$m^2$ per unit of blood at the twentieth hour in excess of that observed with incompatible platelets. A transfusion of platelets with no detectably incompatible antigens but not possessing all the recipient's antigens (B match) gives an increase of only 5300 platelets. It should be noted that platelets in the latter category, except in homozygotes, are probably incompatible at the undetected antigen.

Abbreviation of transfused platelet survival time appears after a varying number of transfusions, depending on the patient. Many factors are involved, including the recipient's HLA type and his ability to form anti-HLA antibodies. In the vast majority of cases, immunization is initially specific, i.e., the platelets of a limited number of donors are rapidly eliminated but other donors' platelets survive normally. Sooner or later, however, immunization seems to become multispecific and the platelets of virtually all donors (except HLA identical sibs) are destroyed in a few hours or even minutes.

To be effective over a long period, platelet transfusions, as far as possible, should not engender immunity in the recipient, especially one whose life depends on this therapy. The first step should be to determine the HLA genotype of members of the immediate family in order to find an HLA identical sib (Yankee *et al.*, 1969). Such a sib is incontest-

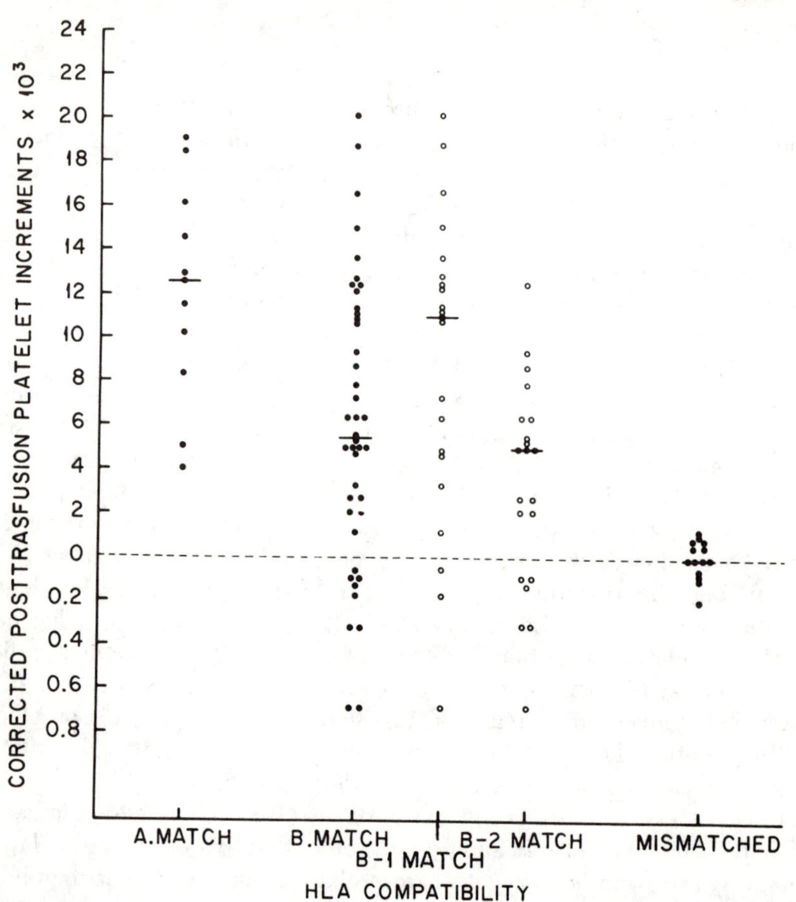


FIG. 10.3. Corrected 20-hour posttransfusion platelet increments (increments × $10^3$/unit) after platelet transfusions in alloimmunized patients, as related to HLA compatibility. Each circle represents a single donor–recipient pair. Donor–recipient pairs of B group have been subdivided into B-1 and B-2 matches, as shown in open circles. B-1 and B-2 indicate, respectively, that 1 or 2 of the antigens found in the recipient could not be detected in the donor. The horizontal lines indicate the medians. (From Lorhmann *et al.*, 1974, courtesy of the *Annals of Internal Medicine.*)

ably the best donor and can be used with a view to hemostasis, even if he is not compatible at the ABO system (Lohrmann *et al.*, 1974). His platelets, collected regularly by plasmapheresis, will continue, as a rule, to have the same efficiency during the entire treatment, no matter how many transfusions are given.

However, in the modern world sibships are frequently small, and it often happens that the patient does not have an HLA identical sib.

An HLA phenotypically identical unrelated individual might be found from a computerized register of blood donors on a national or even international scale. If a phenotypically identical donor is unavailable, the only recourse is to turn to donors who are as compatible as possible and give a negative cross-match. The same donor should be used for as long as possible, until immunization occurs, before going on to another, and so on, making sure that successive donors have the same HLA identities as the recipient, in order to reduce the chances of immunization to a minimum. Thus, long-term transfusion policy for patients with a great risk of prolonged thrombopenia should be carefully planned and strictly adhered to.

It is interesting to note here that one rare but serious type of transfusion accident is not due to HLA incompatibilities but to the platelet system $Pl^{A}$ (Table 10.4). A severe thrombopenia occurs 5 to 7 days after a blood transfusion. Most often this occurs in a $Pl^{A1}$ negative woman, immunized by $Pl^{A1}$ positive platelets. As soon as the antibody reaches a certain titer, the transfused platelets are destroyed. The disappearance of the patient's own platelets remains unexplained. Shulman *et al.* (1961) suggest that this destruction is due to antigen–antibody complexes becoming fixed on the patient's own platelets.

### C. Leukocyte Transfusions

Leukocyte transfusion has assumed an important place in therapeutics. It is mainly indicated for the preventative or curative struggle against infection in cases of severe aplasia or granulopenia. Granulocytes and monocytes are therefore the indicated cell type, but to be effective the quantity transfused must be greatly in excess of the pulmonary capillaries' storage capacity. At least $5 \times 10^{10}$ to $10^{11}$ leukocytes should be transfused at one time. Leukocyte survival is short. Only 10% are circulating at 6 hours in the case of a normal donor and at 24 hours when the donor is a chronic myelocytic leukemia patient. Thus the injection has to be repeated several times, on a daily or even more frequent basis (Graw *et al.*, 1970; Goldstein *et al.*, 1971). This poses a severe supply problem. The use of an HLA identical sib is possible, but not in the same continuous way as for platelet transfusions, since repeated sessions of leukocyte removal by continuous separation are physically exhausting. Several healthy donors are necessary. Although the efficiency of blood from chronic myeloid leukemia patients has been proved, there is a risk that transfused leukemic cells will proprogate. There is also a risk in leukocyte transfusions of a fatal GVH syndrome. This can be avoided by systematic irradiation of the blood prior to injection.

TABLE 10.4
GENE FREQUENCIES OF PLATELET ANTIGENS[a]

| System | Gene | Frequency |
|---|---|---|
| $Pl^A$(Zw) | $Pl^{A1}$($Zw^a$) | 0.845 |
| | $Pl^{A2}$($Zw^b$) | 0.144 |
| $Pl^E$ | $Pl^{E1}$ | Public (only one person without the antigen is known) |
| | $Pl^{E2}$ | 0.025 |
| Ko | $Ko^a$ | 0.074 |
| | $Ko^b$ | 0.920 |

[a] The $Pl^A$(Zw) system was discovered independently by Van Loghem *et al.* (1959) using thromboagglutination and by Shulman *et al.* (1961) using platelet complement fixation. Incompatibilities in this system are responsible for neonatal and posttransfusional purpuras. Anti-$Pl^{E1}$ antibodies can also cause neonatal purpuras (Shulman *et al.*, 1964). Ko antigens can be detected by thromboagglutination (Van der Weerdt, 1965). Anti-Ko antibodies are mostly IgM, which cannot cross the placenta.

The role of the neutrophil blood alloantigens in leukocyte transfusions has not been fully determined. Anti-granulocyte antibodies, demonstrable mainly by leukoagglutination and directed against specific neutrophil antigens of the NA, NB, or 9 systems (Table 10.5) are probably relatively frequent and able to reduce survival and thus the efficiency of this type of transfusion.

## IV. Fetal–Maternal Relationship: Neonatal Thrombopenia and Leukoneutropenia

The possible influence of anti-HLA antibodies on pre-or postzygotic selection has been discussed (Chapter 9, Section II,A). Here we are concerned with the clinical effects of these antibodies on the fetus. In spite of the frequency of maternal immunization, the fetus is normally unharmed, even though HLA antibodies, which are mostly IgG, can cross the placenta.

Various parameters of pregnancy, as related to the presence or absence of anti-HLA antibodies, have been studied exhaustively—abortion, prematurity, the weight of the placenta and of the baby, the number of different varieties of leukocytes and of platelets, the state of pre-

TABLE 10.5
GENE FREQUENCIES OF GRANULOCYTE ANTIGENS[a]

| System | Gene | Frequency | Localization |
|---|---|---|---|
| NA | NA1 | 0.337 | Neutrophils |
| | NA2 | 0.663 | |
| NB | NB1 | 0.83 | |
| 9 | $9^a$ | 0.408 | Neutrophils and eosinophils |

[a] Neutrophil granulocytes possess differentiation antigens that can be detected by leukoagglutination. Anti-NA or-NB antibodies have been found in the mothers of children suffering from newborns' neutropenia. It is, therefore, extremely probable that they play a part in causing this disease (Lalezari and Radel, 1974). $9^a$ is an antigen found on neutrophils and eosinophils (basophils have not been tested) (Van Rood *et al.*, 1966). No newborns' neutropenia attributable to anti-9a has been found.

eclampsia, arterial hypertension, albuminuria, edemia—but no abnormalities have been found (Ahrons, 1971). Jensen (1964) reported a greater number of premature deliveries (17%) in mothers possessing leukoagglutinins, but this observation has not been confirmed.

The usual explanation of the seeming harmlessness of these antibodies is their absorption by the vast mass of HLA antigens present on all the nucleated cells of the placenta and the fetal organism. The number of antibody molecules per cell is thought to be too low to have a deleterious effect. This harmlessness may be contrasted to the severe toxicity of antibodies directed against platelet or granulocyte group antigens. These differentiation antigens are limited to particular blood elements and thus to a considerably smaller number of cells than HLA antigens.

Neonatal purpura by alloimmunization is a relatively rare affliction (approximately 1/10,000 births). Curiously, in half the cases it is the firstborn who is affected. Prior transfusions, causing the mother to be immunized, do not seem to play a major role; it is usually quite harmless, but mortality is nevertheless 11%, mainly due to intracranial hemorrhages.

Anti-HLA antibodies (especially anti-A2) have been held responsible for some cases of neonatal thrombopenic purpura. However there is as yet no biological proof of their role. In no cases are there clear-cut associations between this affliction and the presence or absence of the paternal antigens against which the mother has become immunized (Payne, 1964).

On the other hand, the role of antibodies developed against specifically platelet antigens, such as those belonging to the systems $Pl^A$ and $Pl^E$, has been clearly shown (Shulman *et al.*, 1964). Out of 63 familial cases reported, 17 have been found to be due to an anti-$Pl^{A1}$ and one to an anti-$Pl^{E1}$. The others were due to unknown specificities. The most remarkable fact is doubtless that in many cases the responsible anti-$Pl^{A1}$ antibodies were blocking antibodies, detected because they inhibited a nonblocking antibody of the same specificity in platelet complement fixation. It is now known that similar blocking antibodies exist in the HLA system (Colombani *et al.*, 1973; Sanderson *et al.*, 1972) and could therefore in some rare cases be responsible for newborn thrombopenic accidents. No neonatal purpuras have been attributed to antibodies against a third platelet system, the Ko system, which seems to engender IgM antibodies, detectable by thromboagglutination, which cannot cross the placenta (Table 10.4).

Newborn neutropenia is now well documented (Lalezari and Radel, 1974). In all the cases published, it was due to anti-neutrophil antibodies against two separate systems, NA and NB (Table 10.5). These antibodies can be detected by leukoagglutination. They persist for a long time after parturition, provoking serious accidents when subsequent fetuses are incompatible. Fortunately they rarely appear; occurrence in only about twenty families has been reported. An interesting and unexplained observation is that neutropenia caused by anti-neutrophil antibody occurs between the third and eleventh day after delivery. Antibodies against a fourth system, 9 (Van Rood *et al.*, 1966), are active on neutrophils and eosinophils. No newborn neutropenia due to incompatibility at this system has been reported (Table 10.5).

There is no evidence that anti-HLA antibodies are responsible for isolated newborn neutropenias. Because of the ubiquity of the antigens and the disproportionate size of the leukocyte and platelet reserves, it seems understandable that platelets would be the first structures affected.

## REFERENCES

Ahrons, S. 1971. HL-A antibodies: Influence on the human foetus. *Tissue Antigens* 1:121–128.

Amos, D. B., B. G. Hattler, J. M. MacQueen, I. Cohen, and H. J. Seigler. 1967. An interpretation and application of cytotoxicity typing. Pages 203–212 *in* J. Dausset, J. Hamburger, and G. Mathé, eds. Advances in transplantation. Munksgaard, Copenhagen.

Amos, D. B., H. F. Seigler, J. G. Southworth, and F. E. Ward. 1969. Skin graft rejection between subjects genotyped for HL-A. *Transplant Proc* 1:342–346.

Balner, H., and H. Dersjant. 1965. Iso-antibodies against leukocytes as a tool to study histocompatibility in monkeys. Pages 103–112 *in* H. Balner, F. L. Cleton, and J. G. Eernisse, eds. Histocompatibility Testing 1965. Munksgaard, Copenhagen.

Batchelor, J. R., D. C. Gibbs, T. Casey, A. Werb, and W. Schlesinger. 1976. The influence of HL-A compatibility on the fate of full thickness corneal allografts. In preparation.

Bortin, M. M. 1970. A compendium of reported human bone-marrow transplants. *Transplantation* **9**:571–587.

Ceppellini, R. 1968. The genetic basis of transplantation. Pages 21–34 *in* F. T. Rapaport and J. Dausset, eds. Human transplantation. Grune & Stratton, New York.

Ceppellini, R., E. S. Curtoni, P. L. Mattiuz, G. Leigheb, M. Visetti, and A. Colombi. 1966. Survival of test skin grafts in man: Effect of genetic relationship and of blood group incompatibility. *Ann NY Acad Sci* **129**:421–445.

Ceppellini, R., S. Bigliari, E. S. Curtoni, and G. Leigheb. 1969a. Allotransplantation in man. II. The role of A1, A2, and B antigens. *Transplantation Proc* **1**:390–391.

Ceppellini, R., P. L. Mattiuz, G. Scudeller, and M. Visetti. 1969b. Experimental allotransplantation in man. I. The role of the HL-A system in different genetic combinations. *Transplant Proc* **1**:385–389.

Chambler, K., and J. R. Batchelor. 1969. Influence of defined incompatibilities and area of burn on skin homograft survival in burned subjects. *Lancet* **1**:16–18.

Clark, E. A., P. I. Terasaki, G. Opelz, and M. R. Mickey. 1974. Cadaver-kidney transplant failures at one month. *N Engl J Med* **291**:1099–1102.

Cochrum, K. C., H. A. Perkins, R. O. Payne, S. L. Kountz, and F. O. Belzer. 1973. The correlation of MLC with graft survival. *Transplant Proc* **5**:391–396.

Colombani, J., M. Colombani, and J. Dausset. 1973. Non-complement-fixing IgM antibodies wih anti-HL-A2 specificity and blocking activity. *Transplantation* **16**:257–260.

Dausset, J., and J. Colombani. 1962. Iso-anticorps anti-leucocytaires et anti-plaquettaires. Sérologie et importance pratique en particulier pour les greffes. *Proc Congr Int Soc Blood Transf, 8th, 1960* Pages 324–329.

Dausset, J., and F. T. Rapaport. 1968. Blood group determinants of human histocompatibility. Pages 383–393 *in* F. T. Rapaport and J. Dausset, eds. Human transplantation. Grune & Stratton, New York.

Dausset, J., F. T. Rapaport, P. Iványi, and J. Colombani. 1965. Tissue alloantigens and transplantation. Pages 63–72 *in* H. Balner, F. L. Cleton, and J. G. Eernisse, eds. Histocompatibility Testing 1965. Munksgaard, Copenhagen.

Dausset, J., J. Hors, and J. Bigot. 1969. Etude génotypique de l'histocompatibilité HL-A dans 91 greffes de rein. *Presse Med* **77**:1699–1704.

Dausset, J., F. T. Rapaport, L. Legrand, J. Colombani, and A. Marcelli-Barge. 1970. Skin allograft survival in 238 human subjects: Role of specific relationships at the four gene sites of the first and the second HL-A loci. Pages 381–397 *in* P. I. Terasaki, ed. Histocompatibility Testing 1970. Munksgaard, Copenhagen.

Dausset, J., J. Hors, M. Busson, H. Festenstein, R. T. D. Oliver, A. M. I. Paris, and J. A. Sachs. 1974. Serologically defined HL-A antigens and long-term survival of cadaver kidney transplants. *N Engl J Med* **290**:979–983.

Dausset, J., J. Hors, and M. Busson. 1975. Histocompatibility and kidney transplantation (within the France-Transplant network). *Proc Int Congr Nephrol, 6th, 1975* Karger, Basel.

Dooren, L. J., R. P. Kamphuis, J. DeKoning, and J. M. Vossen. 1974. Bone marrow transplantation in children. *Semin Hematol* **11**:369–382.

Festenstein, H., K. Abbasi, and P. Démant. 1974. The genetic basis of the generation of effector capacity for cell mediated lympholysis in mice. *J Immunogen* **1**:47–51.

Gluckman, E. 1974. Le conditionnement des malades en vue de la transplantation de moelle osseuse. Résultats récents. *Nouv Rev Fr Hematol* **14**:531–533.

Goldstein, I. M., H. J. Eyre, P. I. Terasaki, E. S. Henderson, and R. G. Graw. 1971. Leukocyte transfusions: role of leukocyte allo-antibodies in determining transfusion response. *Transfusion* **11**:19–25.

Graw, R. G., H. J. Eyre, I. M. Goldstein, and P. I. Terasaki. 1970. Histocompatibility testing for leucocyte transfusion. *Lancet* **2**:77–78.

Hamburger, J., J. Crosnier, B. Descamps, and D. Rowinska. 1971. The value of present methods used for the selection of organ donors. *Transplant Proc* **3**:260–267.

Heinrich, D., C. Mueller-Eckhardt, and W. Stier. 1973. The specificity of leukocyte and platelet allo antibodies in sera of patients with nonhemolytic transfusion reactions. Absorption and elution studies. *Vox Sang* **25**:442–456.

Hors, J., N. Feingold, D. Fradelizi, and J. Dausset. 1971. Critical evaluation of histocompatibility in 179 renal transplants. *Lancet* **1**:609–612.

Jeannet, M., A. Rubinstein, and B. Pelet. 1973. Studies on non-HL-A cytotoxic and blocking factor in a patient with immunological deficiency successfully reconstituted by bone marrow transplantation. *Tissue Antigens* **3**:411–416.

Jensen, K. G. 1964. Leucocyte antibodies in serums of pregnant women. Serology and clinic II. *Vox Sang* **9**:315–332.

Joysey, V. C., J. H. Roger, D. B. Evans, and B. M. Herbertson. 1973. Kidney graft survival and matching for HL-A and ABO antigens. *Nature* (*Lond*) **246**:163–165.

Kissmeyer-Nielsen, F., S. Olsen, V. P. Petersen, and O. Fjeldborg. 1966. Hyperacute rejection of kidney allograft associated with pre-existing humoral antibodies against donor cells. *Lancet* **2**:662–665.

Koch, C. T., J. P. Van Hooff, A. Van Leeuwen, J. G. Van den Tweel, E. Frederiks, G. J. Van der Steen, H. M. A. Schippers, and J. J. Van Rood. 1973. The relative importance of matching for the MLC versus the HL-A loci in organ transplantation. Pages 521–526 *in* J. Dausset and J. Colombani, eds. Histocompatibility Testing 1972. Munksgaard, Copenhagen.

Lalezari, P., and F. Radel. 1974. Neutrophil specific antigens: Immunology and clinical significance. *Semin Haematol* **11**:281–290.

Legrand, L., and J. Dausset. 1975a. Immunogenetics of a new lymphocyte system. *Transplant Proc* **7**:5–8.

Legrand, L., and J. Dausset. 1975b. A second lymphocyte system (Ly-Li). Pages 665–668 *in* Kissmeyer-Nielsen, ed. Histocompatibility testing. 1975. Munksgaard, Cophenhagen.

Lohrmann, H. P., M. I. Bull, J. A. Delter, R. A. Yankee, and R. G. Graw. 1974. Platelet transfusion from HL-A compatible unrelated donors to alloimmunized patients. *Ann Intern Med* **80**:9–14.

Mathé, G., J. L. Amiel, L. Schwarzenberg, A. Cattan, M. Schneider, M. J. de Vries, M. Tubiana, M. Papiernik, A. M. Mery, C. Lalanne, G. Seman, W. Schwarzmann, J. L. Binet, M. Matsukura, and A. Flaisler. 1965. Successful allogeneic bone marrow transplantation in man: Chimerism, induced specific tolerance and possible anti-leukemic effects. *Blood* **25**:179–196.

Mawas, C., M. Sasportes, Y. Christen, A. Bernard, J. Dausset, B. J. Alter, and M. L. Bach. 1973. Cell-mediated lympholysis (CML) in the absence of LD2 mixed lymphocyte reaction and CML in the presence of SD1-SD2 identity in two HL-A-genotyped families. *Transplant Proc* **5**:1683–1689.

Mawas, C., D. Charmot, and M. Sasportes. 1975. Is the *LD* region of the human MHC a CML target? Pages 855–857 *in* F. Kissmeyer-Nielsen, ed. Histocompatibility Testing 1975. Munksgaard, Copenhagen.

Nimelstein, S. H., A. R. Hotti, and H. R. Holman. 1973. Transformation of histocompatibility immunogen into a tolerogen. *J Exp Med* **138**:723–733.

Oliver, R. T. D. 1974. Possible evidence for Y-linked histocompatibility antigen in man. *Eur J Immunol* **4**:519–520.

Opelz, G., D. P. S. Sengar, and M. R. Mickey. 1973. Effect of blood transfusions on subsequent kidney transplant. *Transplant Proc* **5**:253–259.

Opelz, G., M. R. Mickey, and P. I. Terasaki. 1974. HL-A and kidney transplants: Reexamination. *Transplantation* **17**:371–382.

Payne, R. 1964. Neonatal neutropenia and leukoagglutinins. *Pediatrics* **33**:194–204.

Rapaport, F. T., L. Thomas, J. M. Converse, and H. S. Lawrence. 1960. The specificity of skin homograft rejection in man. *Ann NY Acad Sci* **87**:217–222.

Rapaport, F. T., J. Dausset, L. Legrand, A. Barge, H. S. Lawrence, and J. M. Converse, 1968. Erythrocytes in human transplantation. Effects of pretreatment with ABO group-specific antigens. *J Clin Invest* **47**:2206–2216.

Sanderson, D. R., E. W. Gelfand, and F. S. Rosen. 1972. A change in HL-A phenotype associated with specific blocking factors in the serum of an infant with severe combined immunodeficiency disease. *Transplantation* **13**:142–145.

Santos, G. W., L. L. Sensenbrenner, P. J. Burke, G. M. Mullins, W. B. Bias, P. J. Tutschka, and R. E. Slavin. 1972. The use of cyclophosphamide for clinical marrow transplantation. *Transplant Proc* **4**:559–564.

Shulman, N. R., R. H. Aster, A. Leitner, and M. C. Hiller. 1961. Immunoreactions involving platelets. V. Post-transfusion due to a complement fixing antibody against a genetically controlled platelet antigen. A proposed mechanism for thrombocytopenia and its relevance in autoimmunity. *J Clin Invest* **40**:1597.

Shulman, N. R., V. J. Marder, M. C. Hiller, and E. M. Collier. 1964. Platelet and leukocyte isoantigens and their antibodies: Serologic, physiologic and clinical studies. *Prog Hematol* **4**:222–304.

Singal, D. P., M. R. Mickey, and P. I. Terasaki. 1969. Serotyping for homotransplantation. XXIII. Analysis of kidney transplants from parental versus sibling donors. *Transplantation* **7**:246–258.

Starzl, T. E., R. A. Lerner, F. J. Dixon, C. G. Groth, L. Brettschneider, and P. I. Terasaki. 1968. Schwartzman reaction after human renal homotransplantation. *N Engl J Med* **278**:642–648.

Storb, R., R. B. Epstein, R. H. Rudolph, and E. Thomas. 1970. The effect of prior transfusion on marrow grafts between histocompatible canine siblings. *J Immunol* **105**:627–633.

Storb, R., E. D. Thomas, C. D. Buckner, R. A. Clift, A. Fefer, H. Glucksberg, and P. E. Neiman. 1974. Transplantation of bone marrow in refractory marrow failure and neoplastic diseases. *Am J Clin Pathol* **62**:212–217.

Thulstrup, H. 1971. The influence of leukocyte and thrombocyte incompatibility on non-haemolytic transfusion reactions. II. A prospective study. *Vox Sang* **21**:434–442.

Ting, A., and P. I. Terasaki. 1975. Lymphocyte-dependent antibody cross-matching for transplant patients. *Lancet* **1**:304–306.

Van der Weerdt, C. M. 1965. Platelet antigens and iso-immunisation. Thesis, Univ. Amsterdam.

Van Hooff, J. P., H. M. A. Schippers, G. J. Van der Steen, and J. J. Van Rood. 1972. Efficacy of HL-A matching in Euro-transplant. *Lancet* **2**:1385–1388.

Van Hooff, J. P., H. M. A. Schippers, G. F. J. Hendriks, and J. J. Van Rood. 1974. Influence of possible HL-A haploidentity on renal-graft survival in Eurotransplant. *Lancet* **1**:1130–1132.

Van Leeuwen, A., J. G. Eernisse, and J. J. Van Rood. 1964. A new leucocyte group with two alleles: Leucocyte group five. *Vox Sang* **9**:431–444.

Van Loghem, J. J., H. Dorfmeier, M. Van der Hart, and F. Schreuder. 1959. Serological and genetical studies on a platelet antigen (Zw). *Vox Sang* **4**:161–169.

Van Rood, J. J., A. Van Leeuwen, A. M. J. Schippers, W. H. Vooys, E. Frederiks, H. Balner, and J. G. Eernisse. 1965. Leucocyte groups, the normal lymphocyte transfer and homograft sensitivity. Pages 37–50 *in* H. Balner, F. L. Cleton, and J. G. Eernisse, eds. Histocompatibility Testing 1965. Munksgaard, Copenhagen.

Van Rood, J. J., A. Van Leeuwen, J. W. Bruning, and J. G. Eernisse. 1966. Current status of human leukocyte groups. *Ann NY Acad Sci* **129**:446–464.

Van Rood, J. J., A. Van Leeuwen, J. W. Bruning, and K. A. Porter. 1967. The importance of leukocyte antigens in renal transplantation. A study of patients of G. R. J. Alexandre, J. Van Geertruyden, W. D. Kelly, J. P. Merrill, J. Morelle, J. P. Nombray, J. Murray, P. S. Russell, T. E. Starzl, C. Toussaint, and M. F. A. Woodruff. Pages 213–219 *in* J. Dausset, J. Hamburger, and G. Mathé, eds. Advances in transplantation. Munksgaard, Copenhagen.

Wachtel, S. S., G. C. Koo, E. E. Zukerman, U. Hammerling, P. P. Scheid, and A. A. Boyse. 1974. Serological cross reactivity between H-Y (male) antigen of mouse and man. *Proc Natl Acad Sci USA* **71**:1215–1218.

Wilbrandt, R., K. S. K. Tung, S. D. Deodar, S. Nakamoto, and W. J. Kolff. 1969. ABO blood group incompatibility in human renal homotransplantation. *Am J Clin Pathol* **51**:15–23.

Yankee, R. A., F. C. Grumet, and G. N. Rogentine. 1969. Platelet transfusion therapy. The selection of compatible platelet donors for refractory patients by lymphocyte HL-A typing. *N Engl J Med* **281**:1208–1212.

Yankee, R. A., K. S. Graff, R. Dowling, and E. S. Henderson. 1973. Selection of unrelated compatible platelet donors by lymphocyte HL-A matching. *N Engl J Med* **288**:760–764.

CHAPTER 11

# BIOCHEMICAL AND STRUCTURAL PROPERTIES OF THE CELL MEMBRANE LOCATED ALLOANTIGENS OF THE MAJOR HISTOCOMPATIBILITY COMPLEX*



* In collaboration with John H. Freed, Department of Microbiology and Immunology, Albert Einstein College of Medicine, New York, New York.

## I. Introduction

As has been amply documented in the previous chapters, the list of defined cell membrane-located alloantigen systems is large and varied. Each is unique with specific genetic and immunological characteristics. The alloantigens which have been most fully characterized chemically are the classical major histocompatibility complex (MHC) glycoproteins: the H-2K and H-2D antigens of the mouse and the first or A series and second or B series antigens of man. A description of the biochemical, immunochemical, and dynamic properties of these antigens forms the major portion of this chapter. The chemical properties of the Tla (also designated TL) and Ia antigens of the mouse, while less well defined, are discussed as well.

## II. Location

The tissue distribution for each of the defined membrane alloantigens is specific and distinctive (Chapter 5). The antigenic products of the classical histocompatibility loci of the MHC, e.g., H-2D and H-2K in the mouse and the A and B series in man, are present in nearly all tissues. On the other hand, the murine Ia antigens, whose genetic determinants map with the *H-2K* and *H-2D* genes, are found mainly on lymphocytes, and the Tla antigens exclusively on thymocytes. Thus, in keeping with the general contention that each *H* gene product must have a unique function, it is reasonable to find that such products have different tissue distributions.

With regard to their subcellular distribution, the antigenic products of the MHC of the mouse and man are situated on the cell surface. However, while it is clear that a large proportion of these antigens are on the cell surface, it is likely that in some cells and possibly at particular stages in the cell cycle, some antigens may also be located on the internal membranes.

The evidence for the location of the H-2 antigens on the cell surface comes from studies visualizing these antigens at the cell membrane by light and electron microscopy (Möller, 1961; Davis and Silverman, 1968; Aoki *et al.*, 1969). Additional evidence comes from studies utilizing proteolytic digestion to remove the antigens from the cell surface. For example, proteolytic treatment of mouse or human lymphoblastoid cell lines can release MHC glycoproteins without killing or lysing the cells (Schwartz and Nathenson, 1971a; Turner *et al.*, 1972). Such an observation suggests a cell surface location. Studies using separated and partially purified membrane fractions also clearly suggest that the H-2 and HLA antigens are located in the membrane fractions isolated from the cell surface (see review by Nathenson, 1970).

The question of the extent to which H-2 alloantigens are found on internal membranes has been difficult to answer quantitatively. Some groups (Palm and Manson, 1968) suggest that a relatively large amount of antigenic activity is found associated with internal membrane systems. Other studies suggest that most of the antigenic activity (with regard to H-2 at least), is found in external membrane fractions (Ozer and Wallach, 1967). In addition it may be that during different periods in the cell cycle, in different cell types, or in cells from different tissues, the H-2 antigen is distributed differently relative to the surface and the internal membranes [see discussion of dynamic properties of these antigen molecules (Section VII)]. For the purpose of our discussion, however, it is important to remember that the external surface is well populated by these antigenic molecules.

The quantity of the H-2 and HLA products on the cell surface can be estimated from several different types of studies. Biochemical isolation studies indicate that the H-2K and H-2D antigens represent about 1% of the protein of the cell surface of lymphocytes (Schwartz and Nathenson, 1971b). These molecules, therefore, form only a small proportion of all cell surface macromolecules. Measurements by labeled antibody binding techniques have placed the number of exposed H-2 antigens per lymphocyte at about 600,000 (Hämmerling and Eggers, 1970) and HLA antigens at not less than 30,000 per lympocyte (Sanderson and Welsh, 1974). In view of the similarity of H-2 and HLA antigens, one would expect these estimates to be closer. The reason for such large differences is not clear. For comparison, amounts of Thy-1 range from 500,000 to 1,000,000 molecules per T lymphocyte (Acton *et al.*, 1974), while B lymphocytes completely lack the Thy-1 antigen. Other antigen systems have much lower densities. For example, the Tla antigen is usually recovered in yields of 0.1% of the total thymocyte membrane protein.

## III. Biochemical and Structural Properties

The molecules determined by the *H-2K* and *H-2D* genes, and the A series and B series HLA genes, are glycoproteins of about 45,000 daltons which are tightly integrated into the matrix of the plasma membrane. *In situ,* the glycoproteins are noncovalently associated with an 11,600 dalton protein, the $\beta_2$-microglobulin. The association is probably in a 1:1 ratio and is thought to be specific (see Section III,D).

According to recent membrane models, the overall general structure of the external or plasma cell membrane of a mammalian cell is that of a fluid bilayer in which the lipid supports or contains protein and glycoprotein molecules. While lateral displacement of these proteinaceous macromolecules is not hindered, they are restricted to the plane of the membrane by their hydrophobic properties. This cell membrane carries many different proteins and glycoproteins in its lipid matrix, each of which may have a different function. The membrane described by such a model is referred to as a fluid mosaic (Singer, 1974).

The hydrophobic character of the membrane and its components makes it necessary to undertake special solubilization steps before each individual macromolecule can be separately isolated for study. Two general techniques have been used successfully to isolate in an immunologically active form the histocompatibility antigens from their membrane sites. One approach is to utilize proteolytic cleavage to release the antigens from the membrane. The second method is to employ detergents to dissolve membrane structure and release the alloantigens.

Both approaches have provided a great deal of information about the basic structure of the H-2 and HLA molecules. The fragments released by limited proteolysis of the membrane of whole cells are biologically active and easily purified by standard biochemical techniques. The plant protease papain is the most widely used for this purpose and was first described for H-2 antigens (Shimada and Nathenson, 1969), and later for HLA (Sanderson, 1968; Mann *et al.*, 1969a; Boyle, 1969; Miyakawa *et al.*, 1971; Cresswell *et al.*, 1973). Ficin and simple autolysis were reported earlier (Nathenson and Davies, 1966) for the *H-2* system, and these methods provide a similar product. KCl extraction (Reisfeld *et al.*, 1971) is included under the proteolytic classification, since it appears that the KCl product is most probably the result of controlled autolysis (Mann, 1972).

The alloantigenic product produced by proteolysis is, of course, only a fragment of the native glycoprotein that is released by detergent, a fact that limits the amount of information that can be obtained by this method. This disadvantage is overcome when the antigenic molecules are solubilized by detergent. Both ionic (deoxycholate) and nonionic (Triton, NP-40, Brij) detergents have been used. The antigenic molecules released by these agents are more difficult to assay and purify, but ultimately these products are needed in order to define the total serological and chemical structure of the H-2 and HLA glycoproteins.

## A. General Chemical Properties

### 1. *Molecules Isolated after Enzymatic Proteolytic Cleavage*

In the method of release by enzyme cleavage, enzymes such as ficin or papain release fragments bearing the intact antigenic sites from their membrane associated state. Either whole cells or membrane fractions can be treated with the proteolytic enzyme, and, after an appropriate time period, the membranes or cells are removed and the soluble supernatant analyzed for antigenic activity. When H-2 alloantigens were solubilized with crystalline papain, two different sized antigenically reactive fragments were recovered after the enzymatic solubilization step (Shimada and Nathenson, 1969). They were purified by a series of fractionation procedures. Analyses of these fragments showed that one series had a molecular weight of approximately 37,000 to 44,000 daltons as shown in Table 11.1. These fragments consisted of 90% protein and 10% carbohydrate. The fragments from two strains differing in their *H-2* haplotype ($H\text{-}2^b$ and $H\text{-}2^d$) had similar overall chemical analysis. The second class of fragments with a molecular weight of approximately 28,000 daltons was not analyzed as thoroughly because only small amounts were available. However, these fragments were also glycoproteins. The molecular weight estimates were established from their relative migration on sodium dodecyl sulfate electrophoresis on polyacrylamide gels of several different pore sizes to overcome possible anomalous migra-

TABLE 11.1
General Chemical and Serological Properties of Papain-Solubilized H-2 Alloantigens[a]

| | Class I | Class II |
|---|---|---|
| Molecular weight (daltons) | | |
| $H\text{-}2^d$ | | |
| $H\text{-}2D^d$ (H-2.4) | 37,000 | Not found |
| $H\text{-}2K^d$ (H-2.31) | 44,000 | 28,000 |
| $H\text{-}2^b$ | | |
| $H\text{-}2D^b$ (H-2.2) | 44,000 | 28,000 |
| $H\text{-}2K^b$ (H-2.33) | 37,000 | Not found |
| Chemical composition | | |
| Protein (%) | 80–90 | 75–85 |
| Neutral carbohydrate (%) | 4–6 | 4–8 |
| Glucosamine (%) | 3–5 | 2–8 |
| Sialic acid (%) | 1 | 0.2–2.5 |

[a] Data taken from Shimada and Nathenson (1969) and Schwartz *et al.* (1973a).

tion due to carbohydrate content. While both the 37,000 to 44,000 dalton and 28,000 dalton fragments were antigenically active, each carried exclusively one private specificity and one or more public specificities.

Papain proteolysis also has been demonstrated to release HLA antigen fragments in antigenically active form (Sanderson, 1968; Batchelor and Sanderson, 1969; Mann *et al.*, 1969b; Boyle, 1969; Miyakawa *et al.*, 1971; Tanigaki *et al.*, 1971; Cresswell *et al.*, 1973). Purification schemes in different laboratories have varied somewhat but have generally included gel filtration, electrophoresis, and in some cases ion exchange chromatography. In some cases preparation of purified membrane fractions preceeded solubilization. While some groups have utilized cell sources internally radiolabeled with amino acids or sugar precursors, others have characterized mainly nonradiolabeled materials or radioiodinated purified antigens.

Each of these laboratories has reported slightly different molecular weights for the purified antigens. However, as indicated in Table 11.2, when fully dissociated, the papain solubilized HLA fragments have molecular weights in the range of 29,000 to 34,000 daltons regardless of whether they belong to the A or B series.

The molecular weight determinations made on the same HLA antigens under nondenaturing conditions, however, vary from 48,000 to 96,000 daltons depending on the exact experimental conditions employed in the determination. This variability almost certainly reflects the amount of quaternary structure preserved during the molecular weight determination. If the 11,600 dalton $\beta_2$-microglobulin subunit (Nakamuro *et al.*, 1973; Peterson *et al.*, 1974; Cresswell *et al.*, 1974b) is present with

TABLE 11.2
MOLECULAR WEIGHT IN DISSOCIATING SOLVENTS OF HLA GLYCOPROTEIN FRAGMENTS SOLUBILIZED BY PAPAIN

| Antigen | Molecular weight and method[a] | Reference |
|---|---|---|
| HLA-A2, HLA-B7 | 34,000 SDS/PAGE | Cresswell *et al.*, 1974a |
| HLA-A2 | 32,000 SDS/gel filtration | Cresswell *et al.*, 1974a |
| HLA-A2, HLA-B7 | 29,000 guanidine/gel filtration | Cresswell *et al.*, 1974a |
| HLA-A1, HLA-A2, HLA-B7 | 33,000 SDS/PAGE | Tanigaki *et al.*, 1974 |

[a] PAGE, polyacrylamide gel electrophoresis.

the larger 34,000 dalton fragment, then a weight of 45,000 to 50,000 daltons is obtained (Mann *et al.*, 1969a; Sanderson *et al.*, 1971; Miyakawa *et al.*, 1973; Cresswell *et al.*, 1974a). On the other hand, use of conditions that prevent dissociation of the dimer formed by the 34,000 dalton chains, allows observation of a 96,000 dalton "tetramer" presumably consisting of two 34,000 dalton fragments combined with two $\beta_2$-microglobulin molecules (Strominger *et al.*, 1974).

Pressman and co-workers have examined the role of quaternary structure in the determination of antigenic sites in papain solubilized HLA molecules. They find that removal of the $\beta_2$-microglobulin subunit exposes an antigenic site that appears to be common to all HLA alloantigens (Tanigaki *et al.*, 1974). Rabbit antibodies directed against this specificity react only weakly with the intact 48,000 dalton molecule and do not react at all with free $\beta_2$-microglobulin. One explanation consistent with these observations is that HLA glycoproteins contain a structurally conserved region that is masked by the binding of $\beta_2$-microglobulin.

In an extension of this work, these authors describe a "primate cross-reacting" determinant detected by the use of rabbit antisera raised against rhesus monkey cell membranes (Katagiri *et al.*, 1974). These antisera detect a common specificity on all intact 48,000 dalton HLA (and RhL-A) alloantigens. This specificity is not found on either the 33,000 dalton or the 11,600 dalton components. These data suggest that separation of the two components results in the modification of the tertiary and quaternary structure of the molecule such that the antigenic sites present on the intact molecule are lost.

Several other laboratories have isolated HLA antigens presumably released from the cell surface *in vivo* or *in vitro* by endogeneous proteolytic enzymes. Billing and Terasaki (1974) have isolated HLA antigens, in soluble form, from serum of normal individuals. The purification sequence used by these workers involved ion exchange chromatography on QAE-Sephadex, lectin affinity chromatography using concanavalin A insolubilized on Sepharose, and preparative polyacrylamide gel electrophoresis. The monomeric molecular weight for HLA-A9 isolated in this manner is 65,000 daltons as established by polyacrylamide gel electrophoresis in the presence of sodium dodecyl sulfate and 2-mercaptoethanol. It is not clear whether the difference between this and the 33,000 to 34,000 dalton antigens obtained by papain solubilization reflects merely a technical difference in procedure or whether soluble HLA molecules from serum are inherently different from those isolated directly from cell surfaces by papain treatment.

The other type of HLA preparation involving proteolytic cleavage is solubilization with 3 *M* KCl (hypertonic extraction). Although a number of laboratories have obtained HLA preparations with this method, the most extensive characterization of 3 *M* KCl-solubilized material has been carried out by Reisfeld and his co-workers (1973). It should be noted that these workers feel that solubilization by 3 *M* KCl occurs *via* "chaotropic disruption" and not by enzymatic cleavage. However, it has been demonstrated that 3 *M* KCl solubilization may be blocked with proteolytic enzyme inhibitors, such as iodoacetamide and diisopropyl phosphofluoridate (Mann, 1972). In addition, electrophoresis of a 3 *M* KCl-solubilized antigen preparation in the presence of SDS shows a MW of 33,000 daltons, which is quite similar to the 33,000–34,000 dalton fragments obtained by papain solubilization (Reisfeld *et al.*, 1974).

The antigenic material obtained by the 3 *M* KCl solubilization was characterized as proteinaceous. Preparations studied by Reisfeld and his co-workers (1973) contained less than 1% carbohydrate as detected by the cysteine-sulfuric acid method, and the preparation did not stain with periodic acid-Schiff (PAS) reagent. The material did not contain lipids as determined by chromatographic characterization of chloroform–methanol extracts of the preparations (Reisfeld *et al.*, 1973). It is not clear why Reisfeld and his co-workers failed to find carbohydrate in their preparations, since these materials appear to have many properties in common with carbohydrate-containing preparations from other laboratories.

### 2. *Molecules Isolated after Membrane Dissolution with Detergent*

The complementary approach to proteolytic solubilization of the MHC alloantigen glycoproteins is the use of detergents that release the molecules in native form. It is generally desirable to use a detergent that preserves antigenic reactivity. Until recently, the detergent-solubilized molecules have been more difficult to assay and purify. However, many of these difficulties have now been solved, and it is finally possible to study the intact molecules in order to define the total chemical structure of the MHC molecules. Both nonionic detergents and ionic detergents (e.g., deoxycholate) have been used.

The general procedure involves a solubilization step in which approximately a 0.1 to 0.5% (v/v) final concentration of the detergent is mixed with the membrane preparations or whole cells. After an appropriate (15 minutes to 1 hour) incubation period, the material not sedimented by centrifugation at 100,000 *g* for 1 hour (i.e., "solubilized") is analyzed for antigenic activity. In many cases radiolabeled antigen has been utilized. Two approaches have been successful in this regard. In one approach the cells are incubated prior to solubilization with either amino acid or sugar precursors, which are then incorporated directly into the MHC glycoproteins. In the second approach, the intact cells are surface-iodinated with lactoperoxidase in the presence of hydrogen peroxide and $Na^{125}I$, which iodinates the tyrosine residues of H-2 or HLA and of other surface proteins.

The glycoprotein nature of the detergent-solubilized, water-insoluble H-2 antigen molecules was confirmed by Schwartz *et al.* (1973a) using double-label experiments in which antigen from cells radiolabeled with both [$^{14}C$]leucine and [$^{3}H$]fucose were solubilized with NP-40 and precipitated with an anti-H-2 alloantiserum and anti-mouse IgG serum. The precipitate was dissolved in sodium dodecyl sulfate (SDS) with 2-mercaptoethanol and subjected to electrophoresis on an SDS-polyacrylamide gel. The amino acid and monosaccharide labels coelectrophoresed as a single peak (Schwartz *et al.*, 1973a). The protein and sugar label could be separated only if the antigenic material was subjected to exhaustive pronase digestion to reduce the protein to dipeptides and amino acids and the carbohydrate chain to glycopeptide(s) containing only one or two attached amino acids. Thus it was concluded that the NP-40 extracted H-2 material was in fact glycoprotein. Additional evidence for the common origin of the glycoproteins solubilized by NP-40 detergent and the fragment released by papain digestion came from experiments showing that the carbohydrate moieties of antigen from these two sources were identical in size when compared by Sephadex G-50 column chromatography (Schwartz *et al.*, 1973a).

An estimate of the molecular size of the H-2 alloantigen complex solubilized by the detergent NP-40 was obtained from measuring its elution position during molecular seive chromatography on BioGel A-5m or A-15m columns in 0.5% NP-40 buffer. A molecular weight of approximately 300,000 to 400,000 daltons was obtained. It is relevant to note, however, that this molecular weight value determined under nondenaturing conditions almost certainly reflects the molecular weight of the complex between the H-2 antigens, the detergent micelle, and possibly other membrane proteins as well and does not reflect the size of the antigen complex *in situ.*

In any event, this complex is broken down to smaller molecular weight units with the strong ionic detergent SDS and a reducing agent (see Fig. 11.1). When reduced samples are analyzed by nondiscontinuous polyacrylamide gel electrophoresis in SDS, they behave as proteins of a molecular size of 45,000 daltons (Schwartz and Nathenson, 1971b). The existence of a dimer form was also suggested by the fact that in unreduced samples two forms were found, one with a molecular size of approximately 90,000 daltons, the other of 45,000 daltons. The 90,000 dalton species could be reduced to the 45,000 dalton form upon reduction

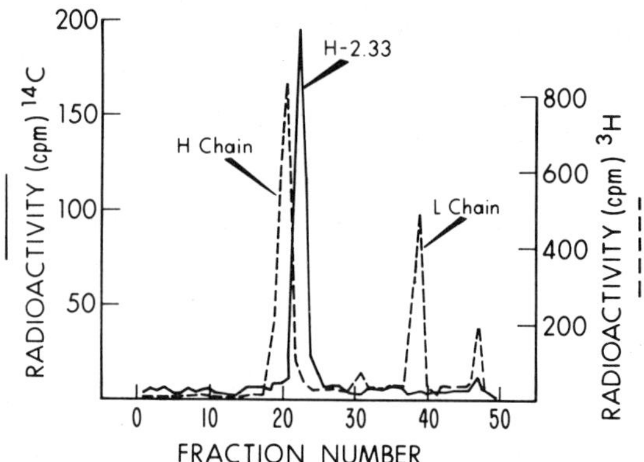


FIG. 11.1. Analysis by discontinuous electrophoresis of a reduced immune precipitate from an NP-40 extract of [$^{14}$C]lysine-labeled C57BL/10 spleen cells. Analysis performed at pH 8.8 on 10% polyacrylamide gels in 0.1% SDS (Davis, 1964; Maizel, 1971). A single peak representing H-2.33 and migrating slightly ahead of the H chain marker may be seen. Solid line, H-2.33; dashed line, H chain and L chain from a [$^{3}$H]leucine, [$^{3}$H]valine, [$^{3}$H]threonine-labeled MPC-11 secretion courtesy of Dr. M. D. Scharff. Analysis courtesy of Dr. J. L. Brown.

with 2-mercaptoethanol. Therefore, the larger form was tentatively called a dimer, while the smaller form was called a monomer.

While the overall molecular size of the monomer H-2 alloantigen glycoprotein was found to be around 45,000 daltons, small molecular weight differences for different allelic products of the *H-2* gene products were noted. For example, H-2D$^{d}$ was found to be around 43,000 daltons while H-2K$^{d}$ was found to be around 47,000 daltons. Products of other haplotypes have also shown small but reproducible differences between themselves as judged by migration behavior during SDS polyacrylamide electrophoresis.

An interesting point arising from a comparison of the two molecular forms available, i.e., the one solubilized by proteolytic digestion and the one solubilized by nonionic detergents, is that the papain solubilized fragment is approximately 80% of the size of the intact NP-40 solubilized molecule (Schwartz *et al.*, 1973a). Thus, the loss of a relatively small portion of the intact molecule confers aqueous solubility on the large glycoprotein fragment remaining. It seems reasonable to assume that this small region, which appears to carry no alloantigenic determinant, is necessary for membrane integration of the molecule and/or for interaction of the molecule with itself to form dimers. The membrane associative properties of this small portion might be due to a particularly hydrophobic region or to a region that is involved or influential in bringing about aggregation into large molecular weight complexes.

The most extensive studies on nonionic detergent solubilized HLA antigens from lymphoid cells have been carried out by Springer *et al.* (1974). Purified membrane fragments from human lymphoblastoid cells were extracted with Brij 99. The soluble extract, after fractionation by affinity chromatography using the lectin from common lentils (LcH) covalently attached to BioGel A, appeared to be 50% pure by polyacrylamide gel electrophoresis in SDS. The gels had two major bands, one at 44,000 daltons and one at 12,000 daltons ($\beta_2$-microglobulin).

These authors also examined the cleavage of detergent solubilized HLA molecules by papain. They found that the 44,000 dalton product is degraded to a 34,000 dalton fragment (presumably very similar to the one obtained directly by papain solubilization) *via* 39,000 and 37,000 dalton intermediates. This observation corresponds to that of Schwartz *et al.* (1973a) that papain cleavage of an H-2 immune precipitate produced an H-2 fragment similar in molecular weight to that obtained directly by papain solubilization (*vide supra*).

In a separate study Colombani, Jollès, and co-workers (Dautigny *et al.*, 1973; Bernier *et al.*, 1974) have used NP-40 to solubilize HLA from platelets. They isolated glycoproteins with molecular weights of 90,000 and 45,000 daltons. This finding appears to be analogous to the observation in the H-2 antigen system of a "dimer-monomer" relationship, since the 45,000 dalton value is in good agreement with the 44,000 dalton figure reported by Strominger and co-workers for reduced, detergent-solubilized HLA molecules.

The *ionic* detergent sodium deoxycholate has also proved to be an extremely effective solubilization agent in studies by Snary *et al.* (1974) and Dawson *et al.* (1974). Both groups made extensive use of lectin affinity chromatography with LcH-Sepharose columns. By sucrose gradient centrifugation in the presence of deoxycholate, Snary *et al.* estimated a molecular weight of 55,000 daltons for HLA-A1 and HLA-A2 and 45,000 daltons for HLA-B8 and HLA-B13. These values depend on the assumption that the HLA glycoproteins bind significant amounts of deoxycholate (e.g., 0.38 gm per gram protein). However, such estimates agree rather well with those obtained for HLA antigens solubilized with the nonionic detergent Brij 99 (Springer *et al.*, 1974). Table 11.3 summarizes the molecular weights of detergent-solubilized HLA preparations.

### B. Carbohydrate Composition and Structure

Shimada and Nathenson (1969) and Muramatsu and Nathenson (1970) showed that the carbohydrate moeity of H-2 alloantigen glyco-

TABLE 11.3
MOLECULAR WEIGHT OF H-2 AND HLA GLYCOPROTEINS SOLUBILIZED BY DETERGENTS

| | Detergent | Antigen | Molecular weight and method[a] | Reference |
|---|---|---|---|---|
| H-2 | NP-40 | $H\text{-}2D^d$ (H-2.4) | 43,000 SDS/PAGE and SDS/gel filtration | Schwartz *et al.*, 1973a |
| | | $H\text{-}2K^d$ (H-2.31) | 47,000 SDS/PAGE | |
| HLA | Brij 99 | HLA-A2<br>HLA-B7<br>HLA-B12 | 43,000–44,000 SDS/PAGE | Springer *et al.*, 1974 |
| | Sodium deoxycholate | HLA-A1<br>HLA-A2 | 54,500 sedimentation centrifugation[b] | Snary *et al.*, 1974 |
| | | HLA-B8<br>HLA-B13 | 45,200 sedimentation centrifugation[b] | Snary *et al.*, 1974 |
| | NP-40 | HLA-A2<br>HLA-B5 | 45,000 SDS/PAGE | Bernier *et al.*, 1974 |

[a] PAGE, polyacrylamide gel electrophoresis.
[b] Calculated from the assumption that 0.38 gm of deoxycholate was bound per gram protein.

protein fragments solubilized by papain contain galactose, glucosamine, mannose, fucose, and sialic acid. The analyses required for this determination were carried out both by paper and gas chromatographic procedures. Confirmatory evidence for these five sugars was also obtained from studies using the incorporation of radiolabeled monosaccharides. In these experiments the H-2 glycoproteins were isolated from tumor or spleen cells previously incubated in tissue culture with radioactive monosaccharides. The papain solubilized alloantigen fragments were recovered from immune complexes and the radioactive sugars present were analyzed by paper chromatography. In separate experiments with different radiolabeled monosaccharides it was clear that galactose, glucosamine, fucose, and mannose were incorporated into the H-2 glycoproteins from two different haplotypes ($H\text{-}2^b$ and $H\text{-}2^d$), but that glucose, rhamnose, arabinose, and zylose, while incorporated by the cells, were absent from the H-2 glycoproteins (Muramatsu and Nathenson, 1970).

The incorporated glucosamine was found 80% as glucosamine and 20% as sialic acid. Galactosamine was absent. These data when taken together with the analyses on nonradiolabeled materials clearly demonstrated that galactose, mannose, fucose, glucosamine, and sialic acid are integral components of the H-2 alloantigens.

For studies on the carbohydrate chains and on the sugars in these chains, the glycopeptides were generated by exhaustive pronase digestion of the protein moiety. These glycopeptides were then chromatographed on Sephadex columns on which they were found to elute in a single peak with a position corresponding to approximately 3300 ± 500 daltons as estimated by comparison with the elution volumes of standard glycopeptides. Thus the H-2 glycopeptide was estimated to carry at most 1 or 2 amino acid residues and from 12 to 15 monosaccharide residues and had a unique size in contrast to the heterogeneous array of sizes observed for glycopeptides from the glycoproteins found in crude membrane fractions of murine cells.

It is of interest that glycopeptides from glycoproteins of different *H-2* haplotypes were found to be indistinguishable by the criteria of gel filtration and DEAE-Sephadex ion exchange chromatography. This similarity was also observed whether the glycopeptides were isolated from H-2 glycoproteins from normal spleen cells or from tumor cells. Thus, easily detectable differences in overall size or charge, dependent on the *H-2* haplotype or on the variations of source (normal versus tumor) were not observed. These results support the contention that the carbohydrate structure does not influence the antigenic properties of the alloantigens, a subject discussed in Section III,E.

A schematic structure of the carbohydrate chain of the H-2 glycopro-

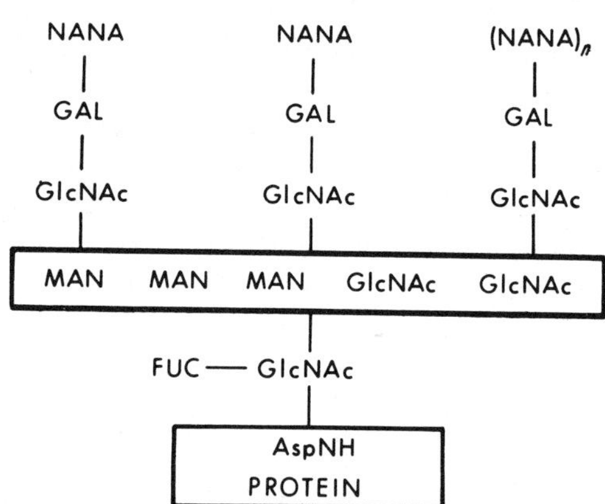


FIG. 11.2. Hypothetical model of the carbohydrate chain of the H-2 glycoproteins. The evidence for this model is discussed in the text and in Nathenson and Muramatsu (1971). Abbreviations: NANA, sialic acid; GAL, galactose; GlcNAc, glucosamine; MAN, mannose; FUC, fucose; AspNH, asparagine. Reprinted from Nathenson and Cullen (1974) by permission of Elsevier Scientific Publishing Company.

teins is shown in Fig. 11.2. This proposed structure was postulated from studies utilizing enzyme digestion and limited chemical hydrolysis (see review in Nathenson and Muramatsu (1971)). It's salient features are the following.

1. The sialic acid residues are located at the termini, a fact which was established because these residues can be easily released by *Vibrio cholerae* neuraminidase.

2. The galactose residues are located immediately internal to the sialic acid residues as judged from evidence that a $\beta$-galactosidase will remove these without releasing mannose or glucosamine.

3. Part of the glucosamine residues are postulated to be located internal to galactose residues, yet external to a core region containing mannose and also some of the glucosamine, since approximately 25% of the glucosamine can be released upon incubation with a mixture of $\beta$-*N*-acetylglucosaminidase, $\beta$-galactosidase, and neuraminidase.

4. The composition of the core sugars, as outlined in heavy lines in Fig. 11.2, was suggested by studies utilizing an endoglycosidase which released this core by cleaving between the *N*-acetylglucosamine and core and leaving fucosyl-*N*-acetylglucosamine attached to an asparagine (or glutamine) of the protein. It is of interest to note that the fucose is attached to an *N*-acetylglucosamine adjacent to the carbohydrate–protein linkage region. This property is true with almost all fucose residues in glycoproteins on the cell surfaces of mammalian cells (Muramatsu *et al.*, 1973a).

Detailed studies on the carbohydrate structure of HLA gene products have not been undertaken. Preliminary compositional evidence suggests that they contain 6–12% carbohydrate and, like the *H-2* gene products, contain sialic acid and neutral monosaccharide residues (Mann *et al.*, 1969a). Studies with biosynthetic precursors further show that HLA gene products incorporate mannose and glucosamine (Cresswell *et al.*, 1973, 1974a). The binding of HLA antigens to LcH affinity columns (Snary *et al.*, 1974; Dawson *et al.*, 1974; Springer *et al.*, 1974) and to concanavalin A (Con A) affinity columns (Billing and Terasaki, 1974) implies the presence of mannose (and/or glucose) residues in the carbohydrate chains of HLA.

### C. Protein Structure

As mentioned previously, the native products of the *H-2K* and *H-2D* genes and the A and B series HLA genes are glycoproteins of approximately 45,000 daltons in molecular weight. For the H-2 products approximately 90% of the weight has been shown to be accounted for by protein, and carbohydrate makes up approximately 10% (Table 11.1). There is no lipid or phospholipid. Since the carbohydrate chain accounts for approximately 10% of the weight, one can calculate that the protein moiety is approximately 40,000 daltons in molecular weight or between 300 to 350 amino acid residues in length. The mouse $\beta_2$-microglobulin, which is found noncovalently linked to the H-2 glycoprotein, is approximately 11,600 daltons in molecular weight and 100 residues long.

Amino acid analyses of the H-2 glycoprotein fragments from two different haplotypes solubilized by papain digestion (Table 11.4) show no unusual amino acids present or absent and a high concentration of glutamic acid and aspartic acid. Both cysteine and methionine are present. Amino acid analysis of two different HLA gene products reveals that these molecules are strikingly similar to H-2 preparations. Such chemical similarities fit with the biological and serological similarities of the *H-2* and HLA systems, and strongly supports the view that these systems are homologous.

An understanding of the primary structure of the polypeptide portion of the MHC glycoproteins is especially important in order to understand the fundamental properties of these molecules. Such information is necessary to determine the basis for their membrane affinity, the basis for their expression of antigenic sites, and the properties of their genetic determinants. For example, such structural information will be indicative

TABLE 11.4
AMINO ACID COMPOSITION OF PAPAIN-SOLUBILIZED H-2 AND HLA ALLOANTIGENS[a]

| Amino acids | H-2[b] | | HLA[c] | |
|---|---|---|---|---|
| | H-2[b] | H-2[d] | HLA-A2 | HLA-A7 |
| Lys | 4.4 | 5.0 | 3.7 | 3.5 |
| His | 3.1 | 2.8 | 4.2 | 4.1 |
| Arg | 4.9 | 5.8 | 8.6 | 9.1 |
| Asp | 9.5 | 9.6 | 8.8 | 9.3 |
| Thr | 7.3 | 7.3 | 7.9 | 7.7 |
| Ser | 6.4 | 5.7 | 5.9 | 5.9 |
| Glu | 12.6 | 13.6 | 14.5 | 15.6 |
| Pro | 6.8 | 6.5 | 4.8 | 5.3 |
| Gly | 7.1 | 7.3 | 7.7 | 7.0 |
| Ala | 7.0 | 7.2 | 9.0 | 8.4 |
| Cys | 2.5 | 2.2 | 1.4 | 1.6 |
| Val | 5.6 | 5.1 | 5.7 | 5.0 |
| Met | 2.1 | 2.1 | 1.4 | 1.0 |
| Ile | 3.8 | 3.2 | 2.5 | 2.7 |
| Leu | 8.3 | 7.6 | 6.7 | 6.8 |
| Tyr | 5.1 | 4.5 | 4.8 | 5.1 |
| Phe | 3.6 | 4.1 | 3.0 | 2.7 |

[a] Expression in moles per 100 moles of amino acids recovered after hydrolysis.

[b] Amino acid analyses were performed on H-2 alloantigens purified by discontinuous polyacrylamide gel electrophoresis as previously described (Shimada and Nathenson, 1969). The H-$2^d$ materials were reactive mostly for the H-$2D^d$ specificity H-2.4, and the H-$2^b$ materials reactive mostly for the H-$2K^b$ specificity H-2.33. No attempts were made to remove murine $\beta_2$-microglobulin.

[c] The $\beta_2$-microglobulin was removed from the HLA preparations by gel filtration at pH 2.3. Data taken from Tanigaki and Pressman (1974).

of the extent of homology between the *K* and *D* genes of the *H-2* system and will indicate whether specific regions of the polypeptide are relatively variable and other regions relatively conserved.

An analysis of the peptides produced by trypsin digestion can provide a qualitative approach to the investigation of the primary structure. In recent studies (Brown *et al.*, 1974) on the *H-2* system the following questions have been examined by comparative techniques.

1. What are the similarities and differences in peptide composition among molecules determined by alleles of the same gene (e.g., *H-$2K^b$* versus *H-$2K^d$*)?
2. What are the similarities and differences in peptide composition

between products of alleles of the *H-2K* and *H-2D* genes of a single haplotype (e.g., *H-2K*$^{b}$ versus *H-2D*$^{b}$)?

Since either one arginine or lysine will be contained in every peptide produced by digestion with the protease trypsin, [$^{3}$H]- or [$^{14}$C]arginine- and [$^{3}$H]- or [$^{14}$C]lysine-labeled, NP-40 solubilized H-2 glycoproteins were used. *H-2* gene products were isolated by indirect immunoprecipitation and purified by SDS gel filtration chromatography. Tryptic peptides of products were compared in a paired-label technique by ion exchange chromatography (Brown *et al.*, 1974).

As an example of such a comparison, an ion exchange chromatogram of a mixture of [$^{14}$C]arginine-labeled H-2K$^{b}$ peptides (private specificity H-2.33) and [$^{3}$H]arginine-labeled H-2K$^{d}$ (private specificity H-2.31) is shown in Fig. 11.3. Approximately eleven peaks from the H-2K$^{b}$ and fifteen peaks from H-2K$^{d}$ antigen are visualized, each peak presumably containing one or at most a few peptides. Only four of the peptide peaks can be said to coincide on this comparative chromatogram, or about 25–35%. Thus, approximately 65–75% of the peptides are unique.

Studies of the products of alleles as shown in this example (Fig. 11.3) have been carried out on all H-2D and H-2K products from two haplotypes, *H-2*$^{d}$ and *H-2*$^{b}$, for both the lysine- and arginine-labeled peptides. A general summary of the results is as follows: peptide comparisons of products of alleles of the same gene (e.g., *K*$^{b}$ versus *K*$^{d}$ and *D*$^{b}$ versus

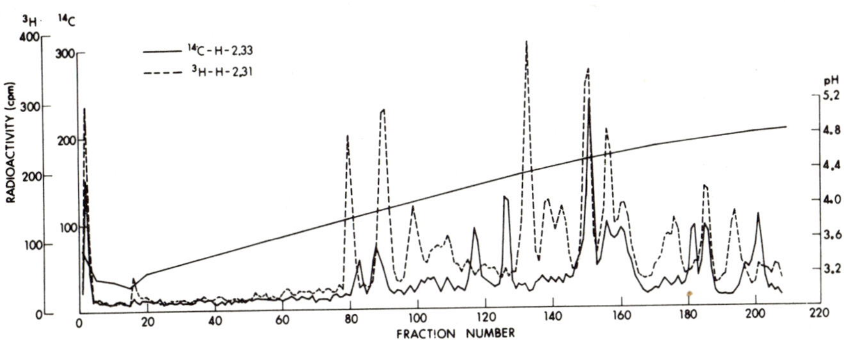


FIG. 11.3. Comparison of the tryptic peptides of two *H-2K* gene products: [$^{14}$C]arginine labeled H-2.33 (H-2K$^{b}$) and [$^{3}$H]arginine labeled H-2.31 (H-2K$^{d}$). The immune precipitates were purified separately on BioGel A-0.5 m. They then were combined, precipitated with 15% trichloroacetic acid, washed, and digested with TPCK-trypsin [L-(tosylamido-2-phenyl)ethyl chloromethyl ketone, an inhibitor of chymotrypsin]. The supernatant containing the acid soluble peptides (recovery of radioactivity was approximately 70–80%) was separated on a column of Spherix XX8-60-0 resin. Methods are described in J. L. Brown *et al.* 1974. *Biochemistry* **13**: 3174. Reprinted by permission of The American Chemical Society.

$D^d$) showed about 35% similarities. Peptide comparisons of the products of alleles of the *H-2K* versus *H-2D* genes showed somewhat divergent results since $K^b$ versus $D^b$ showed 60% similarity, while $K^d$ versus $D^d$ showed about 40% similarities.

These results are most striking, since they demonstrate an extreme degree of diversity between the products of alleles of the same gene. In fact, in some cases there are greater similarities between products of alleles of the *D* and *K* genes than between products of alleles of the same gene. While these are still preliminary studies and pertain to only two haplotypes of the greater than 40 known haplotypes, the results, if they are applicable to other strains, point out the extraordinary uniqueness of the *H-2* gene products, and therefore the diversity of their genes.

It is important to point out, however, that the techniques of peptide mapping lead to overestimates of differences in protein structure. This is the case since a single amino acid exchange can alter the chromatographic behavior of a peptide consisting of many conserved amino acids. For example, peptide maps of the $\kappa$ and $\lambda$ chains can show almost complete nonidentity, while detailed sequence studies show 30–40% homology (Dayhoff, 1972).

The finding of considerable uniqueness for the products of the alleles of the *H-2* genes is possibly not unexpected, since the polymorphism of these genes has been their hallmark. In fact, the complex serological profiles associated with products of different alleles suggests that there must be a complex and variable structural basis. For example, there are at least seven defined antigenic differences between H-2$K^b$ and H-2$K^d$ including their private specificities H-2.33 and H-2.31.

It should be noted that the structural variability observed for these glycoproteins, undisputed products of the *H-2* genes, is in marked contrast to the genetic stability and nonvariability in the putative subunit, the $\beta_2$-microglobulin. As discussed in Section III,D, this 11,600 dalton polypeptide, in contrast to the H-2 glycoproteins, has no known variability among individuals of one species (man) and is almost identical between two species (dog and man) in so far as it has been examined.

### D. $\beta_2$-Microglobulin

The possibility that histocompatibility antigens might have other molecular species specifically associated with them was not given serious consideration until the discovery that papain solubilized HLA antigens frequently contained a 12,000 dalton "fragment." Subsequently it was shown that this "fragment" was actually $\beta_2$-microglobulin, an 11,600 dalton protein initially isolated from urine of patients with certain renal proteinurias (Berggård and Bearn, 1968). It is also found in smaller amounts in the serum and urine of normal individuals, and indeed on the surface of normal lymphoid cells. Homologous proteins have been isolated in the dog and in the mouse. A partial sequence of dog $\beta_2$-microglobulin has been obtained (Smithies and Poulik, 1972b) which shows very close homology with human $\beta_2$-microglobulin, differing in only six of the 42 N-terminal amino acid residues. Surprisingly however, the two proteins are not immunologically cross reactive. The mouse homologue of $\beta_2$-microglobulin has also been isolated; it shows weak serological cross reactivity with human $\beta_2$-microglobulin and has identical mobility with human $\beta_2$-microglobulin on starch gel and polyacrylamide gel electrophoresis (Peterson *et al.*, 1974; Silver and Hood, 1974).

The initial structural studies of $\beta_2$-microglobulin by Smithies and Poulik (1972a), in which a partial amino acid sequence was obtained, led these workers to recognize the sequence homology between $\beta_2$-microglobulin and the $\gamma$ chain from human immunoglobulin. Based on their partial sequence, these workers suggested that the $\beta_2$-microglobulin gene evolved from an immunoglobulin $\gamma$ chain gene due to the genesis of an unusual start signal for initiating protein synthesis.

The complete primary structure has been determined for human $\beta_2$-microglobulin (Cunningham *et al.*, 1973). The protein consists of 100 amino acid residues; no carbohydrate is present. The molecule has two cysteine residues at positions 25 and 81 from the N-terminus which form a single disulfide loop. There are no free sulfhydryl groups. The most striking feature of $\beta_2$-microglobulin is that its overall size and single loop structure is strongly suggestive of an immunoglobulin "domain" (Edelman, 1970). Indeed, Peterson *et al.* (1972) find about 30% sequence homology with the third constant region domain of the $\gamma$ chain ($C_H3$) of the myeloma protein Eu and a lower homology with the other constant region domains of the Eu molecule. This observation led Edelman and his co-workers to postulate that $\beta_2$-microglobulin is not the product of a deletion of an immunoglobulin gene, but rather is a "free" immunoglobulin domain, possibly serving an effector function similar to that of the $C_H3$ domain of $\gamma 1$ chains of immunoglobulin "G" (Peterson *et al.*, 1972). Although the 30% sequence homology found by these workers is not exceptionally high, it is statistically significant and is nearly as high as the sequence homology between the various constant region domains of the protein Eu.

The proof that $\beta_2$-microglobulin is indeed the low molecular weight component associated with the product of the MHC in man and mouse rests on two lines of evidence. The first is the coprecipitation of $\beta_2$-microglobulin with alloantisera directed against histocompatibility antigen specificities, and the second is the "cocapping" of $\beta_2$-microglobulin with human histocompatibility antigens on the lymphocyte surface.

Shortly after the purification and characterization of $\beta_2$-microglobulin, it was shown that the low molecular weight component obtained from papain solubilized HLA gene products precipitated with alloantisera, or from spent lymphoblastoid cell line culture media, were identical to $\beta_2$-microglobulin (Tanigaki *et al.*, 1973; Grey *et al.*, 1973; Peterson *et al.*, 1974; Reisfeld *et al.*, 1974). This identification was based not only on chromatographic and immunological identity but also on the fact that the first 24 amino acid residues at the N-terminus were the same in the two molecules (Tanigaki *et al.*, 1973). $\beta_2$-Microglobulin has also been found in detergent solubilized HLA preparations (Springer *et al.*, 1974), suggesting that the association between $\beta_2$-microglobulin and HLA is not an artifact arising from papain solubilization. Furthermore, since neither solubilization with nonionic detergents nor disaggregation for electrophoresis with the ionic detergent SDS breaks chemical bonds, this experiment strongly suggests that $\beta_2$-microglobulin is *not* a *covalently* attached subunit of HLA.

The mouse homologue of $\beta_2$-microglobulin has been found in detergent and papain-solubilized H-2 preparations (Silver and Hood, 1974; Rask *et al.*, 1974). In both mouse and man, the ratio of the large molecular weight histocompatibility antigen component to $\beta_2$-microglobulin appears to be about 1:1, but the data are not yet firm.

Another set of data that link $\beta_2$-microglobulin with histocompatibility antigens are the immunofluorescence studies carried out with human lymphocytes. Poulik *et al.* (1973), Bismuth *et al.* (1973), Östberg *et al.* (1974), Neauport-Sautes *et al.* (1974), and Solheim and Thorsby (1974) all have shown that treatment of cells with anti-$\beta_2$-microglobulin antisera causes the simultaneous cocapping of $\beta_2$-microglobulin and all of the detectable HLA antigens carried by that cell. The capping of $\beta_2$-microglobulin is specific since it was also shown that $\beta_2$-microglobulin does not cocap with surface immunoglobulins. The converse experiment, however, in which all HLA molecules were capped or aggregated, showed some $\beta_2$-microglobulin still remaining dispersed on the cell surface (Neauport-Sautes *et al.*, 1974). This suggested that possibly all HLA was associated with $\beta_2$-microglobulin but that some $\beta_2$-microglobulin was free or in association with other surface molecules. These experiments are discussed in detail in Section VI.

In agreement with this suggestion of excess $\beta_2$-microglobulin over glycoprotein are the studies on the quantity of these molecules on lymphocyte surfaces. Estimates of the number of $\beta_2$-microglobulin molecules range from $4 \times 10^5$ (Evrin and Pertoft, 1973) to $6 \times 10^6$ (Peterson *et al.*, 1972); the number of HLA molecules per cell varies from $10^4$ to $10^5$ (Sanderson and Welsh, 1973, 1974). Despite the inconsistencies in these estimates, they suggest that in some cases $\beta_2$-microglobulin may be present in a 4 to 600-fold molar excess over HLA. This unequal cell surface distribution implies that, even though $\beta_2$-microglobulin may be intimately associated in a 1:1 complex with HLA at the cell surface, this may not be the sole function for $\beta_2$-microglobulin.

Although there is an intimate molecular association between $\beta_2$-microglobulin and the histocompatibility antigens, Goodfellow *et al.* (1975) have demonstrated, using human–mouse cell hybrids, that the genes coding for $\beta_2$-microglobulin and for HLA are not linked. They showed that the $\beta_2$-microglobulin locus is on human chromosome 15, while the HLA complex is localized on chromosome 6. These results, however, do not bear in any way on the details of the association between $\beta_2$-microglobulin and the histocompatibility antigens nor on their possible evolutionary relationship. Answers to these questions will be obtained only when detailed structural data, comparable to that already obtained for $\beta_2$-microglobulin, are also available for the HLA or H-2 glycoproteins.

### E. The Nature of the Antigenic Sites of the H-2 and HLA Glycoproteins

Since most of the studies directed to the question of the nature of the antigenic sites of the major histocompatibility antigens have been pursued in the *H-2* system, the following discussion will pertain to this system.

The first and most elementary question is whether the antigenic sites are determined by the carbohydrate or protein moieties of the glycoprotein. Several types of studies have been carried out to establish whether or not the carbohydrate could determine antigenic specificity. It was reasoned that if the carbohydrate chains had antigenic activity, one would expect the following.

1. Glycopeptides isolated from H-2 glycoproteins might have antibody binding ability.
2. After removal of some or most of the carbohydrate, the protein portion of the antigen might show lack of antibody binding capacity.
3. Comparative sequencing of the carbohydrate chains from antigen of nonidentical haplotypes might show differences in carbohydrate structure to account for the antigenic differences.

These three approaches were followed, and the results are consistent with the hypothesis that the carbohydrate itself does not directly express the antigenic specificity. Thus, the isolated glycopeptides of H-2 alloantigens have always been inactive when tested for antigenic activity. Enzymatic removal of the carbohydrate, furthermore, was ineffective in destroying antigenic activity. For example, removal of 100% of the sialic acid, 70% of the galactose, and 25% of the glucosamine (or a loss of about 35% of the total carbohydrate) did not produce any change in the antibody binding capacity for the H-2 specificities measured. These results are particularly significant, since the outer sugars are the more likely to be immunodominant residues, and these are the ones which were removed (Nathenson and Muramatsu, 1971).

In addition, comparative structural studies on the carbohydrate chains from different H-2 glycopeptides using a relatively crude enzymic digestion method showed identical patterns for release of sugars. Such studies, of course, are not quantitative, and more precise studies of sequence and linkage may show differences.

Studies on the nature of the determinants of the HLA alloantigens have not been carried out in as much detail as for the H-2 alloantigens. However, one study on the HLA system suggests that while protein structure plays the major role, the carbohydrate moiety may also behave as an antigenic determinant in some cases (Sanderson *et al.*, 1971).

Consistent with the failure of all direct experiments to implicate carbohydrate are considerable data on the protein portion of H-2 which suggest it does determine antigenic reactivity. In these studies it was reasoned that if the protein portion of the H-2 molecule expresses the antigen activity, then

1. Protein denaturants might cause loss of antigen activity due to a change in conformation around the antigen sites
2. Protein modification by reagents affecting specific amino acid residues might cause loss of antigenic activity due to alterations of such residues forming a part of an antigenic site
3. Comparative peptide comparison of molecules from nonidentical haplotypes might show unique peptides, since a model in which antigen activity resides in the protein predicts differences in amino acid sequence which might be revealed in a peptide comparison

The extreme lability of antigen activity to reagents that alter protein conformation was demonstrated in early studies on the H-2 alloantigens (Kandutsch and Reinert-Wenck, 1957). For example, nearly all antigenic activity was lost after treatment with protein denaturants such as 6 *M* urea, or when the antigen was subjected to extremes of pH (below pH 3 and above pH 10), or to proteolytic digestion. Thus protein conformation must be intact in order for the appropriate antigenic activity to be expressed.

When the H-2 glycoproteins were chemically modified by selective reagents that alter only certain amino acid residues, loss of antigenic specificities was found (Pancake and Nathenson, 1973). *N*-Acetylimidazole and tetranitromethane, both of which affect tyrosine residues under the conditions used, caused a loss of all tested antigenic specificities. The use of modification procedures, such as reductive methylation, which affect amino groups rather than tyrosine residues also produced a loss of antigenic activity. However, only certain antigenic specificities were destroyed. With the H-$2^d$ glycoproteins, specificity H-2.4 was almost totally lost, while H-2.31 was nearly completely retained. Such effects were noted under conditions in which 90–95% of the lysine residues were altered to dimethyllysine.

The loss of antibody binding to some antigenic sites upon alteration of lysine amino groups suggests that, for these determinants, a lysine with a free $\epsilon$-amino group is necessary for antigenic activity. Other antigenic sites, however, are not inactivated by reductive methylation and apparently do not contain lysine residues in a critical position for their antigenic activity. Of course, the altered amino group does not necessarily have to be in the antigenic site, but could be located at some distance from the site if it has an effect on the three-dimensional conformation of the polypeptide region bearing the determinant.

These results support the basic hypothesis that protein determines antigenic specificity. In addition, the differential susceptibility of some antigenic sites to lysine modification suggests that these sites are different from unaffected sites.

In studies described in Section III,C, peptide comparisons of the protein portion of antigenically distinct H-2 glycopeptides showed distinct and reproducible differences between products of different *H-2* genes—differences which would be expected to underlie serological differences. Such findings also support the hypothesis that antigenic sites are determined by protein structure.

## IV. Immunochemical–Genetic Relationships of the MHC System

Information on the genetic fine structure of the *H-2* and HLA systems has led to certain predictions concerning the chemical and molecular structure of the gene products. Conversely, a correction of genetic ambiguities and a testing of genetic hypothesis sometimes has been possible from a knowledge of the molecular structure.

In this section, some of the chemical and molecular properties of the *H-2* and HLA systems, insofar as now known, are discussed in relation to the genetics of these systems. Most of the comparisons are based on *H-2*, because of the relatively advanced state of the genetics of this system. But the increasingly refined HLA studies will be cited also, where relevant.

## A. The *H-2* System

Studies revealing recombination between the distal extremes of the *H-2* region were presented shortly after the discovery of the *H-2* locus nearly 40 years ago. Recently, Klein and Shreffler (1972), Shreffler *et al.* (1971), and Snell *et al.* (1971) suggested that *H-2* serology could be best interpreted in terms of two loci, *H-2K* and *H-2D*, mapping in two distinct regions on the chromosome. Verification of this "two gene" hypothesis was possible from immunochemical studies, since the hypothesis implied the presence of two separable gene products, one for the *H-2K* gene and one for the *H-2D* gene. Furthermore, the two gene hypothesis implied that each *H-2* gene product would be multispecific, that is, bear more than one antigenic site, since more than one serological specificity must be determined by one gene. For example, the $H\text{-}2D^d$ gene product has a private specificity H-2.4, but recombination studies suggested that public H-2 specificities 3, 6, 13, 27, 28, 29, 35, 36, 41, 42, and 43 are also determined by this gene.

The distribution of specificities on radiolabeled NP-40 solubilized antigen was analyzed by a coprecipitation technique (Cullen *et al.*, 1972a). An antiserum directed against specificity X was mixed with the antigen preparation, and antigen–antibody complexes were removed by precipitation with anti-mouse γ-globulin antiserum. The supernatant remaining after precipitation was then tested with anti-Y antiserum. If there was no Y specificity remaining in the supernatant, it was presumed to be attached to the X specificity, which had already been removed; that is, both X and Y specificities were on the same antigen fragment or molecule. This type of experiment was always performed in reciprocal order also, using the same antisera and antigen preparations. Appropriate controls were performed to ensure complete precipitation, and H-2 antibody was used in excess, while the anti-mouse γ-globulin was used at equivalence.

*1. Analysis of the $H\text{-}2^b$ Haplotype* (Cullen *et al.*, 1972a)

The private specificities for the $H\text{-}2^b$ haplotype are H-2.33 for the $H\text{-}2K^b$ gene and H-2.2 for the $H\text{-}2D^b$ gene. Specificity H-2.5, a public specificity, could not be assigned to either region from the available recombination data. By the methods outlined in the previous section it was shown that specificities 33 and 2 could be readily separated, an expected finding, since they are associated with different *H-2* genes. When specificity 2 had been removed by precipitation (anti-2 pretreatment), 33 remained in the supernatant. Conversely, when specificity 33 was removed by precipitation, 2 activity remained. When specificity 5 was tested, it was shown to be separable from specificity 2, but was coprecipitated with specificity 33. Thus, specificity 5 could be removed from the antigen preparation by either anti-5 or anti-33 antiserum and, conversely, 33 could be removed by either anti-33 or anti-5 serum. This was evidence that 5 and 33 were parts of the same antigen molecule.

*2. Analysis of the $H\text{-}2^d$ Haplotype* (Cullen *et al.*, 1972a)

The private specificities for the $H\text{-}2^d$ haplotype are H-2.31 in the $H\text{-}2K^d$ region and H-2.4 in the $H\text{-}2D^d$ region. Public specificities studied were H-2.3,42, both of which had been associated with the $H\text{-}2D^d$ gene by genetic recombination. Again it was found that the *H-2K* and *H-2D* gene product private specificities 31 and 4 were readily separated. H-2.4 and H-2.3,42 were precipitated together, and it was concluded that these antigenic specificities reside on the same antigen molecule.

Since the H-2 glycoprotein antigens are primary gene products, it follows that specificities residing on a single molecule are determined by a single gene. However, the number of cases is limited and does not enable us to assume that all the specificities mapping with either the *H-2K* or *H-2D* gene are found together on a single molecule. Nonetheless, the data are consistent with this hypothesis.

*3. Studies to Establish the Number of Molecules in Heterozygotes* (Cullen *et al.*, 1972b)

It has been shown already by the studies discussed above that two H-2 molecules could be found in homozygous cells. Each of these molecules has one of the private specificities, and it was proposed that each was determined by a single structural gene (*H-2K* or *H-2D*). Additional support for this idea was obtained through the use of heterozygous cells as a source for H-2 antigen. In the heterozygous condition, both *H-2* haplotypes are expressed on single cells, and therefore the genes are considered codominant. It was useful to examine the H-2 molecules from such heterozygous cells to determine whether four separate H-2 molecules could be isolated.

For this purpose, spleen cells from $F_1$ animals ($H\text{-}2^a \times H\text{-}2^b$) were radiolabeled in tissue culture, and an NP-40-solubilized antigen preparation was made. The private specificities from the $H\text{-}2^a$ chromosome are H-2.11 ($H\text{-}2K^k$) and H-2.4 ($H\text{-}2D^d$) and from the $H\text{-}2^b$ chromosome are H-2.33 ($H\text{-}2K^b$) and H-2.2 ($H\text{-}2D^b$). Aliquots of antigen were precipitated with one of four monospecific sera and the supernatant remaining was divided and tested with antisera against all four private specificities. When the second set of precipitates was subjected to electrophoresis, the presence or absence of H-2 peaks could be assessed (Fig. 11.4). It was found that all four of these specificities were precipitated independently and hence that all four were on different molecules.

It is worthwhile reiterating that in this type of study, a finding of separation of specificities is only valid when a method that avoids cleavage is used to obtain antigen. Thus, studies with papain solubilized antigen could not be used to show natural separation of specificities conclusively. The reason for the introduction of detergent solubilized antigen was to avoid difficulties introduced by enzymatic cleavage or autolytic processes present in most of the other methods used for solubilization.

It is of significance that these studies carried out on cell extracts were confirmed and extended on living lymphocyte membranes by a series of elegant experiments carried out by Neauport-Sautes *et al.* (1973a). These experiments, which are discussed in more detail in Section VI, examined the redistribution of H-2K and H-2D antigens of ($H\text{-}2^b \times H\text{-}2^a$)$F_1$ hybrids following capping induced with monospecific anti-H-2 antibodies coupled to either tetramethyl rhodamine isothiocyanate or fluorescein isothiocyanate. By comparing all antigens in pairs, with one antibody labeled with fluorescein and another with rhodamine, they showed independent migration of H-2K and H-2D glycoproteins. Such results support the conclusion that these glycoprotein gene products exist *in vivo* in separate units on the cell membrane and have independent mobility within the lateral plane of the membrane.

### B. The HLA System

Several sets of experiments have also been carried out to elucidate the immunochemical genetic relationships of the HLA system. Unfortunately, these studies suffer the limitation that papain solubilization was used to produce the antigenic material. However, since the results obtained have been confirmed by membrane rearrangement techniques

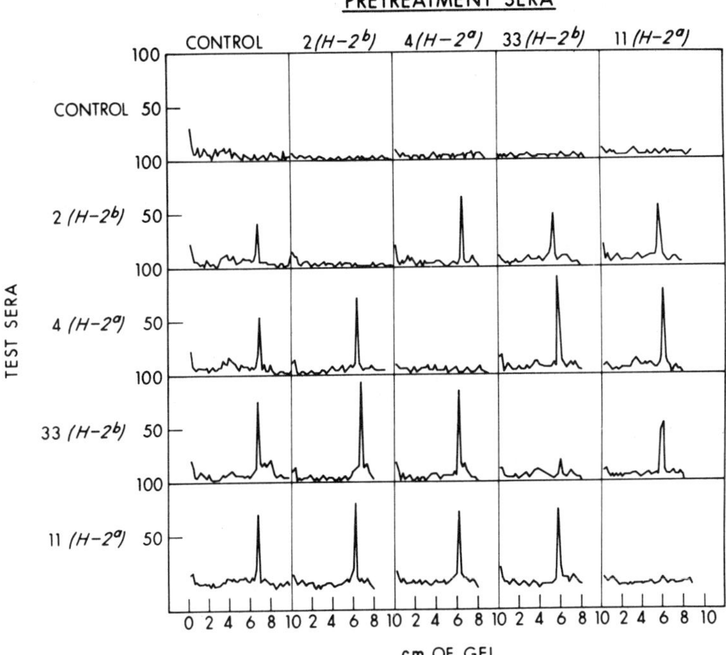


Fig. 11.4. Analysis by immunoprecipitation of antigen extracts solubilized with NP-40. This figure shows the dodecyl sulfate–polyacrylamide gel patterns of precipitates from the reactions of test antisera (shown on the left of the figure) with the supernatant fraction remaining after reaction with the pretreatment antisera (shown across the top of the figure) and removal of the resultant precipitate. The cpm of [$^{3}$H]fucose-labeled antigen are plotted along the ordinate of each graph. In each case, completeness of the treatment is shown by the lack of a specific H-2 peak when the sera are tested for the same antigen putatively removed by the antiserum pretreatment. The presence of the other three gene products after removal of one gene product by pretreatment is demonstrated by the observation of specific antigen peaks when the remaining three specificities are tested (see text for discussion). Reprinted from Cullen *et al.* (1972b) by permission of the United States National Academy of Sciences.

and are parallel to the results obtained with NP-40 solubilized H-2 antigens, they can be considered as supportive of the model in which antigenic specificities coded for by genes of the two segregant series are carried on separate molecules.

In one study (Mann *et al.*, 1969b), gel filtration was used to separate papain solubilized fragments into two peaks of HLA activity, one reactive for the A and the other reactive for the B series antigens. These results fit with the findings of similar separations of H-2 fragments of different sizes.

In other experiments, Cresswell *et al.* (1974a) were able to separate the HLA-B7 and HLA-A2 antigen bearing molecules which were of the same size. They formed a soluble immune complex by combining an anti-HLA-A2 alloantiserum with a radiolabeled, papain solubilized preparation from the RPMI 4265 (HLA-A2, B7, B12, and AW32) lymphoblastoid line. Gel filtration chromatography was used to separate the immune complex from the bulk of the radiolabeled material that was then pooled and concentrated. The material that was nonreactive with the anti-HLA-A2 was treated with either the same anti-HLA-A2 alloantiserum (as a control) or with an anti-HLA-B7 alloantiserum. The gel filtration chromatography was repeated; in the case of the control (HLA-A2) no immune complex was obtained, but with the anti-HLA-B7 antiserum a new immune complex was formed.

Similar studies by Fahey and his co-workers (Thieme *et al.*, 1974) showed that all four HLA antigenic specificities from the same RPMI 4265 cell line can be separated. These workers used discontinuous electrophoresis to separate the specific immune complex from the other unbound HLA glycoproteins. Bands were cut from the gels and eluted; the presence or absence of an antigenic specificity was assayed for by inhibition of cytotoxicity. Using this technique, Fahey and his co-workers were able to show that in this heterozygous cell line each HLA specificity resided on a molecule that could be separated from the molecules bearing the other specificities.

As discussed in detail in Section VI, the membrane rearrangement studies of Kourilsky (Neauport-Sautes *et al.*, 1973b) and Ceppelini (Bernoco *et al.*, 1973) fully confirm the separability of the HLA gene products on the lymphocyte membrane.

## V. Biochemical and Structural Properties of Other MHC Products

### A. The Immune Response Region Associated Antigens (Ia) of the *H-2* Complex

As noted in Chapter 6, a new system of cell surface antigens determined by one or more genes of the *I* region of the murine MHC has recently been defined by cytotoxic antisera (see review by David and Shreffler, 1975). These antigens have been found mainly on lymphoid cells, and most studies so far have suggested that they are mainly on B cells. The *I* region, of course, is of particular interest because it contains genes controlling several immune functions. Included, among others, are the *Ir-1A* and *Ir-1B* loci controlling the capacity to respond to certain antigens (Benacerraf and McDevitt, 1972), the locus or loci controlling the mixed lymphocyte reaction or MLR (Chapter 8, Section I; Démant, 1973), and a gene that is important in leukemagenesis (Lilly, 1973).

Several groups have carried out studies using available anti-Ia sera and the technique of indirect precipitation of detergent solubilized antigen extracts of radiolabeled cells. In one series of studies by Cullen *et al.* (1974), the Ia antigens were isolated using A.TL anti-A.TH ($I^k$ versus $I^s$) antisera with NP-40 solubilized [$^3$H]leucine-labeled spleen cells from B10.S ($I^s$) mice. The immune precipitates, solubilized and analyzed by electrophoresis in SDS on polyacrylamide gels, showed two specific radioactive peaks of approximately 60,000 and 30,000 daltons. The controls containing either normal serum or antisera with an inappropriate specificity showed no such peaks. When the 60,000 dalton peak was isolated by gel filtration chromatography, reduced with 2-mercaptoethanol and reanalyzed by electrophoresis, only a 30,000 dalton peak was found. This finding suggested a possible dimer–monomer relationship.

The experiments carried out so far have suggested that the Ia antigens are glycoproteins (Cullen and Nathenson, 1974). These data came from experiments in which spleen cell extracts were labeled with the radioactive monosaccharide precursors, fucose, galactose, and mannose. All three sugars were incorporated into protein-containing materials that precipitated with the specific antiserum and were found to migrate as proteins of approximately 30,000 daltons upon electrophoresis. The Ia antigens were also shown to be membrane located by the demonstration that spleen cell membrane preparations contained molecules of the expected electrophoretic mobility which were reactive with the anti-Ia sera. These molecules were absent from the cell sap.

A great deal of heterogeneity both in the antibody response and in the molecular product detected by the antibodies has been revealed. The heterogeneity was demonstrated by subjecting immune precipitates to new biochemical fractionation methods, and by the application of the indirect immune coprecipitation technique. In the former type of experiments, the use of improved discontinuous SDS electrophoresis (S. E. Cullen, J. H. Freed, and S. G. Nathenson, unpublished data) has shown that what previously was thought to be a rather broad 30,000 dalton peak could be fractionated into three peaks of approximately 35,000, 30,000, and 26,000 daltons. Thus many molecular species are detected by most of the Ia antisera presently being utilized.

Based on the observations by David *et al.* (1973) that absorption techniques revealed different specificities in a single antiserum, Cullen *et al.* (1974) used the indirect immune coprecipitation technique to examine the possibility that more than one antigen molecule could be present. The homozygous recombinant mouse strain B10.HTT was utilized as antigen source. Radiolabeled antigen preparations were treated with two reciprocal anti-Ia sera, A.TL anti-A.TH ($I^k$ versus $I^s$) and A.TH anti-A.TL ($I^s$ versus $I^k$). Sequential indirect precipitation with these sera in different combinations revealed the presence of at least two populations of molecules. Thus, not only are there Ia reactive molecules of different sizes but also separable molecules of identical electrophoretic mobility.

In summary therefore, the Ia antigen system has been shown to be extremely complex. The antigen-bearing gene products of the *Ia* genes are glycoproteins of at least three molecular weight classes, 35,000, 30,000 and 26,000 daltons. They are found mainly on the cell membrane of lymphocytes of the B cell series. This complicated system is a subject of extreme activity at present and the situation will undoubtedly be clarified as new data are revealed.

### B. Thymus Leukemia (Tla) Antigens

The Tla alloantigens have been isolated and examined by both proteolytic cleavage with papain (Muramatsu *et al.*, 1973b) and by NP-40 solubilization methods (Vitetta *et al.*, 1972; Yu and Cohen, 1974a). The Tla antigen isolated by papain digestion was found to be a glycoprotein fragment of approximately 38,000 daltons. The carbohydrate moiety of the Tla antigen was shown to slightly larger in size than that from H-2, with a molecular weight of 4500 daltons as compared with 3300 daltons for the H-2 carbohydrate. The findings thus underscored the chemical similarity of the Tla and H-2 antigens, a similarity that was noted in previous studies by Davies *et al.* (1969).

The Tla alloantigen isolated by NP-40 solubilization (Vitetta *et al.*, 1972) was approximately 45,000 daltons, and thus was of the same size as the H-2 glycoprotein when similarly isolated. In view of the genetic linkage of the *H-2* and *Tla* genes and the striking similarities of their products, it would be of interest to establish whether the murine $\beta_2$-microglobulin component also is associated with the Tla glycoprotein. Such an association has been suggested (J. W. Uhr and E. S. Vitetta, unpublished communication).

## VI. Membrane Arrangement

Since the cell membrane is a mosaic structure consisting of many different proteins or glycoproteins imbedded in fluid bilayer, it is important to establish whether there are defined topographical associations between these membrane components. Two approaches that have provided information on the membrane arrangements of molecular components are the antibody blocking method and the capping method. The antibody blocking method predated the capping technique, and the results in part may be explicable in terms of the processes that underlie capping. In the antibody blocking technique, antigen associations are inferred from the inhibition of the cytolytic effect of specific antibody directed against one antigenic determinant due to prior incubation of target cells with antibodies directed against another antigenic determinant. In the capping (or membrane rearrangement) technique, addition of bivalent antibodies against determinants carried by one set of molecules causes rearrangement of the immune complexes into aggregates (patches) or caps. Membrane associations can be deduced if capping of one set of molecules by specific antibody also causes capping of the other molecules (cocapping). Alternately, cytotoxicity techniques can be used to test for the removal of a second molecule after capping of the first ("lysostrip"). The "lysostrip" or clearance technique differs from the antibody blocking method in that the conditions used during the first antiserum treatment are chosen to maximize membrane rearrangements.

## A. Antibody Blocking

In an elegant series of studies utilizing the antibody blocking technique, Boyse *et al.* (1968) examined the spatial association of selected membrane antigenic sites. They studied the relationships between the antigenic sites determined by the *H-2D* and *H-2K* genes relative to one another, and relative to several other alloantigenic specificities. The major premise of these experiments was that if one antiserum coated the cell and prevented the uptake of the second antiserum, it could be concluded that there was a geographical relationship between the antigenic determinants detected by these two separate antibodies. Specifically, it was reasoned, the two antigenic sites were close enough that Ig bound to the first site would cover the second site. An equally plausible explanation would be that addition of the first Ig may have caused aggregation or capping of the molecules bearing the first antigenic site, and, by virtue of coaggregation or cocapping of the second set of molecules, removed them and their antigenic sites from the surface or in some way made them unavailable for reaction with antibody.

Whatever, the physical explanation, the experimental facts show that antibodies against the *Tla* gene products blocked the uptake of alloantibodies against the products of the *H-2D* gene but not those of the *H-2K* gene. The reciprocal experiment confirmed these observations, and further it was found that antisera to the H-2D and H-2K specificities did not block one another. These observations thus fit with the independent capping of H-2K and H-2D (Neauport-Sautes *et al.*, 1973a) and with the findings on the chemical separation of NP-40 solubilized H-2K and H-2D antigen extracts (Cullen *et al.*, 1972a,b). Other studies using antibodies directed against the Ly-1 alloantigen showed blocking of uptake of antibodies against the *H-2K* but not the *H-2D* gene products. Thus, there appears to be a geographical relationship between Tla and H-2D molecules and between the Ly-1 and H-2K molecules. Further studies with anti-Thy-1 antisera showed an inhibition of uptake of anti-Tla, anti-H-2D, and anti-Ly-2 antisera, but no blocking of the uptake of anti-H-2K serum.

### B. Capping (Membrane Rearrangement)

The phenomenon of capping refers to the rearrangement and then aggregation of membrane macromolecules under the influence of reagents that bind them, such as antibodies, lectins, or antigens. This phenomenon was first discovered in 1971 and 1972 (Taylor *et al.*, 1971; Loor *et al.*, 1972), using the technique of fluorescence microscopy with fluorescein- or rhodamine-linked antibodies. When these workers studied the effects of labeling surface immunoglobulin with anti-immunoglobulin antisera, three types of labeling patterns were observed. (1) Cells labeled with specific anti-immunoglobulin reagents at 0°C exhibited a diffuse labeling pattern. (2) When the cells with a diffuse label were allowed to incubate for a short while at 37°C, the anti-immunoglobulin label and the bound surface immunoglobulin gathered into spots or patches. This spotting or patching process required only that the labeling reagent be divalent, since monovalent Fab fragments did not form patches. It was not affected by inhibitors of metabolic processes, but was inhibited by substances or conditions that changed the fluidity of the lipid bilayer. (3) When the labeled cells were held at warmer temperatures for longer times, the patches or spots aggregated into caps, or concentrated regions, over one pole of the cell. Capping required that the cell be metabolically active and was inhibited by azide, cyanide, dinitrophenol, and other metabolic inhibitors.

The current interpretation of the capping is as follows. The applied antibodies bind the cell surface component against which they are directed. Under conditions in which the antibodies are divalent and the membrane is sufficiently fluid to allow lateral diffusion of its components, the antibodies eventually form an antibody–antigen matrix based on random collision and binding of the components of the membrane. This membrane rearrangement is called *patching* or *spotting*. Under conditions in which the cell is metabolically active, these patches are collected at one pole of the cell and the antigen–antibody complexes may be extensively internalized by endocytosis. This is called *capping*.

As mentioned previously, capping can be used to explore the relationship between various antigenic structures on the membrane surface. The first antigen is treated with labeled (e.g., fluorescein) antibody under conditions which permit cap formation; then the second antigen is treated with a differently labeled (tetramethyl rhodamine) antibody under conditions which prevent cap formation. If, when the cell is examined, both labels are found in the same polar cap, it can be concluded that treatment with the first antibody caused capping of both substances and that they must therefore be intimately associated on a membrane. If the first label is found in a polar cap and the second is spread evenly over the cell in a diffuse pattern, then the antigens do not cocap and they must not have been intimately associated. Such an experiment, taken from a paper by Neauport-Sautes *et al.* (1973a), is shown in Fig. 11.5.

A variation of the capping method (lysostrip) makes use of the fact that capping of one molecule induces a specific unresponsiveness to cytolysis by antibodies against the molecule, presumably due to the movement of the macromolecule into the polar capped position. This clearance, as measured by loss of sensitivity to complement, can also be used as a measure of association between membrane components.

The studies carried out on the question of capping of HLA and H-2 antigens have been referred to briefly in previous sections of this chapter. Kourilsky and his co-workers (Preud'homme *et al.*, 1972; Kourilsky *et al.*, 1972) first demonstrated by fluorescent microscopy that HLA antigens and surface immunoglobulins cap independently of each other and hence are separate. The HLA antigens of the A series and the B series have also been shown to be independent of one another (Neauport-Sautes *et al.*, 1973b). In these studies the investigators directly coupled fluorescein and tetramethyl rhodamine to anti-HLA-A2 and anti-HLA-B5 antibodies. They showed that HLA-A2 and HLA-B5 capped independently of one another when the normal double label protocol was followed. Ceppelini and his co-workers (Bernoco *et al.*, 1973) obtained similar results using anti-HLA-A1 and anti-HLA-B8 antibodies in studies which were carried out using the indirect staining method in which

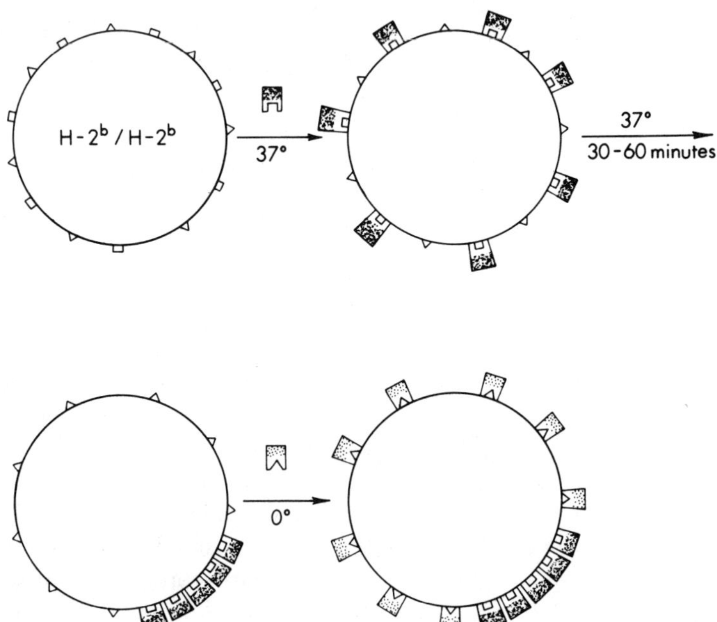


FIG. 11.5. Two-stage capping experiments demonstrating independent capping of $H\text{-}2K^b$ and $H\text{-}2D^b$ gene products. C57BL/6 lymph node cells bearing $\text{H-2K}^b$ (H-2.33, □) and $\text{H-2D}^b$ (H-2.2, △) antigens were incubated first at 37°C with tetramethyl rhodamine-labeled anti-H-2.33 (stippled) and second at 0°C with fluorescein-labeled anti-H-2.2 (dotted). Microscopic examination of the cells then showed that in most cells the red fluorescence appeared in discrete clusters, whereas the green fluorescence appeared diffusely over the entire cell surface. Modified from Neauport-Sautes *et al.* (1973c) with permission of Grune and Stratton, Inc.

the anti-human Ig carried the two different fluorescent labels. These results were confirmed by the clearance method.

In studies on H-2, immunoglobulin and the H-2 antigens (H-2D and H-2K) were found to be distinct by the capping procedure (Unanue *et al.*, 1972; Karnovsky *et al.*, 1972) using both immunoelectron and fluorescein microscopy. That H-2K and H-2D cap independently of one another was demonstrated by Neauport-Sautes *et al.* (1973a) in a study of $F_1$ hybrid cells (C57BL/6 × C3H)$F_1$ using sera identical to those used by Cullen *et al.* (1972b) in the study of noncoprecipitation of NP-40 solubilized *H-2K* and *H-2D* gene products. The results of Neauport-Sautes clearly show that the *H-2* gene products cap independently of one another whether they are coded for by genes in the cis position (e.g., $H\text{-}2K^k$ and $H\text{-}2D^k$) or in the trans-homologous position (e.g., $H\text{-}2K^b$ and $H\text{-}2K^k$), or in the trans-nonhomologous position (e.g., $H\text{-}2D^b$

and *H-2K*$^k$). In a series of studies carried out to map H-2 antigens, but performed under conditions that would measure capping by the clearance method, Krištofová *et al.* (1970) presented data which can be interpreted to mean that some public specificities cap together with private specificities carried by the same gene product. Thus H-2.5 and H-2.11, both of which are carried by H-2K$^k$, were cleared together. Independent clearing was also demonstrated for other specificities when carried on separate gene products, e.g., H-2K$^k$ and H-2D$^d$.

Evidence from chemical studies concerning the association between $\beta_2$-microglobulin and the HLA alloantigens (Section III,D) has been confirmed by capping. A number of investigators (Fanger and Bernier, 1973; Poulik *et al.*, 1973; Bismith *et al.*, 1973, 1974; Solheim and Thorsby, 1974; Neauport-Sautes *et al.*, 1974) have studied the capping of $\beta_2$-microglobulin on human lymphocytes. The techniques have included both direct and indirect immunofluorescence, immunoelectron microscopy, and resistance to complement-dependent lysis. These studies showed that $\beta_2$-microglobulin capped independently of surface immunoglobulin, but capping of $\beta_2$-microglobulin caused the cocapping of all defined HLA antigens. In the reverse experiment, in which capping of HLA antigens is carried out first, there was a cocapping of only part of the $\beta_2$-microglobulin. Hence all $\beta_2$-microglobulin does not appear to be associated with HLA.

### C. Antigenic Modulation

Antigenic modulation was originally demonstrated *in vivo* (Boyse *et al.*, 1963) and *in vitro* (Old *et al.*, 1968) in the *Tla* (thymus leukemia) system, and while some features are similar to those described for capping, the *Tla* system manifests specific and unique properties. The original *in vitro* observation was that exposure of *Tla*+ cells to Tla antibody in the absence of lytic complement causes disappearance of the antigen. This disappearance is clearly a membrane rearrangement. It is not a simple capping phenomenon, however, since the modulation is inhibited by actinomycin, an inhibitor of messenger RNA synthesis. It is also accompanied by an increase in H-2D alloantigen expression and, most important, can occur even with monovalent Fab fragments of anti-Tla antibodies.

Studies by Yu and Cohen (1974b) on the metabolism of Tla antigen have supported the observations of the serological findings. Their results suggest that cells undergoing modulation lose radiolabeled Tla more rapidly than normal controls, although synthesis of Tla molecules is not altered. Other studies (Stackpole *et al.*, 1974), however, suggest that modulation is much more complicated, since Tla antigen–antibody complexes appear not to be lost from cells when examined by immunoelectron microscopy.

## VII. Dynamic Properties of the MHC Products of the Membrane

Studies on the biogenesis of membrane molecules have established that different components of the cell membrane are renewed and degraded at different rates. For example, different enzymes of liver cell membranes turn over at different rates, and lipids also show variable turnover properties (Omura *et al.*, 1967; Schimke and Dehlinger, 1972). Studies on the turnover or biosynthesis and degradation of the antigenic products of the major histocompatibility loci have been carried out for both H-2 glycoproteins and HLA glycoproteins (Schwartz and Nathenson, 1971a; Turner *et al.*, 1972; Schwartz *et al.*, 1973b). Since these glycoproteins can be readily labeled and isolated in a pure form, it is possible to assess the biosynthetic and degradative steps which involve these integral components of the membrane. Several types of experiments have been carried out to determine the H-2 turnover rate. In a study on the H-2 antigens by Schwartz and Nathenson (1971a), papain was used to destroy the antigen on the surface of intact cells and the reappearance of the antigen in the cell membrane was assessed. Tumor cells bearing the H-2D$^d$ alloantigen were treated with papain until only about 40% of the H-2 antigen was left. The cells were suspended in growth medium and the reappearance of antigenic activity was monitored. While the antigen in the control cells remained at a constant level for the entire experimental time, the antigenic activity on the papain treated cells began to increase after a lag of about 60 minutes. It rose from a base line value of 40 to 100% by 6 hours. The level of antigenic activity remained constant after 100% of normal activity had been achieved. This study shows that the reappearance of antigenic activity in these tumor cells is quite rapid. The 6 hours required is much less than the 24 hours time that the cells need for division. In a study done with HLA antigens on lymphoblastoid cell lines (Turner *et al.*, 1972), 6 hours were required for the establishment of the normal levels of HLA. Thus the kinetics were identical to those found for the *H-2* system.

In another study (Schwartz *et al.*, 1973b), turnover rates were determined in two different types of $H\text{-}2^d$ tumor cells. As shown in Fig. 11.6, radiolabel in specific cell surface H-2 antigen decayed with a $t_{1/2}$ (half-time) of about 7 hours, whereas the radiolabel in the crude membrane fraction decayed with a $t_{1/2}$ of about 24 hours. Since the doubling

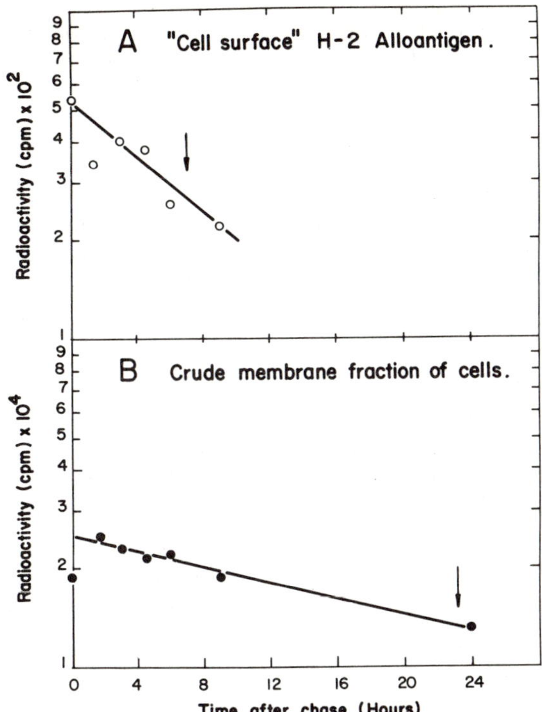


FIG. 11.6. Turnover of H-2 alloantigens in external cell surface fraction. Cells labeled with [$^{14}$C]leucine for 24 hours were transferred to chasing medium and aliquots collected at the same points indicated. In (A) are plotted the results of the membrane-filtration assay for specific H-2 alloantigenic activity in the "cell surface" material obtained by papain digestion of intact cells. In (B) the measurements of total radioactivity in the crude membrane fraction are plotted. This figure is reprinted with permission of Grune and Stratton from Schwartz *et al.* (1973b), which should be consulted for further details.

time for the cells under these experimental conditions is about 48 hours, the turnover rate for the H-2 antigen is 4 to 5 times faster than the rate of cell division.

One interesting question is whether the disappearance of radiolabeled H-2 antigen is due to (1) actual degradation, (2) sequestration of the molecules in a place not accessible to antibody, or (3) the secretion from the cell, possibly in an antigenic form. An answer to this question is not yet available; however, studies on the phenomenon of aggregation and capping may give some clue to the actual fate of the H-2 antigens and other membrane molecules during their lifetime on the cell surface.

A rapid turnover rate, as noted for both H-2 and HLA antigens, would be consistent with recent findings of a marked variation in the amount of H-2 and HLA on cells in different phases of the cell cycle (Cikes and Friberg, 1971; Pasternak *et al.*, 1971; Pellegrino *et al.*, 1972). Since the cell volume and hence the membrane area varies during different phases of the cell cycle, particular periods of intense biosynthetic and degradative activity might be expected. Further investigations are needed to answer the questions about the biosynthetic pathway of the H-2 and HLA glycoproteins, such as details of the synthesis at the polysome level, the mode and sites of addition of the carbohydrate residues, the transport of partially or fully completed glycoprotein to the cell surface membrane, and the mode of exteriorization.

From recent results (Uhr and Vitetta, 1973), it has been postulated that the pathway for the H-2 glycoproteins is very similar to that for the IgG glycoproteins, i.e., from the polysomes to the Golgi apparatus and finally to the cell exterior by fusion of the Golgi vesicles with surface membranes. H-2 glycoproteins that are tightly bound to the membrane remain in the cell surface, however, while the soluble IgG glycoproteins are secreted. Of interest with regard to the major MHC antigenic products are recent observations (Vitetta *et al.*, 1974) that the Ia glycoproteins, in contrast to the H-2 glycoproteins, are easily lost from the cell surface and possibly can be recovered in the supernatant fraction of lymphocytes growing in culture. These findings suggest that Ia products may have distinct and unique biosynthetic properties.

## VIII. A Hypothetical Model for the Classical MHC Antigens

The H-2 and HLA antigens appear to contain a highly polymorphic glycoprotein unit of approximately 45,000 daltons, the product of structural genes located in the MHC, and, in noncovalent association, a highly conserved, low molecular weight protein of 11,600 daltons called $\beta_2$-microglobulin.

Some hypothetical features of the H-2 antigen complex are presented in Fig. 11.7. Most of the predicted features apply also to HLA molecules and, in fact, some of them were demonstrated first with human material. The antigen complex is shown to consist of two chains—the glycoprotein and the $\beta_2$-microglobulin. Some preliminary evidence (Schwartz *et al.*, 1973a) suggest that larger forms of the antigens may also exist. Consistent with these data would be the existence of a tetrameric structure consisting of two disulfide-linked glycoprotein chains each with an associated $\beta_2$-microglobulin molecule. However these data must be interpreted with caution, and further experimentation is needed. The suggestion

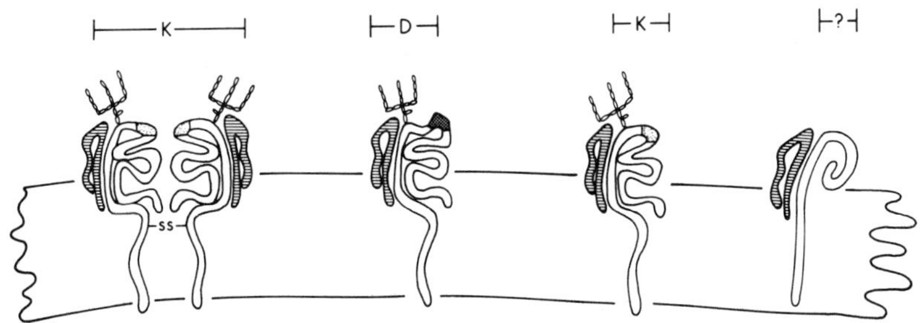


FIG. 11.7. Hypothetical model of H-2 antigens. This figure depicts the H-2 antigens visualized in a schematic cross section through the plasma membrane. The glycoprotein (45,000 daltons) and the noncovalently associated murine $\beta_2$-microglobulin (11,600 daltons) are shown. The H-2 glycoproteins are represented by long convoluted tubular-shaped structures with a globular region at the external surface of the lipid bilayer. One end of the molecule is depicted as passing entirely through the membrane bilayer into the inside of the cell. Stippled areas reflect antigenic sites at which K and D molecules differ. The carbohydrate chains (3300 daltons) are depicted by the small, branched chain structures. The figure also shows an example of a possible H-2 "tetramer" consisting of two disulfide-linked glycoprotein chains each with its associated $\beta_2$-microglobulin chain. The murine $\beta_2$-microglobulin protein, which is noncovalently associated with the H-2 glycoprotein, is depicted by the shaded tubular structure. The $\beta_2$-microglobulin, which exists in excess of the H-2 glycoproteins chains, is shown schematically to be associated with other unspecified membrane proteins and glycoproteins.

that the glycoprotein and $\beta_2$-microglobulin moeities exist in a noncovalent association comes from the HLA field.

According to the model, the protein backbone extends through the membrane for possible interaction with internal structures such as microfilaments. In support of an extensive penetration of the membrane is the finding that H-2 and HLA structures can be considered integral proteins (Singer, 1974) as they are not easily removed from the membrane unless the membrane itself is dissolved or the protein itself is cleaved proteolytically.

With regard to primary structure, the $\beta_2$-microglobulin is partially homologous to immunoglobulin constant region domains and has an intrachain disulfide configuration similar to that of the immunoglobulin domains. This "immunoglobulinlike" structure suggests a relationship with the immunoglobulins either in the sense that the $\beta_2$-microglobulin might have immunological function or in the sense that it might have been derived from the same ancestor precursor genes from which immunoglobulins evolved.

With regard to the H-2 glycoprotein, relatively little information is available about its primary structure. It is shown that the peptide profile comparisons between products of alleles of the same *H-2* gene, as well as between products of alleles of *D* or *K* genes, reveal extraordinary differences. Judging from the H-2 peptide comparisons and hypothetical comparisons constructed for selected immunoglobulins (B. M. Ewenstein, unpublished observations) one would expect a maximum of 80–85% homology between products of alleles of one gene. Such a substitution of one or two amino acid residues out of each ten residues constitutes an amazing level of variability for the allelic products of one locus.

Each glycoprotein is multispecific since it carries at least several antigenic sites determined by the primary protein structure. This suggestion of several variable or antigenic regions of the H-2 glycoproteins is in accord with serological evidence that suggests the existence of several distinct antigenic sites. Thus, it is tempting to speculate that the polypeptide chain configuration that gives rise to the private antigenic sites is coded by a genetic region that has an effective high mutation rate. The existence of such a region would explain the high number of unique private specificities among the presently available laboratory strains and is further supported by the finding of a large number of new unique private specificities among wild mice, which, on the other hand, have tended to have the same public specificities as found in known laboratory strains (Klein, 1972). In view of the vast polymorphism or diversity of these sites in the species, such regions might possibly bear some resemblance to the immunoglobulin variable region genes.

On the other hand, the polypeptide regions that determine the public or common specificities, which are more widespread among haplotypes, appear to be more conserved among the strains of the species. For example, recombination data show that the public specificity H-2.3 sometimes maps in the *K* gene, sometimes in the *D* gene, and perhaps in both genes in some strains. Lower effective variability in the genetic region underlying these polypeptide areas might explain the wider distribution of these specificities, the fact that the specificities map in both *D* and *K* genes, and the generally lower titer of antisera directed against the public specificities. Such genetic regions that tend to conserve structure during evolution might be similar to the immunoglobulin constant region genes.

The carbohydrate site as outlined in Fig. 11.7 is entirely hypothetical at present. At least one but not more than two carbohydrate molecules of 3300 daltons could be attached. This follows from the evidence that approximately 10% of the dry weight of the molecule is carbohydrate.

Another point depicted in Fig. 11.7 is that the *D* gene products and the *K* gene products of the *H-2* system exist as separate entities. This is the case since, when isolated by indirect immune precipitation, the

H-2 glycoprotein consists of only D or K molecules, but not both. It is of course possible that larger aggregates containing both D and K dimer molecules can exist on the cell surface. However, the capping studies show that treatment with one antiserum leaves the molecules reacting with the other antisera in a diffuse staining pattern.

## REFERENCES

Acton, R. T., R. J. Morris, and A. F. Williams. 1974. Estimation of the amount and tissue distribution of rat Thy 1.1 antigen. *Eur J Immunol* **4**:598.

Aoki, T., U. Hämmerling, E. de Harven, E. A. Boyse, and L. J. Old. 1969. Antigenic structure of cell surfaces. An immunoferritin study of the occurrence of topography of H-2, $\theta$, and TL alloantigens on mouse cells. *J Exp Med* **130**:979.

Batchelor, J. R., and A. R. Sanderson. 1969. HL-A substances: Properties and immunization of rabbits. *Transplant Proc* **1**:489.

Benacerraf, B., and H. O. McDevitt. 1972. Histocompatibility-linked immune response genes. *Science* **175**:273.

Berggård, I., and A. G. Bearn. 1968. Isolation and properties of a low molecular weight $\beta_2$-globulin occurring in human biological fluids. *J Biol Chem* **243**:4095.

Bernier, I., A. Dautigny, J. Colombani, and P. Jollès. 1974. Detergent solubilized HL-A antigens from human platelets: A comparative study of various purification techniques. *Biochim Biophys Acta* **356**:82.

Bernoco, D., S. Cullen, G. Scudeller, G. Trinchieri, and R. Ceppellini. 1973. HL-A molecules at the cell surface. Page 527 *in* J. Dausset and J. Colombani, eds. Histocompatibility Testing 1972. Munksgaard, Copenhagen.

Billing, R. J., and P. I. Terasaki. 1974. Purification of HL-A antigen from normal serum. *J Immunol* **112**:1124.

Bismuth, A., C. Neauport-Sautes, F. M. Kourilsky, Y. Manuel, and T. Greenland. 1973. Association entre les antigènes HL-A et la $\beta_2$-microglobuline detéctée par immunofluorescence sur la membrane des lymphocytes humains. *C R Acad Sci* [D] (*Paris*) **277**:2845.

Bismuth, A., C. Neauport-Sautes, F. M. Kourilsky, Y. Manuel, T. Greenland, and D. Silvestre. 1974. Distribution and mobility of $\beta_2$-microglobulin on the human lymphocyte membrane: Immunofluorescence and immunoferritin studies. *J Immunol* **112**:2036.

Boyle, W. 1969. Soluble HL-A iso-antigen preparations. *Transplant Proc* **1**:491.

Boyse, E. A., L. J. Old, and S. Luell. 1963. Antigenic properties of experimental leukemias. II. Immunological studies *in vitro* with C57BL/6 radiation-induced leukemias. *J Natl Cancer Inst* **31**:987.

Boyse, E. A., L. J. Old, and E. Stockert. 1968. An approach to the mapping of antigens on the cell surface. *Proc Natl Acad Sci USA* **60**:886.

Brown, J. L., K. Kato, J. Silver, and S. G. Nathenson. 1974. Notable diversity in peptide composition of murine H-2K and H-2D alloantigens. *Biochemistry* **13**:3174.

Cikes, M., and S. Friberg, Jr. 1971. Expression of H-2 and Moloney leukemia virus-determined cell-surface antigens in synchronized cultures of a mouse cell line. *Proc Natl Acad Sci USA* **68**:566.

Cresswell, P., M. J. Turner, and J. L. Strominger. 1973. Papain-solubilized HL-A antigens from cultured human lymphocytes contain two peptide fragments. *Proc Natl Acad Sci USA* **70**:1603.

Cresswell, P., R. J. Robb, M. J. Turner, and J. L. Strominger. 1974a. Papain solubilized HL-A antigens. Chromatographic and electrophoretic studies of the two subunits from different specificities. *J Biol Chem* **249**:2828.

Cresswell, P., T. Springer, J. L. Strominger, M. J. Turner, H. M. Grey, and R. T. Kubo. 1974b. Immunological identity of the small subunit of HL-A antigens and $\beta_2$-microglobulin and its turnover on the cell membrane. *Proc Nat Acad Sci USA* **71**:2123.

Cullen, S. E., and S. G. Nathenson. 1974. Further characterization of Ia (immune response region associated) antigen molecules. Page 191 *in* C. F. Fox, ed. The immune system: genes, receptors, signals. Academic Press, New York.

Cullen, S. E., B. D. Schwartz, and S. G. Nathenson. 1972a. The distribution of alloantigen specificities of native H-2 products. *J Immunol* **108**:596.

Cullen, S. E., B. D. Schwartz, S. G. Nathenson, and M. Cherry. 1972b. The molecular basis of codominant expression of the histocompatibility-2 genetic region. *Proc Natl Acad Sci USA* **69**:1394.

Cullen, S. E., C. S. David, D. C. Shreffler, and S. G. Nathenson. 1974. Membrane molecules determined by the *H-2* associated immune response region: Isolation and some properties. *Proc Natl Acad Sci USA* **71**:648.

Cunningham, B. A., J. L. Wang, I. Berggård, and P. A. Peterson. 1973. The complete amino acid sequence of $\beta_2$-microglobulin. *Biochemistry* **12**:4811.

Dautigny, A., I. Bernier, J. Colombani, and P. Jollès. 1973. Purification and characteristization of HL-A antigens from human platelets, solubilized by the nonionic detergent NP-40. *Biochim Biophys. Acta* **298**:783.

David, C. S., and D. C. Shreffler. 1975. The *H-2* major histocompatibility complex and the *I* immune response region: Genetic variations, functions and organization. *Adv Immunol* **20**:125.

David, C. S., D. C. Shreffler, and J. A. Frehlinger. 1973. New lymphocyte antigen system (*Lna*) controlled by the *Ir* region of the mouse *H-2* complex. *Proc Natl Acad Sci USA* **70**:2509.

Davies, D. A. L., B. J. Alkins, E. A. Boyse, L. J. Old, and E. Stockert. 1969. Soluble TL and H-2 antigens prepared from a TL positive leukemia of a TL negative mouse strain. *Immunology* **16**:669.

Davis, B. D. 1964. Disc electrophoresis. II. Method and application to human serum proteins. *Ann NY Acad* Sci **121**:404.

Davis, W. C., and L. Silverman. 1968. Localization of mouse H-2 histocompatibility antigen with ferritin-labeled antibody. *Transplantation* **6**:536.

Dawson, J. R., J. Silver, L. B. Sheppard, and B. D. Amos. 1974. The purification of detergent-solubilized HL-A antigens by affinity chromatography with the hemagglutinin from lens culinaris. *J Immunol* **112**:1190.

Dayhoff, M. 1972. Atlas of protein sequence and structure, 1972. Vol. 5, pages D375–D376. National Biomedical Research Foundation, Silver Springs, Maryland.

Démant, P. 1973. *H-2* gene complex and its role in alloimmune reactions. *Transplant Rev* **15**:164.

Edelman, G. M. 1970. The covalent structure of a human $\gamma$G-immunoglobulin. XI. Functional implications. *Biochemistry* **9**:3197.

Evrin, P.-E., and H. Pertoft. 1973. $\beta_2$-Microglobulin in human blood cells. *J Immunol* **111**:1147.

Fanger, M. W., and G. M. Bernier. 1973. Subpopulations of human lymphocytes defined by $\beta_2$-microglobulin. *J Immunol* **111**:609.

Goodfellow, P. N., E. A. Jones, V. van Heyningen, E. Solomon, M. Bobrow, V. Miggiano, and W. F. Bodmer. 1975. The $\beta_2$-microglobulin gene is on chromosome 15 and not in the HL-A region. *Nature (Lond)* **254**:267.

Grey, H. M., R. T. Kubo, S. M. Colon, M. D. Poulik, P. Cresswell, T. Springer, N. Turner, and J. L. Strominger. 1973. The small subunit of HL-A antigens is $\beta_2$-microglobulin. *J Exp Med* **138**:1608.

Hämmerling, U., and H. J. Eggers. 1970. Quantitative measurement of uptake of alloantibody on mouse lymphocytes. *Eur J Biochem* **17**:95.

Kandutsch, A. A., and U. Reinert-Wenck. 1957. Studies on a substance that promotes tumor homograft survival (the "enhancing substance"). Its distribution and some properties. *J Exp Med* **105**:125.

Karnovsky, M. J., E. R. Unanue, and J. Leventhal. 1972. Ligand-induced movement of lymphocyte membrane macromolecules. II. Mapping of surface moieties. *J Exp Med* **136**:907.

Katagiri, M., N. Tanigaki, V. P. Kreiter, and D. Pressman. 1974. Common antigenic structures of HL-A antigens. III. An HL-A common antigenic marker closely associated with HL-A alloantigenic activity and detected by use of rabbit anti-rhesus monkey cell membrane antibodies. *Immunology,* **27**:487.

Klein, J. 1972. Histocompatibility-2 system in wild mice. I. Identification of five new *H-2* chromosomes. *Transplantation* **13**:291.

Klein, J., and D. C. Shreffler. 1972. Evidence supporting a two-gene model for the *H-2* histocompatibility system of the mouse. *J Exp Med* **135**:1972.

Kourilsky, F. M., D. Silvestre, C. Neauport-Sautes, Y. Loosefelt, and J. Dausset. 1972. Antibody-induced redistribution of HL-A antigens at the cell surface. *Eur J Immunol* **2**:249.

Krištofová, H., A. Lengerová, and J. Rejzková. 1970. Indirect mapping of spatial distribution of some H-2 antigens on the cell membrane. *Folia Biol (Praha)* **16**:81.

Lilly, F. 1973. Mouse leukemia: A model of multiple-gene disease. *J Natl Cancer Inst* **49**:927.

Loor, F., L. Forni, and B. Pernis. 1972. The dynamic state of the lymphocyte membrane. Factors affecting the distribution and turnover of surface immunoglobulins. *Eur J Immunol* **2**:203.

Maizel, J. V. 1971. Polyacrylamide gel electrophoresis of viral proteins. *Methods Virol* **5**:179.

Mann, D. L. 1972. The effect of enzyme inhibitors on the solubilization of HL-A antigens with 3 *M* KCl. *Transplantation* **14**:398.

Mann, D. L., G. N. Rogentine, J. L. Fahey, and S. G. Nathenson. 1969a. Human lymphocyte membrane (HL-A) alloantigens: Isolation, purification and properties. *J Immunol* **103**:282.

Mann, D. L., G. N. Rogentine, Jr., J. L. Fahey, and S. G. Nathenson. 1969b. Molecular heterogeneity of human lymphoid (HL-A) alloantigens. *Science* **163**:1460.

Miyakawa, Y., N. Tanigaki, Y. Yagi, and D. Pressman. 1971. An efficient method for isolation of HL-A antigens from hematopoietic cell lines. *J Immunol* **107**:394.

Miyakawa, Y., N. Tanigaki, Y. Yagi, and D. Pressman. 1973. Common antigen structures of HL-A antigens. I. Antigenic determinants recognizable by rabbits on papain-solubilized HL-A molecular fragments. *Immunology* **24**:67.

Möller, G. 1961. Demonstration of mouse isoantigens at the cellular level by fluorescent antibody technique. *J Exp Med* **114**:415.

Muramatsu, T., and S. G. Nathenson. 1970. Studies on the carbohydrate portion of membrane-located mouse H-2 alloantigens. *Biochemistry* **9**:4875.

Muramatsu, T., P. Atkinson, C. Cecarrini, and S. G. Nathenson. 1973a. Cell-surface glycopeptides: Growth-dependent changes in the carbohydrate–peptide linkage region. *J Mol Biol* **80**:781.

Muramatsu, T., S. G. Nathenson, E. A. Boyse, and L. J. Old. 1973b. Some biochemical properties of thymus leukemia antigens solubilized from cell membranes by papain digestion. *J Exp Med* **137**:1256.

Nakamuro, K., N. Tanigaki, and D. Pressman. 1973. Multiple common properties of human $\beta_2$-microglobulin and the common portion fragment derived from HL-A antigen molecules. *Proc Natl Acad Sci USA* **70**:2863.

Nathenson, S. G. 1970. Biochemical properties of histocompatibility antigens. *Annu Rev Genet* **4**:69.

Nathenson, S. G., and S. E. Cullen. 1974. Biochemical properties and immunochemical-genetic relationships of mouse H-2 alloantigens. *Biochim Biophys Acta* **344**:1.

Nathenson, S. G., and D. A. L. Davies. 1966. Solubilization and partial purification of mouse histocompatibility antigens from a membraneous lipoprotein fraction. *Proc Natl Acad Sci USA* **56**:476.

Nathenson, S. G., and T. Muramatsu. 1971. Properties of the carbohydrate portion of mouse H-2 alloantigen glycoproteins. Page 245 *in* G. A Jamieson and J. Greenwalt, eds.) Glycoproteins of blood cells and plasma. Lippincott, Philadelphia, Pennsylvania.

Neauport-Sautes, C., F. Lilly, D. Silvestre, and F. M. Kourilsky. 1973a. Independence of *H-2K* and *H-2D* antigenic determinants on the surface of mouse lymphocytes. *J Exp Med* **137**:511.

Neauport-Sautes, C., D. Silvestre, F. M. Kourilsky, and J. Dausset. 1973b. Independence of HL-A antigens from the first and second locus at the cell surface. Page 539 *in* J. Dausset and J. Colombani, eds. Histocompatibility Testing 1972. Munksgaard, Copenhagen.

Neauport-Sautes, C., D. Silvestre, F. Lilly, and F. M. Kourilsky. 1973c. Molecular independence of H-2K and H-2D antigens on the cell surface. *Transplant Proc* **5**:443.

Neauport-Sautes, C., A. Bismuth, F. M. Kourilsky, and Y. Manuel. 1974. Relationship between HL-A antigens and $\beta_2$-microglobulin as studied by immunofluorescence on the lymphocyte membrane. *J Exp Med* **139**:957.

Old, L. J., E. Stockert, E. A. Boyse, and J. H. Kim. 1968. Antigenic modulation. Loss of TL antigen from cells exposed to TL antibody. Study of the phenomenon *in vitro*. *J Exp Med* **127**:523.

Omura, T., P. Siekevitz, and G. E. Palade. 1967. Turnover of constituents of the endoplasmic reticulum membranes of rat hepatocytes. *J Biol Chem* **242**:2389.

Östberg, L., J. B. Lindblom, and P. A. Peterson. 1974. Subunit structure of HL-A antigens on cell surfaces. *Nature* (*Lond*) **249**:463.

Ozer, J. H., and D. F. H. Wallach. 1967. H-2 components and cellular membranes: Distinctions between plasma membrane and endoplasmic reticulum governed by the *H-2* region of the mouse. *Transplantation* **5**:652.

Palm, J., and L. Manson. 1968. Immunogenetic analysis of microsomal and nonmicrosomal lysoproteins from normal and malignant mouse tissues for histocompatibility-2 (H-2) antigens. *J Cell Comp Physiol* **68**:207.

Pancake, S. J., and S. G. Nathenson. 1973. Selective loss of H-2 antigenic reactivity after chemical modification. *J Immunol* **11**:1086.

Pasternak, C. A., A. M. H. Wormsley, and D. B. Thomas. 1971. Structural alterations in the surface membrane during the cell cycle. *J Cell Biol* **50**:562.

Pellegrino, M. A., S. Ferrone, P. G. Natali, A. Pellegrino, and R. A. Reisfeld. 1972. Expression of HL-A antigens in synchronized cultures of human lymphocytes. *J Immunol* **108**:573.

Peterson, P. A., B. A. Cunningham, I. Berggård, and G. M. Edelman. 1972. $\beta_2$-microglobulin—A free immunoglobulin domain. *Proc Natl Acad Sci USA* **69**:1697.

Peterson, P. A., L. Rask, and J. B. Lindblom. 1974. Highly purified papain-solubilized HL-A antigens contain $\beta_2$-microglobulin. *Proc Natl Acad Sci USA* **71**:35.

Poulik, M. D., M. Bernoco, D. Bernoco, and R. Ceppellini. 1973. Aggregation of HL-A antigens at the lymphocyte surface induced by anti-serum to $\beta_2$-microglobulin. *Science* **182**:1352.

Preud'homme, J. L., C. Neauport-Sautes, S. Piat, D. Silvestre, and F. M. Kourilsky. 1972. Independence of HL-A and immunoglobulin determinants on the surface of human lymphoid cells. *Eur J Immunol* **2**:297.

Rask, L., J. B. Lindblom, and P. A. Peterson. 1974. Subunit structure of H-2 alloantigens. *Nature* (*Lond*) **249**:833.

Reisfeld, R. A., M. A. Pellegrino, and B. D. Kahan. 1971. Salt extraction of soluble HL-A antigens. *Science* **172**:1134.

Reisfeld, R. A., M. A. Pellegrino, S. Ferrone, and B. D. Kahan. 1973. Chemical and molecular nature of HL-A antigens. *Transplant Proc* **5**:447.

Reisfeld, R. A., E. D. Sevier, M. A. Pellegrino, S. Ferrone, and M. D. Poulik, 1974. Association of HL-A antigens and $\beta_2$-microglobulin at the cellular and molecular level. *Immunogenetics* **2**:183.

Sanderson, A. R. 1968. HL-A substances from human spleens. *Nature* (*Lond*) **220**:192.

Sanderson, A. R., and K. I. Welsh. 1973. Quantitative measurement of the transplantation (HL-A) antigen sites on peripheral human lymphocytes. *Biochem Soc Trans* **1**:956–958 (abstr).

Sanderson, A. R., and K. I. Welsh. 1974. Properties of histocompatibility (HL-A) determinants. I. Site density of antigens of the two HL-A segregant series on peripheral human lymphocytes. *Transplantation* **17**:281.

Sanderson, A. R., P. Cresswell, and K. I. Welsh. 1971. Involvement of carbohydrate in the immuno-chemical determinant area of HL-A substances. *Nature* (*Lond*), *New Biol* **230**:8.

Schimke, R. T., and P. J. Dehlinger. 1972. Turnover of membrane proteins of animal cells. Page 115 *in* C. F. Fox, ed. Membrane research. Academic Press, New York.

Schwartz, B. D., and S. G. Nathenson. 1971a. Regeneration of transplantation antigens on mouse cells. *Transplant Proc* **3**:180.

Schwartz, B. D., and S. G. Nathenson. 1971b. Isolation of H-2 alloantigens solubilized by the detergent NP-40. *J Immunol* **107**:1363.

Schwartz, B. D., K. Kato, S. E. Cullen, and S. G. Nathenson. 1973a. H-2 histocompatibility alloantigens. Some biochemical properties of the molecules solubilized by NP-40 detergent. *Biochemistry* **12**:2157.

Schwartz, B. D., S. Wickner, T. V. Rajan, and S. G. Nathenson. 1973b. Biosynthetic properties of H-2 alloantigens: Turnover rate in $H\text{-}2^d$ tumor cells. *Transplant Proc* **5**:439.

Shimada, A., and S. G. Nathenson. 1969. Murine histocompatibility-2 (H-2) alloantigens. Purification and some chemical properties of soluble products of $H\text{-}2^b$ and $H\text{-}2^d$ genotypes released by papain digestion of membrane fractions. *Biochemistry* **8**:4048.

Shreffler, D. C., C. S. David, H. C. Passmore, and J. Klein. 1971. Genetic organization and evolution of the mouse *H-2* region: a duplication model. *Transplant Proc* **3**:176.

Silver, J., and L. Hood. 1974. Detergent-solubilized H-2 alloantigen is associated with a small molecular weight polypeptide. *Nature (Lond)* **249**:764.

Singer, J. S. 1974. The molecular organization of membranes. *Annu Rev Biochem* **43**:805.

Smithies, O., and M. D. Poulik. 1972a. Initation of protein synthesis at an unusual position in an immunoglobulin gene. *Science* **175**:187.

Smithies, O., and M. D. Poulik. 1972b. Dog homologue of human $\beta_2$-microglobulin. *Proc Natl Acad Sci USA* **69**:2914.

Snary, D., P. Goodfellow, M. J. Hayman, W. F. Bodner, and M. J. Crumpton. 1974. Subcellular separation and molecular nature of human histocompatibility antigens (HL-A). *Nature (Lond)* **247**:457.

Snell, G. D., M. Cherry, and P. Démant. 1971. Evidence that H-2 private specificities can be arranged in two mutually exclusive systems possibly homologous with two subsystems of HL-A. *Transplant Proc* **3**:183.

Solheim, B. G., and E. Thorsby. 1974. $\beta_2$-Microglobulin. Part of the HL-A molecule in the cell membrane. *Tissue Antigens* **4**:83.

Springer, T. A., J. L. Strominger, and D. L. Mann. 1974. Partial purification of detergent-soluble HL-A antigen and its cleavage by papain. *Proc Natl Acad Sci USA* **71**:1539.

Stackpole, C. W., J. B. Jacobson, and M. P. Lardis. 1974. Antigenic modulation *in vitro*. I. Fate of thymus–leukemia (TL) antigen–antibody complexes following modulation of TL antigenicity from the surfaces of mouse leukemia cells and thymocytes. *J Exp Med* **140**:939.

Strominger, J. L., P. Cresswell, H. Grey, R. E. Humphreys, D. Mann, J. McCune, P. Parham, R. Robb, A. R. Sanderson, T. A. Springer, C. Terhorst, and M. J. Turner. 1974. The immunoglobulin-like structure of human histocompatibility antigens. *Transplant Rev* **21**:126.

Tanigaki, N., and D. Pressman. 1974. The basic structure and the antigenic characteristics of HL-A antigens. *Transplant Rev* **21**:15.

Tanigaki, N., Y. Miyakawa, Y. Yagi, and D. Pressman. 1971. HL-A antigens from hematopoietic cell lines: Molecular size and electrophoretic mobility. *J Immunol* **107**:402.

Tanigaki, N., K. Nakamuro, E. Appella, M. D. Poulik, and D. Pressman. 1973. Identity of the HL-A common portion fragment and human $\beta_2$-microglobulin. *Biochim Biophys Acta* **55**:1234.

Tanigaki, N., K. Nakamuro, T. Natori, V. P. Kreiter, and D. Pressman. 1974. Common antigenic structures of HL-A antigens. V. An antigenic determinant characteristic of a 33,000 dalton fragment of HL-A antigen molecules. *Transplantation* **18**:74.

Taylor, R. B., W. P. H. Duffus, M. C. Raff, and S. de Petris. 1971. Redistribution and pinocytosis of lymphocyte surface immunoglobulin molecules induced by anti-immunoglobulin antibody. *Nature (Lond), New Biol* **233**:225.

Thieme, T. R., R. A. Raley, and J. L. Fahey. 1974. Demonstration of molecular individuality of HL-A antigens. *J Immunol* **113**:323.

Turner, M. J., J. L. Strominger, and A. R. Sanderson. 1972. Enzymic removal and re-expression of a histocompatibility antigen, HL-A2, at the surface of human peripheral lymphocytes. *Proc Natl Acad Sci USA* **69**:200.

Uhr, J. W., and E. S. Vitetta. 1973. Synthesis, biochemistry and dynamics of cell surface immunoglobulins on lymphocytes. *Fed Proc* **32**:35.

Unanue, E. R., W. D. Perkins, and M. J. Karnovsky. 1972. Ligand-induced movement of lymphocyte membrane macromolecules. I. Analyses by immunofluorescence and ultrastructural radioautography. *J Exp Med* **136**:885.

Vitetta, E. S., J. W. Uhr, and E. A. Boyse. 1972. Isolation and characterization of H-2 and TL alloantigens from the surface of mouse lymphocytes. *Cell Immunol* **4**:187.

Vitetta, E. S., J. Klein, and J. W. Uhr. 1974. Partial characterization of Ia antigens from murine lymphoid cells. *Immunogenetics* **1**:82.

Yu, A., and E. P. Cohen. 1974a. Studies on the effect of specific antisera on the metabolism of cellular antigens. I. Isolation of thymus leukemia antigens. *J Immunol* **112**:1285.

Yu, A., and E. P. Cohen. 1974b. Studies on the effect of specific antisera on the metabolism of cellular antigens. II. The synthesis and degradation of TL antigens of mouse cells in the presence of TL antisera. *J Immunol* **112**:1296.

CHAPTER 12

# HISTOCOMPATIBILITY GENES AND DISEASE



All immunogenetic systems are biological markers. The discovery of erythrocyte polymorphism in man inspired much research into possible associations with disease, but with only limited results in spite of considerable effort. Some associations have nevertheless been confirmed, such as that of duodenal ulcers with blood group O and stomach cancers with blood group A. In addition, many linkages have been clearly established, e.g., elliptocytosis with the rhesus locus and genes responsible for several hereditary diseases with the X chromosome, Xg locus.

Notable results have already been obtained from similar research in connection with the HLA system. The studies grew out of experimental evidence indicating that MHC genes show substantial correlations with viability, in general, with susceptibility to certain oncogenic viruses, and with the immune response.

After a survey of the experimental findings we shall indicate the current, rapidly advancing state of our knowledge concerning associations between the HLA system and disease. We shall look at the various mechanisms that have been suggested to explain these associations. Finally we shall consider the consequences of these discoveries, from the points of view of both medical practice and basic science. The implications are potentially of extreme interest.

## I. Experimental Bases

### A. Correlation between Histocompatibility Antigens and Susceptibility to Viruses

An area of medical significance where the MHC plays a role is resistance to oncogenic viruses. Gorer and Boyse (quoted by Lilly, 1971) were the first to point out that each of the four inbred strains used by Gross in demonstrating his leukemogenic virus possess the $H\text{-}2^k$ haplotype. Experimental proof of the role of the *H-2* genes or of a closely linked locus in this susceptibility was obtained by Lilly *et al.* (1964) and Lilly (1966) from crosses of the susceptible C3H ($H\text{-}2^k$) and resistant C57BL ($H\text{-}2^b$) strains. Resistance to the virus was dominant in the $F_1$. Results in $F_2$ and backcross generations showed that susceptibility is associated with the $H\text{-}2^k/H\text{-}2^k$ constitution. The gene linked to the *H-2* complex that is responsible for this effect was called *Rgv-1* (resistance to Gross virus). On statistical grounds, the intervention of another gene (*Rgv-2*), not linked to the *H-2* complex was also postulated. The existence of *Rgv-1* was amply confirmed in studies of congenic mice that differ from one another only at the *H-2* locus. Such animals differed radically in their susceptibility to the Gross virus. Subsequent studies with mice bearing recombinant *H-2* haplotypes showed that *Rgv-1* is associated with the *Ir-1* loci at the *K* end of the *H-2* complex. More recent studies have shown that the most probable number of genes involved in susceptibility to the Gross virus is three, thus adding a third locus *Rgv-3*, independent of *H-2*. The *H-2* system thus does not appear to be an all or nothing determinant of susceptibility.

The situation is different in connection with another leukemogenic agent, the Tennant virus. In this case, strains bearing the $H\text{-}2^d$ allele are the most susceptible. Tennant and Snell (1965), using strains congenic for the *H-2* complex, showed that although susceptibility to the virus is always greater in mice bearing the $H\text{-}2^d$ allele, several non-*H-2* genes must be postulated. In the case of the Friend virus complex, an influence of the *H-2* system, possibly through *Rgv-1*, has been demonstrated (Lilly, 1968). The role of *H-2* in this case seems to be limited to the ability of some mouse strains to recover from early lesions caused by the spleen focus-forming virus (SFFV) (Chesebro *et al.*, 1974), a neoplastic proliferation of erythropoietic cells in the spleen. Again, several loci not linked to *H-2* have been shown to be involved in the induction of both early splenomegaly due to the SSFV and in the later lymphatic leukemia attributed to the lymphoid leukemia virus (LLV). The two viruses form a complex in which LLV may work as a helper for SFFV.

A correlation, probably of entirely different type, has been established between the *H-2* complex and susceptibility to the erythrocyte-borne Bittner virus (R-MTV), which is responsible for mammary tumors in mice. Nandi (1967) showed that, unlike the mammary tissue-borne virus (M-MTV), viral activity associated with erythrocytes is highly strain-specific and is capable of consistently infecting only those strains that are compatible at the *H-2* locus with the R-MTV donors. Other results (Nandi *et al.*, 1971) indicate that R-MTV from C3H ($H\text{-}2^k/H\text{-}2^k$) mice was virtually incapable of infecting *H-2* incompatible strains and hybrids, although it infected 66% of $H\text{-}2^k/H\text{-}2^d$ mice and 89% of $H\text{-}2^k/H\text{-}2^k$) mice. Similarly, R-MTV from mice with the $H\text{-}2^d/H\text{-}2^d$ genotype could infect 50% or more of mice that were either heterozygous or homozygous for $H\text{-}2^d$. Conversely, only 0–22% of *H-2*-incompatible mice were susceptible to the same R-MTV. These observations support the hypothesis that the virus envelope contains parts of the host cell membrane. Testing congenic resistant strains on the C57BL/10 background for susceptibility to C3H-MTV showed that $H\text{-}2^b$ strains were less susceptible than $H\text{-}2^a$, $H\text{-}2^d$, $H\text{-}2^k$ or $H\text{-}2^m$ strains. The presence of different non-*H-2* alleles at histocompatibility loci had no effect on the resistance of $H\text{-}2^b$ mice to the virus.

Other correlations with *H-2* genotypes have been reported. Duran-Reynals and Lilly (1971) studied inbred strains and found a close correlation between susceptibility to vaccinia virus infection of the skin and tumorogenesis by methyl cholanthrene painting. Further analysis of the data collected in backcrosses shows a significant correlation between the *H-2* type and the occurrence of skin tumors. Seventy-five percent of the $H\text{-}2^d/H\text{-}2^d$ homozygotes developed skin tumors that were malignant in 33%, whereas only 34% of the $H\text{-}2^d/H\text{-}2^k$ heterozygotes developed skin tumors, malignant in 21%.

These different approaches have clearly shown that susceptibility to various oncogenic viruses is somehow associated with the mouse MHC, although the role of the *H-2* genes themselves in this connection has not been demonstrated. Perhaps these effects are determined by a gene or genes very closely linked to the *H-2* region, possibly by the *Ir* genes. It must be emphasized that these experiments can be applied to human pathology by analogy only. No human oncogenic virus is presently known, despite highly suggestive evidence.

## B. Correlation between Histocompatibility Antigens and Immune Response

Considerable evidence has been accumulated showing that immune response is genetically controlled. Two different mechanisms seem to be involved.

### 1. *General Ability to Mount a Humoral Immune Response*

A limited number of genes appear to control *general* ability to produce an antibody response. The work of Biozzi *et al.* (1971) on mice indicate that a limited number of generations of selective breeding is sufficient to provide populations of uniformly good or poor responders to several antigens. In mice these antigens are varied, including sheep and pigeon red cells, ovalbumin, and histocompatibility antigens. It has been calculated that this effect is due to the selection of 10–18 genes. One of them, accounting for 20% of this effect, is situated in the *H-2* complex (Stiffel *et al.*, 1974). The differences in response capability do not extend to histocompatibility antigens, since the average survival time of skin grafts between good and poor responders is approximately the same in both directions. Studies with infectious bacteria have shown, paradoxically, that it is the good responders that are most susceptible to gram-negative organisms (*Salmonella, Yersinia, Pasteurella pestis*), which are phagocytized by macrophages. The authors interpret this observation in terms of enhancing antibodies (Howard *et al.*, 1972).

### 2. *Specific Immune Response*

Immune response or *Ir* have been shown by studies with mice (Chapter 7) to control *specific* responses to a variety of antigens. The intervention of *Ir* genes in the response to a pathogenic agent, the murine lymphocytic choriomeningitis virus, has been demonstrated (Olstone *et al.*, 1973).

### 3. *Other Genes in the H-2 Complex*

Other genes, present in the MHC of vertebrates, may intervene in various ways in the immune response. To the two categories already mentioned should doubtless be added a gene or genes that control complement components, also localized in the *H-2* complex (Démant *et al.*, 1973). Finally, as reported in Chapters 8 and 9, genes in the MHC govern cell proliferation during the mixed lymphocyte reaction (MLR). This is a very specialized response since it includes only to a limited extent an anamnestic recall. It possibly represents an archaic form of the immune response, associated mainly with recognition of allogeneic cells. It cannot be excluded, however, that the same mechanism also controls reactions with other structures, especially those of infectious agents such as viruses or bacteria, possibly through recognition of the carrier in T–B lymphocyte collaboration.

### 4. *Histocompatibility Antigens and Autoimmune Diseases*

Another possible relationship between histocompatibility antigens and susceptibility to illness can be found in autoimmune diseases. It is well known that autoimmune hemolytic anemia of the acquired type is due to autoimmunization against diverse components of the rhesus antigenic system. Likewise, the antibody found in paroxysmal hemoglobinuria is directed against antigens of the P system. It is thus possible to foresee the existence of autoimmune diseases in man due to autoimmunization against histocompatibility antigens or against organ-specific antigens. This autoimmune state could be either cellular, or humoral, or both. Models of this type are well known. Chronic allogeneic disease has been produced by the injection of parental lymphoid cells from inbred animals into their $F_1$ hybrids. A chronic disorder resembling an autoimmune disease often develops (Armstrong *et al.*, 1970). Three immunologic syndromes have been described: immunohemolytic anemia and glomerulonephritis in mice and polyarthritis with dermatitis and carditis in rats. In other experiments a high incidence of lymphoma and reticulum cell sarcoma developed (Walford, 1966). It has also been reported that the ability to produce autoimmune thyroiditis in mice is closely linked to the H-2 type of the mouse (Vladutiu and Rose, 1971). In rats, susceptibility to the development of experimental allergic encephalomyelitis has been shown to be linked to, but not identical with, the Rt *H-1* histocompatibility locus (Gasser *et al.*, 1973).

Some autoimmune disorders in man may be provoked by similar mechanisms, a state of immunity being established against some of the normal components of the histocompatibility mosaic, possibly modified by a virus. It is interesting, in this connection, that Milgrom *et al.* (1970) have demonstrated the possibility of autoimmune response against renal tissue, provoked by an incompatible kidney graft.

It will be seen below (Section II,E) that several autoimmune diseases involving various tissues are associated with HLA-B8. Therefore, the defect seems to be rather at the HLA complex than at the tissue level.

### C. Modification of Endocrine Regulation by the MHC

Another aspect of the intervention of the MHC in physiology, and doubtless in pathology, concerns endocrine regulation. Several hormonally influenced traits, such as the relative weights of seminal vesicles, testes, and thymuses, were shown to be influenced by the *H-2* genotype. The genetic factor linked to *H-2* which is responsible for these differences was shown to be situated close to *H-2K* and was named *Hom-1* (hormone metabolism).

The *H-2* genotype also influences the plasma testosterone level and the plasma level of testosterone-binding globulin. It should be noted that, because of the varying sensitivity of different subpopulations of lymphoid cells to hormone action, immune responsiveness could be altered by the effect of hormones on the composition of lymphoid tissues (Iványi *et al.*, 1972). The influence of endocrines is also shown by the fact that cortisone-induced cleft palate is linked to the maternal $H\text{-}2^a$ haplotype (Bonner and Slavkin, 1975).

We have tried to show, from the various examples given, that MHC's intervene in many biological processes. However, the most striking fact that emerges is the concentration of genes governing the immune response in this chromosomal region. Their intervention in pathology, therefore, is easily conceivable.

## II. Associations between HLA and Disease

These studies led investigators to search for correlations between HLA antigens and certain diseases. This type of research holds many pitfalls, not the least of which is the scarcity of good HLA reagents and the problems that this creates in HLA typing. The problem is exaggerated when abnormal cells are being tested. The choice of control populations is vitally important. For each patient, at least one, and preferably several normal unrelated individuals of the same age and genetic background should be selected at random, and serological typing should be done with the same sera, using the same technique and ideally by the same technician. In theory, studies should be prospective rather than retrospective, since this eliminates any selective bias due to resistance to the disease. The method of statistical analysis is also important, and the reader is referred to a warning paper by Wiener (1970) on this subject. For at least the first series of cases, *all* comparisons should be taken into account, i.e., the $p$ value obtained for a given antigen must be multiplied by the number of antigens tested to give the corrected $p$ value.

Such rigorous standards have often been ignored. However strong correlations have been found independently by several teams and can be considered as firmly established. Many others are still uncertain, either because the correlation is borderline or because the results obtained by different teams do not agree.

A wide assortment of results has nevertheless been obtained. Because this is only the beginning, a meaningful classification of observed facts is difficult. The classification we have adopted is arbitrary. We shall discuss first malignant diseases that, by analogy with what was then known about mice, were the first to be studied. Nonmalignant diseases are classified by gross clinical syndromes. The literature on this subject is expanding rapidly, and for this reason we can only give the most striking and potentially instructive facts and quote only key references. The reader is referred to the reviews which have already been published (McDevitt and Bodmer, 1974; Svejgaard *et al.*, 1975). Precise data can be found in Ryder *et al.* (1974).

## A. HLA and Malignant Disease

### 1. *Leukemia and Burkitt's Disease*

Because of the demonstrated influence of *H-2* on leukemia in mice, it seemed logical to start research into associations between HLA and disease with the acute leukemias. The first study was done in 1967 by Kourilsky *et al.*, who investigated HLA types of 116 patients with acute leukemia—all of them in remission (102 acute lymphoblastic leukemias and 14 acute myeloblastic leukemias). They found a normal distribution of the ten antigens studied, including A2, 3 + 11, B5, 7, 8, and 12. Since that time, several reports with conflicting results have appeared, the most provocative of which was that of Walford *et al.* (1970). This report stressed the importance of looking for correlations on the basis of genotypic, as well as phenotypic data, and found in a small number of cases that there was an excess of the hapotype A2, B12. Many other series have since been done, some finding no deviation from controls and others noting an excess, whether or not statistically significant, of A2 and sometimes of B12.

In attempts to explain these discrepancies, the heterogeneity of the disease (as proved by two frequency peaks according to age), the geographical area of study (supposing the existence of viruses varying according to the region), and, more prosaically, technical factors (some sera appear to react more frequently on leukoblasts than on normal cells) have all been invoked at one time or another. Attention has been drawn to another cause of error introduced by retrospective studies. Rogentine *et al.* (1973) noted that A2 was abnormally high (84%) in his retrospective series but lower in his prospective series (53% versus 44% in controls). When the 18 survivors of the two series were considered, it was noted that 83% of those surviving more than 1500 days possessed A2 and 94% possessed one of the three cross-reacting antigens A2, A28 or A9. Lawler *et al.* (1974) took a similar approach. In their series, the antigens A2 and A28 were not more frequent among the survivors, but those individuals possessing A9 had the best estimated median survival time, the highest ratio of survivors to nonsurvivors, and the lowest median age at diagnosis. Finally studying again the 1967 series of Kourilsky *et al.*, a slight, but not significant, increase of A2 among the 25 survivors was found (Dausset and Hors, 1975). These facts require confirmation, but we have emphasized them because they suggest a new point of view, namely, that an increase in the frequency of an antigen may not signify special susceptibility to leukemic or other diseases, but, on the contrary, may signify increased *resistance*. We shall return to this point later.

Other acute (myeloblastic and monocytic) and chronic (lymphocytic and myelocytic) leukemias have been the object of several studies, but no evident conclusions could be drawn. In each of the laboratories the series was relatively small, and an attempt to pool them would be unwise owing to racial and technical variations.

Anti-HLA test sera showed frequent unexpected reactions in tests on chronic lymphocytic leukemia patients (Jeannet and Alberto, 1972; Walford *et al.*, 1973). The most probable interpretation is that they are due to antibodies directed toward B lymphocyte specificities, the equivalent of the mouse Ia specificities. It is also known that chronic lymphocytic leukemia sometimes occurs in families. The disease can attack several sibs [up to five in the case reported by Schweitzer *et al.* (1973)]. The results with this and one other family (Delmas-Marsalet *et al.*, 1974) do not exclude the possibility that susceptibility to this disease is linked to HLA. Results with multiple myeloma are inconclusive.

Another example of malignant hemopathy, Burkitt's disease, can be taken as a model of disease caused by an infectious, probably viral, agent. Three studies have been devoted to it. Although the series were short and the results not entirely in agreement, there does not seem to be any obvious difference in the distribution of HLA antigens in relation to the controls taken from the same populations as the patients.

### 2. *Hodgkin's Disease, Lymphosarcoma, and Reticulosarcoma*

The most disputed association concerns Hodgkin's disease. Since Amiel's provocative report in 1967, many series of patients have been studied, but the heterogeneity of the serology as well as, possibly, that of the disease itself, results in a confused picture. During the Fifth Histocompatibility Workshop (Morris *et al.*, 1973), 523 patients were tested with the same sera; 303 of these were blindly classified by an international board of pathologists. No associations were found, except for a possible excess of A10 in patients over 45 years old. Falk and Osoba (1974), in a prospective series of 113 patients, attributed a certain resistance to patients possessing A3 and A11 who less frequently developed the severe, rapidly evolving forms, and similarly an increased survival to B8 found more frequently in patients who survived over five years.

Hodgkin's disease should be dissociated from other forms of sarcoma such as lymphoma, reticulosarcoma and lymphocytic lymphosarcoma. No evident correlation has emerged from the study of these various forms.

### 3. *Epithelial Cancers*

Of the epithelial cancers, breast cancer has been the most thoroughly studied because this disease tends to cluster in families, suggesting that genetic factors may play a role in its etiology. It does not appear that the few deviations observed are significant. It would be desirable to study families in which there are several cases of breast cancer, but in one case the two girls afflicted did not possess a common HLA haplotype (Dausset and Hors, 1975).

A large-scale study was organized by Takasugi *et al.* (1973) on cancers of the lung, the bladder, the colon, the stomach, the prostate, the cervix, the endometrium of the uterus, and the ovaries. A significant deviation was only found in cancers of the cervix (increased A1, decreased A9).

The authors observed that these two antigens varied similarly in Israelis, among whom the incidence of cancer of the cervix is in fact higher.

### 4. *Other Tumors*

An especial emphasis has been laid on melanoma. Eight different studies have failed to establish a clear association. The study of Clark *et al.* (1975) should, however, be quoted since it puts forward a hypothesis to explain a decrease in the antigen B5 which these authors observed. It appears that the serum of the more severly ill patients is capable of partially blocking the lymphocytotoxic activity of anti-B5 serum. This masking activity is thought to be relatively specific and does not seem to be due to an anti-complementary effect. It is found not only in the serum but also in the supernatant of melanoma cells in culture. A study of the patients' families showed that this is an acquired factor. The failure to note a deficiency of B5 in the other series may be explained by differences in interpretation—most teams may not have counted partial blocking as negative. This study has yet to be confirmed, but it does offer a possible interpretation of the decrease in frequency of an antigen.

Nasopharyngocarcinoma has an especial interest because of its geographical and racial localization in the Chinese of southeast Asia. A study by Simons *et al.* (1974) showed an increase in a new antigen, SIN-2 or Hs found in the Chinese population (40 versus 25%).

A detailed study of 64 families suffering from retinoblastoma, known to run in families, has been reported. No correlation with HLA haplotypes was found, but Bw35 was present in excess in the patients; five Bw35 homozygotes were found where only 1.90 were predicted (Bertrams *et al.*, 1973a).

One study has implicated HLA homozygosity in the development of cancer. Among normal and cancerous individuals aged over 75 and under 36, heterozygosity was highest in the elderly normal and lowest in the cancerous young. Thus, 73% of normal elderly people had four discernible antigens as opposed to only 58% of young people with cancer (Gerkins *et al.*, 1974). Another study compared children with cancer to healthy individuals over 70 years old. More possible homozygotes (the genotype was not determined) were found among the children (Bender *et al.*, 1973).

The observation that healthy individuals manifest more HLA heterozygosity than people of the same age with cancer seems to indicate that HLA heterogeneity is associated with lowered susceptibility to overt cancer. Survival to old age may thus be correlated with heterogeneity, and lack of such heterogeneity may increase the risk of cancer.

## B. Arthropathies

### 1. *Ankylosing Spondylitis*

The outstanding example of an association between HLA and disease is indubitably that between ankylosing spondylitis (AS) and the antigen B27 (Brewerton *et al.*, 1973a; Schlosstein *et al.*, 1973). This disease has the strongest association. Up to 96% of the patients possess B27, in contrast to only 3–7% in the controls. This is an overwhelming correlation; the antigen occurs 15 to 20 times more frequently in patients than in controls. AS is predominantly a disease of males, about eight men being afflicted for every woman. Its frequency in Caucasoids is about 1 or 2 per thousand. A much higher figure was found in a study where x-ray diagnosis was used (Calin and Fries, 1975). We may take AS as a model for the analysis of disease incidence in different groups.

It is interesting to study the risk of this disease among B27 positive individuals compared to that among non-B27 individuals. This can be done using Woolf's formula (1955):

$$x = \frac{pd(1 - pc)}{(1 - pd)pc}$$

in which $pd$ is the frequency of the antigen in patients and $pc$ in the controls. Where several studies are available, the combined relative risk can be calculated using the standard weighing procedure and its heterogeneity can be determined (Svejgaard *et al.*, 1974, 1975). In the case of AS, the combined relative risk is 120.9 (both sexes) (Table 12.1) with virtually no heterogeneity between the various studies. This risk is much greater when sex is taken into consideration.

It is also interesting to know the personal risk of contracting the disease run by a B27 individual. This risk, $R$, can be obtained from the formula

$$R = \frac{pd \times F}{pc}$$

in which $F$ is the frequency of the disease in the population. For an $F$ of 1/1000, 3% of B27 men will contract AS and only 0.4% of B27 women. The frequency of the disease among the patients' first-degree relatives can also be calculated, and its relationship to the presence of the incriminated antigen. For example, about 50% of these relatives have B27 if the proband is B27 positive (Feldmann, 1974).

A study of a presumed genetic component in a disease should be completed by family studies. These show whether or not the disease is always transmitted with the antigen in question, and whether the

TABLE 12.1
MOST EVIDENT ASSOCIATIONS BETWEEN HLA SPECIFICITIES AND DISEASE[a]

| Disease | Antigen | Antigen frequencies: In controls (%) | Antigen frequencies: In patients (%) | Combined relative risk |
|---|---|---|---|---|
| Arthropathies | | | | |
| (and associated syndromes) | | | | |
| Ankylosing spondylitis | B27 | | 90 | 120.9 |
| Reiter's syndrome | B27 | | 76 | 40.3 |
| Acute anterior uveitis | B27 | 4 to 8 | 55 | 30.7 |
| Juvenile rheumatoid arthritis | B27 | | 47 | 11.5 |
| Psoriatic arthritis | | | | |
| with sacroileitis | B27 | | 27 | 4.7 |
| | Bw38 | 3 | 27 | 11.5 |
| Skin diseases | | | | |
| Psoriasis vulgaris | Bw17 | 7 | 26 | 5.0 |
| | B13 | 5 | 19 | 4.8 |
| Behçet's disease | B5 | 13 | 71 | 16.4 |
| Intestinal diseases (and associated syndromes) | | | | |
| Celiac disease | B8 | | 57 | 8.3 |
| Dermatitis herpetiform | B8 | | 60 | 4.3 |
| Autoimmune and endocrine diseases | | 14 to 25 | | |
| Myasthenia gravis | B8 | | 45 | 4.4 |
| Active chronic hepatitis | B8 | | 37 | 3.6 |
| Grave's disease | B8 | | 37 | 3.5 |
| Addison's disease | B8 | | 80 | 6.4 |
| Diabetes (juvenile) | B8 | | 54 | 2.1 |
| | Bw15 | 12 | 36 | 3.0 |
| Neurological diseases | | | | |
| Multiple sclerosis | B7 | 22 | 42 | 1.4 |
| | Dw2 | 16 | 70 | 5.0 |

[a] Most data from Svejgaard *et al.* (1975).

disease can occur independently of the antigen. The genetical analysis is, in many cases, rendered difficult when the disease does not develop until adulthood.

AS is rarely observed in families. However, well-conducted family studies have shown that not all B27 children are afflicted, at any rate clinically, and that the disease can occur in a non-B27 child. A family with 13 children was especially instructive in this respect, since not only were three B27 children afflicted, but also a fourth child was afflicted who did not possess this antigen (Strosberg *et al.*, 1973; see also Dick *et al.*, 1975). A family of this kind indicates that the gene involved is not identical to B27. The simplest explanation of course, is that the non-B27 child was derived from a recombination between the B locus and an AS-causing gene. However, if enough cases were observed, this hypothesis would be incompatible with the close association of the disease with B27 and another interpretation would be necessary. Be that as it may, these observations indicate that AS, like other diseases associated with HLA, is polygenic or otherwise complex in its determination.

Another instructive comparison concerns the racial and geographic distribution of the disease in relation to that of B27. Curiously, B27 is found mainly in the Northern Hemisphere, in both Caucasoids and Mongoloids. It is encountered most frequently (13–20%) among North American Indians. It is absent from South American Indians, Australian aboriginals, and African Negroes. The disease has a high frequency among North American tribes (650 cases per 10,000 among Pimas) and is very rare in Negroes. It is about ten times less frequent among Japanese than French (4/10,000 versus 50/10,000), which corresponds to the frequency of B27 (0.8 and 5%, respectively). There is, therefore, a correlation in the geographical distribution of the disease and the suspect genotype.

### 2. *Reiter's Syndrome*

Reiter's syndrome has several features in common with ankylosing spondylitis, such as male predominance, young age at onset, ocular inflammation, spondylitis, and aortic regurgitation. Moreover, in certain patients who have an acute form of the disease, chronic sacroileitis and spondylitis develop which are indistinguishable from ankylosing spondylitis. Because of these close links, an association with HLA was sought, and a similar association with B27 was found (Brewerton *et al.*, 1973b). Seventy-two percent of the patients possessed B27, and the combined relative risk is 40.3. In males, related sacroileitis was found in 14% and AS in 4%.

The special interest attached to Reiter's syndrome is that, of all the diseases showing associations with HLA, it is the one most likely to have an infectious etiology, since it appears to begin with genitourinary (urethritis) and gastrointestinal (diarrhea) involvement. The role of *Bedsonia* as an infectious agent has been suggested. An excess of B27 has also been found in patients with *Yersinia* arthritis. It would be extremely interesting to know whether this microorganism possesses an antigenic structure similar or identical to that of B27. Absorption of anti-B27 on *Yersinia enterolitica,* cultivated from a patient with B27, was nonspecific (Dausset and Hors, 1975).

### 3. *Associated Syndromes (Uveitis, Ulcerative Colitis)*

Acute anterior uveitis is an inflammation mainly confined to the anterior segment of the eye, often associated with several systemic disorders. It is also frequently associated with AS (18%) and Reiter's syndrome (28%), but 45% of the cases are of unknown etiology. The discovery that 55% of patients possess the antigen B27 suggests that certain symptoms, even when characteristic of different diseases, may be associated with a particular HLA profile.

But AS and Reiter's syndrome are also accompanied by other pathological symptoms such as aortitis, diarrhea, and more specifically, ulcerative colitis. Taken separately, these disorders are not accompanied by a significant increase in B27. It is only in the forms associated with sacroileitis or spondylitis that B27 is frequent.

In summary, the frequency of the antigen B27 in diseases giving pelvirachidian articular problems permits a whole series of separate conditions to be grouped into a large, polygenically controlled syndrome. It is probable that juvenile rheumatoid arthritis (Thomsen *et al.*, 1975), psoriatic arthritis, and the reactive arthritises (*Yersinia*, gonococcal, and *Salmonella* arthritis), in which B27 is also increased, are also part of this syndrome. It should, however, be noted that B27 is increased in juvenile rheumatoid arthritis, although sacroiliac articulation is not affected.

### 4. *Rheumatoid Arthritis*

In spite of many studies of the genetics of rheumatoid arthritis, it is still difficult to state whether or not there is an association with HLA. However, an increase in Bw40 or an associated antigen (and possibly B13) has been noted by several authors (Seignalet *et al.*, 1972; Nyalassy *et al.*, 1974).

## C. Skin Diseases

### 1. *Psoriasis vulgaris*

Psoriasis poses a complex problem. Two HLA antigens have been found to be associated with this disease, Bw17 and B13 (Russell *et al.*, 1972; White *et al.*, 1972). This asociation has been confirmed by many teams and can be accepted as proved. B13 occurs in about 20% of patients (versus 5% in controls) and Bw17 in 26% (versus 7%) (Table 12.1).

A more detailed study of the material seems to indicate that the association with Bw17 occurs mainly in the familial forms of this disease, while B13 is commonest in the nonfamilial acquired forms. The overall frequency of psoriasis in close relatives was 8.8% for all subjects, 20% for Bw17 subjects, and only 2% for B13 subjects.

In nonfamilial cases, the infection is said to be more easily reversible, the onset to occur later, and streptococcal infection to be more frequently observed. A cross-reaction between the antigen B13 and the M protein of group A hemolytic *Streptococcus* has been observed (Hirata *et al.*, 1973).

The immunological symptoms that often accompany psoriasis are noteworthy. These are a great increase in salivary and serum IgA, a slight increase in serum IgG, and the presence of rheumatoid rosettes and anti-IgG activity in the serum (Seignalet *et al.*, 1974).

Another facet of psoriasis is the frequent appearance of articular manifestations. In psoriatic arthritis not only are Bw17 and B13 increased, but also B27, mostly when sacroiliac articulation is involved, as it is in AS and Reiter's syndrome, or Bw38 mostly in polyarticular forms (Dausset and Hors, 1975). It would, therefore, appear that several very different syndromes are grouped under the title of psoriasis, and it may be that their individual characterization will be aided by their association with different HLA antigens.

#### 2. *Other Skin Diseases*

Reports on pemphigus are confusing. Some have indicated that B13 is increased, but others contradict this. A10 is said to be greatly increased in Jewish patients. Behçet's disease seems to be associated with B5 (Ohno *et al.*, 1973). Tests with systemic sclerodermia have been negative (Crouzet *et al.*, 1975).

Herpetiform dermatitis will be considered in the next section because of its close relationship with intestinal diseases.

### D. Intestinal Diseases

#### 1. *Celiac Disease*

Celiac disease, or gluten enteropathy, which is a form of specific gluten intolerance, is one of a series of illnesses linked to B8 (Stokes *et al.*, 1972; Falchuk *et al.*, 1972). This antigen is present in approximately 60% of patients versus only 14% of controls. The antigen A1 is only present in proportion to its gametic association with B8. It is accordingly not involved. A number of immunological abnormalities have been demonstrated in this disease. Patients in relapse have increased serum IgA levels associated with increased mucosal synthesis of IgA. They respond to gluten challenge with an increase in mucosal IgA and IgM immunoglobulin synthesis, mainly due to the synthesis of anti-gluten antibodies (Falchuk *et al.*, 1972). These antibodies are thought to be responsible for the mucosal injuries observed in this disease. Celiac enteropathy is characterized by an abnormal tendency to respond to the ingestion of gluten with local synthesis of anti-gluten antibodies. It has also been demonstrated by immunofluorescence that the intestinal epithelial cells of patients bind gluten.

Family studies have shown that children with B8 are not regularly afflicted, although B8 is transmitted according to Mendelian laws. Although B8 is predominantly a Caucasian antigen, there is no special racial distribution of the disease. Perhaps other specificities are associated with the disease in other populations.

### 2. *Other Intestinal or Associated Diseases*

There are close links between celiac disease and herpetiform dermatitis. Approximately two out of three patients suffering from this disease develop gluten enteropathy. In both gluten enteropathy and herpetiform dermatitis, there is considerable evidence that immunological mechanisms are important primary pathogenic factors. IgA and occasionally IgG and complement are found to be deposited near the basal membrane adjacent to the skin lesions. B8 is found in 60% of the patients with an average relative risk of 4.3. Undoubtedly the increase in B8 in herpetiform dermatitis and celiac disease is additional evidence that the two diseases are associated. It also provides a genetic basis for the link. Among other intestinal diseases studied, ulcerative colitis and Crohn's disease do not show any HLA deviation. In pernicious anemia an excess of B7 was noted (Mawhenney *et al.*, 1975; Zittoun *et al.*, 1975).

## E. Autoimmune and Endocrine Diseases

Studies of systemic diseases, especially autoimmune diseases, are considered together because the antigen B8 is very often involved (reviewed by Morris, 1973; Marchalonis *et al.*, 1974).

### 1. *Myasthenia Gravis*

In myasthenia gravis, 45% of the patients possess B8 and the average relative risk is 4.4% (Pirskanen *et al.*, 1972). Sex is also a factor, the disease occurring considerably more frequently in women than in men. Moreover, the form of the disease is relevant, since B8 is found far more frequently in the early feminine forms occurring prior to the age of

40, which are not accompanied by thymomas or antibodies to skeletal muscles (Fritze *et al.*, 1974).

It seems that there are two different forms of myasthenia gravis. In patients with autoimmune phenomena, i.e., antibodies to skeletal muscles, or thymomas, or both, the prevalence of B8 is less, and that of A2 more, than in patients with no such phenomena (Feltkamp *et al.*, 1974).

An important genetic notion, new to the associations between HLA and disease, has been announced but not yet fully published. B8 heterozygotes are 5 times as likely to become myasthenic and B8 homozygotes are 25 times as likely. This fact is the first example of a quantitative effect of an allelic gene (Feltkamp *et al.*, 1974).

### 2. *Systemic Lupus Erythematosus*

The problem of systemic lupus erythematosus (SLE), the classic example of an autoimmune systemic disease, is a difficult one. Some studies have suggested an increase in B8 and Bw15 (Grumet *et al.*, 1971), but others have not found any deviation. One study indicates an increase in B8 in North American Caucasians (19 versus 8%) and A1 in Negroes (22 versus 9%). These results require confirmation, but are particularly interesting since they show a possible difference in association according to racial group.

### 3. *Other Autoimmune Diseases*

It is noteworthy that increased frequency of B8 has been reported in several other autoimmune diseases, of various clinical manifestations, involving the thyroid and adrenal glands and the liver. This has been found in Grave's disease (Grumet *et al.* 1973), autoimmune chronic active hepatitis (Mackay and Morris 1972), idiopathic Addison's disease (Platz *et al.* 1974), and Sjögren's disease (D. Ivanyi, personal communication). It seems that a gene closely linked to B8 and Dw3 is involved in the genesis of autoimmunity. B8 and Dw3 belong to the haplotype A1, B8, Dw3 which manifests the strongest known linkage disequilibrium. However, other well-characterized autoimmune diseases, such as Hashimoto's disease, acquired hemolytic anemia, and idiopathic thrombopenic purpura, do not show any HLA association. The B8 association, although very frequent in autoimmune disease, is not, therefore, always the rule.

### 4. *Diabetes Mellitus*

Diabetes mellitus is a genetically determined metabolic disorder in which inherited susceptibility plays an important part. In juvenile diabetes, certain studies indicate that there may be an association with

B8 and Bw15. Bw15 is present with significantly higher frequency in insulin-dependent diabetic patients than in either the non-insulin-dependent diabetic patients or in the controls (Cudworth and Woodrow, 1974; Nerup *et al.*, 1974). Patients possessing both B8 and Bw15 have a higher risk. The effect of these two associations seems to be cumulative. Recent work has also shown that there is an association with the D alleles Dw3 and Dw6, which are themselves in disequilibrium with B8 and Bw15, respectively.

### F. Neurological Diseases

#### 1. *Multiple Sclerosis*

Studies of multiple sclerosis (MS) have introduced a new dimension into our concepts of the association between HLA and disease. For if a strong association exists with an A or B HLA specificity, it is even stronger with a D gene defined by the mixed lymphocyte reaction, as later discovered for diabetes. The gradual accumulation of evidence pinning down a specific genetic factor in this disease provides an interesting example of HLA research.

The first publications (Naito *et al.*, 1972; Bertrams *et al.*, 1972) noted an increased frequency of A3 (37 versus 25%). Later, an association with B7 was reported (40 versus 22%) in some (Bertrams *et al.*, 1974), but not all, publications. B7 was thought to be increased only where there were no anti-cerebral white matter antibodies, demonstrable by the leukocyte migration test. In this situation, B7 was found to be present in 55% of the patients (Finkelstein *et al.*, 1974).

In a third stage, HLA-D typing was performed. Normal, homozygous Dw2 (one of the D alleles frequently associated with B7) cells were used as stimulating cells in mixed lymphocyte reaction (MLR) against which the patients' cells were allowed to react. If the patient was at least heterozygous for Dw2, the results were negative or very weak. A strong association of MS was found with the Dw2 gene (70% versus 16%) (Jersild *et al.*, 1973a,b). Out of the 28 randomly selected patients, 19 were both B7 and Dw2 positive, which is significantly different from the frequency of Dw2 in normal B7 individuals (56%). Of the remaining 15 patients, six were Dw2. Family studies showed that the Dw2 characteristic is not acquired. It would appear that the presence of Dw2 presages the diseae in its early, rapidly-evolving forms.

It is striking that this association is found with HLA-B or D genes that are frequently associated in the haplotype A3, B7, Dw2. Using the available data and considering the number of recombinations that would be necessary to explain the associations found, it seems likely that the postulated MS gene is situated outside the A3–Dw2 interval on the Dw2 side (Degos and Dausset, 1974a).

The geographical distribution of MS corresponds with that of the A3, B7 linkage disequilibrium, which is known to be at its maximum in northern Europe (Scandinavia). It is not found in other populations. In the same way MS is most frequent in that area of the world. However, it is clear that an allele other than Dw2 can accompany the postulated MS gene and consequently the disease can occur in populations where Dw2 is not found.

Multiple sclerosis is also interesting from another point of view. The role of the measles virus or a similar agent is suspected because of the frequency of a high antibody titer against this virus in patients. Jersild *et al.* (1973a) reported a significant association between the antigens A3, B7, and B18 and anti-measles antibody titers in MS patients. However, Bertrams *et al.* (1973b) were unable, in a large sample, to confirm this association.

### 2. *Paralytic Poliomyelitis*

The problem becomes more intriguing with the results obtained in a study of patients who contracted paralytic poliomyelitis prior to the introduction of the Salk vaccine. An increase in B7 (38 versus 19%) was found by Morris and Pietsch (1973). Thus association with HLA antigens seems to influence development of paralysis rather than susceptibility to the initial infection.

Use of the Salk vaccine resulted in the development of anti-poliovirus antibodies in the entire population, and hence independently of HLA genotypes. Morris and Pietsch (1973) compared their observations to those of Jersild *et al.* (1973a) and proposed the concept that B7 "might be linked to an immune response gene which determines the response to a common product of viral infection of central nervous tissue, namely the poliovirus in poliomyelitis and perhaps the measles virus in MS."

## G. Allergic Diseases

Data concerning allergic diseases are still too incomplete to permit a comprehensive synthesis. Levine *et al.* (1972) have shown that hay fever and IgE antibody production specific for the allergic antigen E are in close correlation with particular HLA haplotypes in successive generations in seven families (different haplotypes in each family). This fact has been confirmed in a large family with three generations (Blumenthal *et al.*, 1974). In the light of these studies, therefore, this is not an association with a given HLA antigen, but a linkage with the HLA complex.

Marsh *et al.* (1973) have found that the ability to produce a reagenic IgE antibody to a low molecular weight, naturally-occurring human pollen antigen (Ra5) is linked to the presence of B7 or cross-reacting specificities. Similarly, the frequency of B8 or the cross-reacting specificity B14 is increased in subjects sensitive to Rye-1 compared to insensitive subjects. It is interesting to note than in mice there is an *Ir* gene linked to *H-2* which governs IgE and IgG response to ragweed extract (*Ir-RE*) (Dorf *et al.*, 1974). Several studies failed to correlate the atopy with HLA.

### H. Various Diseases

It is not possible to give here an exhaustive list of the diseases for which an association with HLA has been sought, but some should be mentioned. Of infectious diseases, infectious mononucleosis, leprosy, tuberculosis, and sarcoidosis have not shown any significant deviation. An increase in A2 in glomerulonephritis has been indicated. Familial hemochromatosis is associated with A3 (Simon *et al.*, 1975).

### I. Congenital Diseases

Congenital abnormalities are more interesting, especially spina bifida. This affliction can be likened to tail and vertebral abnormalities in mice, produced by the *T* locus, one of the loci linked to the *H-2* complex (Chapter 5, Section II,C). Some alleles at this locus not only lead to spinal defects but also inhibit crossing over in the *T* region. If there is a locus with similar effects in man, a familial association between spina bifida and an HLA haplotype might be expected. Amos *et al.* (1975) studied a large family of 200 members, some of whom had clinical cases of mild spina bifida and others infraclinical cases, detectable only by X-ray examination. The abnormality followed the haplotypes A2, B12 and A2, B18. The recombination frequency between HLA and spina bifida is thought to be about 0.27, which is of the same order as that between *H-2* and *T*. These data require confirmation.

Rapaport and Bach's observation (1973) of MLR abnormalities in families with harelips or cleft palates deserves to be mentioned. Chromosomal abnormalities such as 21 trisomy (Down's syndrome) do not appear to be associated with HLA.

To summarize, the association of certain diseases with HLA antigens is well established. In most cases this association is with an antigen determined by the B locus. Possible associations with the A locus still require confirmation. In multiple sclerosis, diabetes, and Addison's disease, the association is even stronger with an allele at the main D locus. The strength of the association varies from almost complete, e.g., ankylosing spondylitis and B27, to the barely significant. The antigen B27 does not belong, in Caucasoids, to a haplotype with a linkage disequilibrium, but there are many associations with B and D locus antigens which are in disequilibrium with a A locus antigens (A1, B8, Dw3 and A3, B7, Dw2). This seems to indicate that the entire chromosomal region is in disequilibrium. The possible significance of this fact will be discussed later.

The diseases showing an HLA association are very varied. Contrary to expectation, no certain association has been found in malignant diseases. Most of the proved correlations are with diseases whose physiopathology is uncertain, which cannot be clearly classified as infectious or tumoral. Many of them have an immunological factor, either overtly, as in autoimmune diseases, or more implicitly. A characteristic common to all is their hereditary tendency, although it has not yet been possible to define exactly the gene or genes responsible. Most of the diseases are therefore probably under polygenic control.

## III. Physiology of the Association

The discovery of these now undoubted associations will probably contribute to our understanding of fundamental causes of disease. It is now clear that the HLA genes themselves, or very closely linked genes, favor, in one way or another, the appearance of the known symptoms. Their intervention in different stages by means of very different mechanisms can be imagined.

### A. Is It the HLA Genes Themselves?

#### 1. *Receptor Hypothesis*

The possibility that the HLA molecules themselves can act as receptors, more particularly viral receptors, has been suggested. In weighing the possibility, we must remember that the genetic control of viral infection can occur at various stages of virus–cell interactions: (1) penetration of an exogenous virus into a cell, (2) replication of this virus by the exploitation of the cell's own machinery, (3) use of endogenous information for virus synthesis and/or for its expression, and (4) possibly, malignant transformation of the cell by the viral genome. The intervention of the HLA molecules can most easily be envisaged at the stage of adsorption on to the cell surface, an event necessary for penetration.

The receptor hypothesis seems scarcely probable. In view of the extreme polymorphism of the HLA system, it is incompatible with the ability of many viruses, e.g. influenza and measles, to infect almost everyone. Moreover, the absorption and replication of four viruses (two RNA viruses: echovirus and measles virus; and two DNA viruses: *Herpesvirus hominis* and adenovirus) on fibroblasts genotyped for HLA, was found to be unrelated to the HLA type (Dausset *et al.*, 1972). Similarly three enteroviruses (poliovirus, coxsackie B3, and echovirus 11) are able to replicate on man–mouse hybrid cells that have lost their HLA antigens (Couillin and Fellous, 1974). In these situations, at any rate, it does not appear that the A or B locus of the HLA complex influence adsorption or viral replication.

### 2. *Mimicry Hypothesis*

A similarity of structure between the HLA molecules and the structures of the infectious agents could make it impossible for the organism to mount an immune response. An identical structure would lead to tolerance. This hypothesis has solid support. Brent *et al.* (1961) have described a cross-reaction between pneumococcal polysaccharides and the transplantation antigens of A strain mice. Rapaport and Chase (1964) have shown that the membranes of heat-killed group A streptococci induce a state of hypersensitivity to skin allografts in mice, rats, guinea pigs, and rabbits which is indistinguishable from that resulting from pretreatment of the recipients with allogeneic tissue. This capacity was shared by all types of group A streptococci tested, but was absent from other groups (B, C, D, E, G, H, L and O). Tests of a wide variety of other gram-positive, gram-negative, and acid-fast bacteria for their ability to induce allograft sensitivity were positive only with *Straphylococcus aureus* and *Staphylococcus albus*.

Cross-reaction has been described by Hirata and Terasaki (1970) between the streptococcal $M_1$ protein (from $\beta$-hemolytic group A *S. pyrogenes* type 1) and human transplantation antigens. Analogous M protein from streptococci types 3, 4, 5, 6, 12, and 14 had little or no inhibitiory activity. Streptococcal polysaccharide and 73 other polysaccharides were inactive. The authors concluded from the specific inhibition of all anti-HLA sera tested (directed against seven specificities) that $M_1$ protein has a structure common to human histocompatibility antigens.

The hypothesis of mimicry between the infectious agents and HLA structures would necessarily entail dominant susceptibility. This has, in fact, been observed in man in all the associated diseases for which family studies have been done (myasthenia gravis, psoriasis, etc.). However, this conflicts with information concerning the leukemogenic viruses in mice. Although dominant resistance to Gross virus is definite, it is less so for the Bittner, Friend, and Tennant viruses (reviewed by Iványi, 1970). Hence different mechanisms could be involved.

### 3. *Viral Modification of HLA Antigens*

A study of the mechanics of T cell-mediated cytotoxicity in lymphocytic choriomeningitis (LCM) has led to the suggestion of another hypothesis. LCM was known to be associated with *H-2.* Zinkernagel and Doherty (1974) showed that the T cells of mice immunized against the LCM virus could kill cells infected with this virus *in vitro,* but only on condition that these cells were syngeneic or semisyngeneic for *H-2.* Similar observations have been made with other viruses [ectromelia virus (Blanden *et al.* 1975), vaccinia virus (Koszinowski and Ertl 1975)] as well as with chemically induced antigens [TNP, Shearer *et al.* 1974)].

This interesting observation has at least two possible interpretations. The first is that the T cells are indeed immunized against the virus, but in order to lyse a cell bearing it an intimate contact between the two cells is necessary. This contact can only exist if they have at least one *H-2* complex in common.

The second interpretation is that the T cells are immunized against a slight modification of the H-2 antigens caused by the virus. In short, this is an autoimmunization against a modified histocompatibility antigen. Integration of the virus into the genome at the level of the *H-2* genes, for example, or its acting on the mRNA designed for the histocompatibility antigens could have provoked this modification.

In order to apply these facts to human diseases, it is necessary to consider that some viruses, e.g., a hypothetical virus for ankylosing spondylitis, have a selective localization in certain tissues (sacroiliac articulation) and preferentially modify the gene or gene product B27. Such a supposition cannot be dismissed *a priori.* Nevertheless this mechanism does not appear to be applicable to all known associations, e.g., the association of HLA with multiple sclerosis seems to be more closely associated with a D gene than with a B gene.

## B. Is It Genes Closely Linked to the HLA Gene?

The many dissociations that have been observed, in population and family studies between the presence of an HLA gene and the accompanying disease, lead us to suspect, not the HLA genes themselves, but genes closely linked to them. If this suspicion is correct, there must be a strong linkage disequilibrium between the associated loci.

*1. Immune Response Gene Hypothesis*

A tempting hypothesis attributes variations in disease resistance to immune response (*Ir*) genes in man similar to those known in mice. We have seen (Section I,B) that a distinction must be made between two types of genetic control of the immune response.

1. A nonspecific control conditioning the intensity of the humoral response. This control is polygenic, but at least one gene is in the *H-2* region. No control of this kind has yet been found in man. Nevertheless a preliminary observation by Hors *et al.* (1974) deserves mention. An excess of A1 (47 versus 21%) was found in patients with immune deficiencies, mainly IgA deficiencies.
2. A specific control, similar to the mouse *Ir* genes (Chapter 7). *Ir* genes have been found linked to the MHC of several different species, and it is therefore probable that they also exist in man, although direct proof of this is lacking. No relationship was found between the ability to develop anti-Rh(D) antibodies and HLA types, but family studies have not yet been done. The other antigens studied were the Australian antigen and *Salmonella* flagellins. The results so far have been negative or conflicting, but this by no means excludes *Ir* genes in man. It merely indicates that the effect of these genes is extremely difficult to prove except in inbred animals.

With respect to cellular immunity, there are no data from man relevant to genetic control. However, a study by Buckley *et al.* (1973) suggests that the specificity of delayed hypersensitivity against several common bacterial antigens segregates in families with HLA haplotypes.

*Ir* genes in mice are situated within the *H-2* complex, in the *I* region. The same region governs the strongest MLR. In man, the main MLR locus, D, is situated outside the interval between the A and B loci. It is therefore possible that human *Ir* genes are located in the same HLA-D region. This situation would be compatible with the frequent association of diseases with a B locus antigen. It is also indicated in multiple sclerosis (MS) by the greater strength of the association of the MS gene with the D allele Dw2, than with the B allele B7. A close correlation with a serologically defined antigen specific for B lymphocytes (Ia human analogue) has been found in multiple sclerosis (Winchester *et al.*, 1975) and in celiac disease (Mann *et al.*, 1975; Van Rood *et al.*, 1976).

The first impulse is to attribute susceptibility to a lack of immune response to the responsible agent. But the absence of a favorable *Ir* allele should in most cases be compensated by the *Ir* allele on the other chromosome. Contrary to the dominant resistance to Gross virus in mice, susceptibility is usually dominant in humans. Accordingly, if *Ir* genes are to have a place, it is necessary to postulate some anomaly in their function (as opposed to a simple lack). Hyperresponse could perhaps lead to the appearance of enhancing antibodies, which would prevent cellular immunity from intervening. Another explanation is that autoimmunization is involved. This is tempting because of the number of autoimmune disorders in the list of diseases associated with HLA, especially with B8. We have already mentioned the possibility that viruses can modify a product on the cell surface. Here, we may assume that only individuals possessing certain *Ir* alleles respond to immunization against this autoantigen. This mechanism would lead to a dominant susceptibility.

The dominance of susceptibility requires further examination. As already stated (Section II,A), the association between acute leukemia and A2 has been interpreted as due to enhanced resistance to the disease. In this case, a favorable *Ir* gene would be present. It seems difficult to generalize this concept to include other diseases, such as ankylosing spondylitis, which is not fatal and therefore for which there is no bias from retrospective studies. Moreover, dominance is not universal. Thus in myasthenia gravis, for example, B8 homozygotes contract the disease five times more frequently than heterozygotes (Feltkamp *et al.*, 1974). It has also been observed that there is a greater number of potential homozygotes (increased frequency of "blank" antigens) in patients suffering from tumors (Gerkins *et al.*, 1974).

### 2. *Metabolic Gene Hypothesis*

Although *Ir* genes are likely candidates for a role in disease processes, we must also admit a possible role for other genes with no immunological function that might be present close to the HLA complex. Such genes could intervene in the metabolic processes connected with the polygenic diseases with which we are concerned. A gene could be a link in a chain of reactions, an interruption or alteration of which would cause the disease. We can easily imagine a gene of this sort being either dominant or recessive.

Whatever the details of the interpretation, in all probability it is not the HLA genes themselves, but very closely linked genes, which account for the associations. This implies that there are linkage disequilibria between the responsible genes and the HLA genes, especially those at the B locus. How have these disequilibria developed?

## C. Formation of Linkage Disequilibria ($\Delta$)

If the genes responsible for a disease (e.g., the *Ir* genes) are closely linked to the B locus, a new allele formed by mutation will be associated with the same B locus allele, provided that the time that has elapsed since the mutation is insufficient for recombination to have occurred, and provided that it has escaped elimination by selection. If the new allele has a favorable selective action, the combination will be spread and a positive $\Delta$ will be found in healthy individuals. On the other hand, if the new allele produces pathological effects, but has not been eliminated, the $\Delta$ will also be found in sick people. To explain the persistence of an unfavorable gene it must be supposed either that the mutation is recent, or that it has been maintained in a small population (by gene drift), or that it is in fact favorable in other circumstances.

It should be noted that a transitory selection on an *Ir* gene alone due to environmental factors (e.g., an epidemic) cannot lead to a gametic association with a particular haplotype. Indeed, prior to selection, *Ir* genes do not show any preferential associations. If the frequency of a given *Ir* gene increases with selection, the proportion of HLA genes associated therewith on the same chromosome will be the same as before. No disequilibrium will therefore occur. However, external selective pressure may create a linkage disequilibrium, but only when the selection is active on the two genes simultaneously. This could happen if the *Ir* and HLA genes form a functional unit. Fisher (1958) has stated that natural selection is expected to maintain close linkage between genes whose interaction can increase fitness. This law should not apply to genes with an unfavorable effect, such as those with which we are dealing. They could, however, possibly be favorable at another stage of life or in a different environment.

There is another situation that could have led to the association between *Ir* genes and the B locus, namely, the occurrence of migrations. When two populations, one with a high frequency of two closely linked genes and the other lacking these genes, or possessing them at a lower frequency, are mixed, a linkage disequilibrium is formed which will disappear only many generations later (Degos and Dausset, 1974b). The migration of Indo-European populations from the East is a plausible explanation of the formation of some of the high deltas in Caucasoids (e.g., A1 and B8) (Fig. 12.1).

It has been seen that these associations with diseases are often with B8 and B7 which are on the two chromosomes (A1, B8 and A3, B7) that have the strongest linkage disequilibria in Caucasians. On the other hand, there are no known disequilibria with B27 which is strongly associated with ankylosing spondylitis.

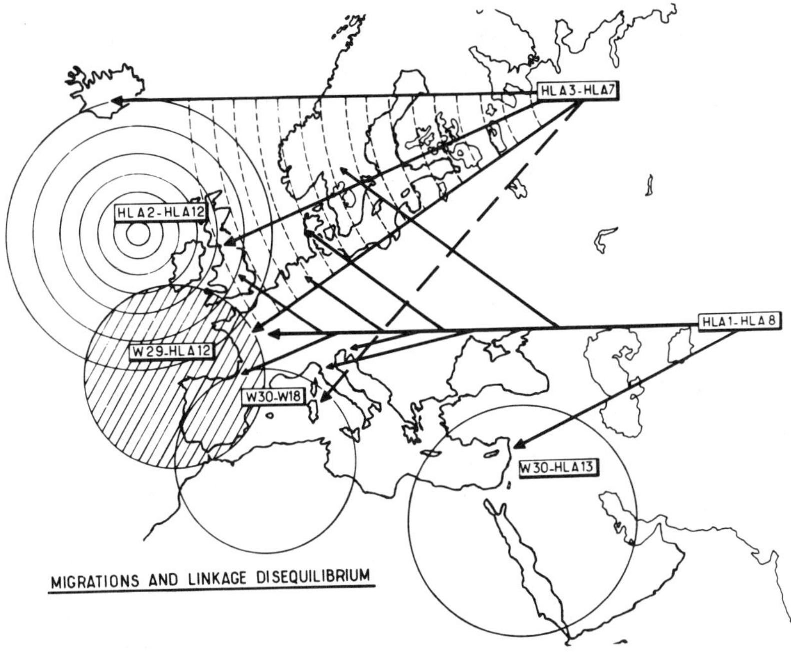


FIG. 12.1. HLA linkage disequilibria produced by fusion of two populations, one of them possessing an HLA-A and an HLA-B allele in high frequency and the other with lower frequency or lacking them altogether. One case illustrated concerns the Indo-European invaders of Europe. These people possessed A1 and B8 with no gametic association. Fusion with the indigenous populations led to a disproportionate frequency of the A1, B8 haplotype. In the same way other disequilibria were formed between genes existing in the original population (e.g., A29, B12). (From Degos and Dausset, 1974b, courtesy of *Immunogenetics.*)

## IV. Concluding Remarks

For several years, the attention of HLA system specialists was exclusively concentrated on the practical applications of this system in transplantation. It is now apparent that the chromosomal area marked by these genes is vitally important in pathology and probably in immune response in general.

From a practical point of view, the HLA markers permit the dissection of certain heterogeneous clinical entities and the reclassification of various diseases that are often clinically associated. Typical examples are ankylosing spondylitis, Reiter's syndrome, anterior uveitis, aortitis, and associated intestinal symptoms. Rheumatology is already benefiting from this new classification tool.

Epidemiological research should also benefit. Doctors and patients could be warned of the risks run in each particular situation. Earlier diagnoses could often be made and hence the appropriate treatments administered from the first symptoms onward. More enlightened genetic counseling could also be given. In the extreme case of a very serious familial affliction strongly associated with a given HLA haplotype, it is even foreseeable that therapeutic abortion will be suggested after determination of the fetal HLA type by amniocentesis. The probably haploid presence of HLA antigens on spermatozoa also opens up the possibility of artificial insemination by spermatozoa that are free from the trait, those bearing the afflicted chromosome having been eliminated by the cytotoxic action of anti-HLA antibodies (Dausset *et al.*, 1970).

From a basic point of view, the exploitation of HLA markers should lead to a better understanding of the role of the HLA complex whose genes probably make up a functional unit. Its intervention in a large number of normal, and therefore of pathological, immune response mechanisms already suggests its importance. Our growing knowledge of HLA should clarify the genetic control of immune responses in man.

The contributions of the HLA complex to medical genetics will doubtless be considerable. In familial diseases that typically show polygenic control, it should become possible to separate and analyze the function of individual loci. Medical genetics, long confined to the description of rare or abnormal genes, whould find relevance in far more widespread genes. The penetrance of some HLA-associated phenotypes is variable, especially in the two sexes. Ankylosing spondylitis mainly attacks men, and myasthenia gravis mainly women. Weakly penetrating genes of this kind should become more amenable to analysis.

Finally the branch of medical genetics concerned with the distribution of diseases in different populations and environments will be enriched by the realization and exploitation of HLA's extraordinary polymorphism.

More basic still will be the study of the biological advantages of individual HLA haplotypes. New light will be shed on the crucial problems of selection and the origins and maintenance of polymorphism.

## REFERENCES

Amiel, J. L. 1967. Study of the leukocyte phenotypes in Hodgkin's disease. Pages 79–81 *in* E. S. Curtoni, P. L. Mattiuz, and R. M. Tosi, eds. Histocompatibility Testing 1967. Munksgaard, Copenhagen.

Amos, D. B., N. Ruderman, N. Mendell, and A. H. Johnson. 1975. Linkage between HL-A and spinal development. *Transplant Proc* 7:93–95.

Armstrong, M. Y. K., E. Gleichmann, M. Gleichmann, L. Beldotti, J. Schwartz, and R. Schwartz. 1970. Chronic allogeneic diseases. II. Development of lymphoma. *J Exp Med* 1:417–439.

Bender, K., G. Rutter, A. Mayerová, and C. Hiller. 1973. Studies on the heterozygosity at the HL-A gene loci in children and old people. Pages 287–290 Int. Symp. HL-A reagents. Karger, Basel.

Bertrams, J., E. Kuwert, and U. Liedke. 1972. HL-A antigens and multiple sclerosis. *Tissue Antigens* **2**:405–408.

Bertrams, J., P. Schilberg, W. Hopping, U. Bohme, and E. Albert. 1973a. HL-A antigens in retinoblastoma. *Tissue Antigens* **3**:78–87.

Bertrams, J., E. Von Fisenne, P. G. Hoher, and E. Kuwert. 1973b. Lack of association between HL-A antigens and measles antibody in multiple sclerosis. *Lancet* **2**:441.

Bertrams, J., P. G. Hoher, and E. Kuwert. 1974. HL-A antigens in multiple sclerosis. *Lancet* **1**:1287.

Biozzi, G., C. Stiffel, D. Mouton, Y. Bouthillier, and C. Descrousefond. 1971. Genetic regulation of the function of antibody-producing cells. *Progr Immunol* **1**:529.

Blanden, R. V., P. C. Doherty, M. B. C. Dunlop, I. D. Gardner, R. M. Zinkernagel, and C. S David, 1975. Genes required for cytotoxicity against virus-infected target cells in *K* and *D* regions of *H-2* complex. *Nature (Lond)* **254**:269–270.

Blumenthal, M. N., D. B. Amos, H. Noreen, and E. J. Yunis. 1974. Genetic mapping of the Ir locus in man: Linkage to second locus of *HL-A*. *Science* **184**:1301–1303.

Bonner, J. J., and H. C. Slavkin. 1975. Cleft palate susceptibility linked to histocompatibility-2 (*H-2*) in the mouse. *Immunogenetics* **2**:213–218.

Brent, L., P. B. Medawar, and M. Ruskiewicz. 1961. Serological methods in the study of transplantation antigens. *Br J Exp Pathol* **42**:464–477.

Brewerton, D. A., M. Caffrey, F. D. Hart, A. Nicholls, D. C. O. James, and R. D. Sturrock. 1973a. Ankylosing spondylitis and HL-A27. *Lancet* **1**:904–907.

Brewerton, D. A., A. Nicholls, J. R. Oates, M. Caffrey, D. Walters, and D. C. O. James. 1973b. Reiter's disease and HL-A27. *Lancet* **2**:996–998.

Buckley, C. E., F. C. Dorsey, W. B. Ralph, M. A. Woodbury, and D. B. Amos. 1973. HL-A linked human immune-response genes. *Proc Natl Acad Sci USA* **70**:2157–2161.

Calin, A., and J. F. Fries. 1975. Striking prevalence of ankylosing spondylitis in "healthy" W27 positive males and females. A controlled study. *N Engl J Med* **293**:835–839.

Chesebro, B., K. Whehrly, and J. Stimpfling. 1974. Host genetic control of recovery from Friend leukemia virus-induced splenomegaly. *J Exp Med* **140**:1457–1467.

Clark, D. A., T. Necheles, L. Nathanson, and E. Silverman. 1975. Apparent HL-A5 deficiency in malignant melanoma. *Transplantation* **15**:326–328.

Couillin, P., and M. Fellous. 1974. Recherche d'une corrélation entre le système antigénique HL-A et les récepteurs viraux de 3 entéro-virus à l'aide de l'hybridation cellulaire. *C R Soc Biol* **168**:180–186.

Crouzet, J., M. C. Marbach, J. P. Camus, P. Godeau, G. Herreman, D. Richier, and J. Dausset. 1975. Recherche d'une association entre antigènes HL-A et sclérodermie systématique. *Nouv Presse Med* **4**:2489–2492.

Cudworth, A. G., and J. C. Woodrow. 1974. HL-A antigens and diabetes mellitus. *Lancet* **2**:1153.

Dausset, J. 1972. Correlation between histocompatibility antigens and susceptibility to illness. Pages 183–210 *in* R. S. Schwartz, ed. Progress in clinical immunology. Grune & Stratton, New York.

Dausset, J., J. Colombani, L. Legrand, and M. Fellous. 1970. Genetics of the HL-A system: Deduction of 480 haplotypes. Pages 53–77 *in* P. I. Terasaki, ed. Histocompatibility Testing 1970. Munksgaard, Copenhagen.

Dausset, J., and J. Hors. 1975. Some contributions of the HL-A complex to the genetics of human diseases. *Transplant Rev* **22**:44–74.

Dausset, J., A. L. Florman, R. Bachvaroff, G. Y. Kanra, M. Sasportes, and F. T. Rapaport. 1972. *In vitro* approach to a correlation of cell susceptibility to viral infection with HL-A genotypes and other biological markers. *Proc Soc Exp Biol Med* **140**:1344–1349.

Dausset, J., L. Degos, and J. Hors. 1974. The association of the HL-A antigens with disease. An interpretative review. *J Clin Immunopathol* **3**:127–149.

Degos, L., and J. Dausset. 1974a. Histocompatibility determinants in multiple sclerosis. *Lancet* **1**:307–308.

Degos, L., and J. Dausset. 1974b. Human migrations and HL-A linkage disequilbrium. *Immunogenetics* **1**:195–210.

Delmas-Marsalet, Y., J. Hors, J. Colombani, and J. Dausset. 1974. Study of HL-A genotypes in a case of familial chronic lymphocytic leukemia (C. L. L). *Tissue Antigens* **4**:441–445.

Démant, P., J. Capková, E. Hinzová, and B. Vorácová. 1973. The role of the histocompatibility-2-linked *Ss-Slp* region in the control of mouse complement. *Proc Natl Acad Sci USA* **70**:863–864.

Dick, H. M., R. D. Sturrock, G. K. Goel, N. Henderson, B. Canesi, P. J. Rooney, W. C. Dick, and W. W. Buchanan. 1975. The association between HL-A antigens, ankylosing spondylitis and sacro-ileitis. *Tissue Antigens* **5**:26–32.

Dorf, M. E., P. E. Newburger, T. Hamaoka, D. H. Katz, and B. Benacerraf. 1974. Characterization of an immune response gene in mice controlling IgE and IgG antibody responses to ragweed pollen extract and its 2,4-dinitrophenylated derivative. *Eur J Immunol* **4**:346–349.

Duran-Reynals, M. L., and F. Lilly. 1971. The role of genetic factors in the combined neoplastic effects of vaccinia virus and methylcholanthrene. *Transplant Proc* **3**:1243–1246.

Falchunk, Z. M., G. N. Rogentine, and W. Strober. 1972. Predominance of histocompatibility antigen HL-A8 in patients with gluten-sensitive enteropathy. *J Clin Invest* **51**:1602–1605.

Falk, J. A., and D. Osoba. 1974. The association of the human histocompatibility system with Hodgkin's disease. *J Immunogen* **1**:39–47.

Feldmann, J. L. 1974. Les antigènes HL-A dans la spondylarthrite ankylosante et le syndrome de Fiessinger–Leroy–Reiter. Thesis, Univ. Paris.

Feltkamp, T. E. W., P. M. Van den Berg-Loonen, C. P. Engelfriet, A. L. Van Rossum, J. J. Van Loghem, and H. J. G. H. Dosterhuis. 1974. Myasthenia gravis, autoantibodies, and HL-A antigens. *Brit Med J* **1**:131–133.

Finkelstein, S., R. L. Walford, L. W. Myers, and G. W. Ellison. 1974. HL-A antigens and hypersensitivity to brain tissue in multiple sclerosis. *Lancet* **1**:736.

Fisher, R. A., 1958. The genetical theory of natural selection. Dover, New York.

Fritze, D., C. Herrman, F. Naeim, G. S. Smith, and R. L. Walford. 1974. HL-A antigens in myasthenia gravis: Relation to sex, age and thymic pathology. *Lancet* **1**:240–242.

Gasser, D. L., C. M. Newbin, J. Palm, and N. K. Gonatas. 1973. Genetic control of susceptibility to experimental allergic encephalomylitis in rats. *Science* **181**:873–874.

Gerkins, V. R., A. Ting, H. T. Menck, P. I. Terasaki, M. C. Pike, and B. E. Henderson. 1974. HL-A heterozygosity as a genetic marker of long-term survival. *J Natl Cancer Inst* **52**:1909–1911.

Grumet, F. C., A. Coukell, J. G. Bodmer, W. F. Bodmer, and H. O. McDevitt. 1971. Histocompatibility (HL-A) antigens associated with systemic lupus erythematosus. A possible genetic predisposition to disease. *N Engl J Med* **4**:193–196.

Grumet, F. C., J. Konishi, R. Payne, and J. P. Kriss. 1973. Association of Grave's disease with HL-A8. *Clin Res* **21**:439.

Hirata, A. A., and P. I. Terasaki. 1970. Cross-reactions between streptococcal M proteins and human transplantation antigens. *Science* **168**:1095–1096.

Hirata, A. A., F. C. McIntire, P. I. Terasaki, and K. K. Mittal. 1973. Cross-reactions between human transplantation antigens and bacterial lipopolysaccharides. *Transplantation* **15**:441–445.

Hors, J., C. Griscelli, M. Schmid, and J. Dausset. 1974. Letter to the editor: HL-A antigens and immune deficiency states. *Br Med J* **4**:5935.

Howard, J. G., G. H. Christie, B. M. Courteney, and G. Biozzi. 1972. Studies on immunological paralysis. VIII. Pneumococcal polysaccharide tolerance and immunity differences between the Biozzi high and low responder lines of mice. *Eur J Immunol* **2**:269–273.

Iványi, P. 1970. The major histocompatibility antigens in various species. *Curr Top Microbiol Immunol* **53**:1–90.

Iványi, P., R. Hampl, L. Stárka, and M. Micková. 1972. Genetic association between *H-2* genes and testosterone metabolism in mice. *Nature (Lond), New Biol* **238**:280–281.

Jeannet, M., and P. Alberto. 1972. HL-A antigens in chronic lymphocytic leukemia: Preliminary evidence for the existence of leukemia-specific antigens. *Schweiz Med Wochenschr* **102**:1170–1172.

Jersild, C., T. Ammitzbøll, J. Clausen, and T. Fog. 1973a. Association between HL-A antigens and measles antibody in multiple sclerosis. *Lancet* **1**:151–152.

Jersild, C., T. Fog, G. S. Hansen, A. Svejgaard, M. Thomsen, and B. Dupont. 1973b. Histocompatibility determinants in multiple sclerosis, with special reference to clinical course. *Lancet* **2**:1221–1224.

Koszinowski, U., and H. Ertl. 1975. Lysis mediated by T cells and restricted by *H-2* antigen of target cells infected with vaccinia virus. *Nature (Lond)* **255**:552–554.

Kourilsky, F. M., J. Dausset, N. Feingold, J. M. Dupuy, and J. Bernard. 1967. Étude de la répartition des antigènes leucocytaires chez des malades atteints de leucemie aigue en rémission. Pages 515–522 *in* J. Dausset, J. Hamburger, and G. Mathé, eds. Advances in transplantation. Munksgaard, Copenhagen.

Lawler, S. D., P. T. Klouda, P. G. Smith, M. M. Till, and R. M. Hardistry. 1974. Survival and the HL-A system in acute lymphoblastic leukaemia. *Br Med J* **1**:547–548.

Levine, B. B., R. H. Stember, and M. Fotino. 1972. Ragweed hay fever: Genetic control and linkage to HL-A haplotypes. *Science* **178**:1201–1203.

Lilly, F. 1966. The histocompatibility-2 locus and susceptibility to tumor induction. *Natl Cancer Inst Monogr* **22**:631.

Lilly, F. 1968. The effect of histocompatibility-2 type on response to the Friend leukemia virus in mice. *J Exp Med* **127**:465–473.

Lilly, F. 1971. The influence of *H-2* type on Gross virus leukemogenesis in mice. *Transplant Proc* **3**:1239–1241.

Lilly, F., E. A. Boyse, and L. J. Old. 1964. Genetic basis of susceptibility to viral leukemogeneses. *Lancet* **2**:1207–1209.

McDevitt, H. O., and W. F. Bodmer. 1974. HL-A, immune-response genes and disease. *Lancet* **1**:1269–1275.

Mackay, I. R., and P. Morris. 1972. Association of autoimmune active chronic hepatitis with HL-A1, 8. *Lancet* **2**:793–795.

Mawhinney, H., J. W. M. Lawton, A. G. White, and W. J. Irvine. 1975. HL-A3 and HL-A7 in pernicious anemia and autoimmune atrophic gastritis. *Clin Exp Immunol* **22**:47–53.

Marchalonis, J. J., P. J. Morris, and A. W. Harris. 1974. Speculation on the function of immune response genes. *J Immunogen* **1**:63–67.

Marsh, D. G., W. B. Bias, and S. H. Hsu. 1973. Association of the HL-A7 cross-reaction group with a specific reaginic antibody response in allergic man. *Science* **179**:691–693.

Mann, D. L., S. Hsia, and D. B. Amos. 1976. Br and Wh, B cell antigens in gluten sensitive enteropathy and dermatitis herpetiformis. *In* D. H. Katz and B. Benacerraf eds. The role of the products of the histocompatibility gene complex in immune responses. Academic Press, New York.

Milgrom, F., J. Klassen, and K. Kano. 1970. Auto-immunity and homograft rejection. *J Reticuloendothel Soc* **7**:264–279.

Morris, P. J. 1973. Histocompatibility systems, immune response and disease in man. *Contemp Top Immunobiol* **3**:141–169.

Morris, P. J., and M. C. Pietsch. 1973. A possible association between paralytic poliomyelitis and multiple sclerosis. *Lancet* **2**:847–848.

Morris, P. J., S. Lawler, and R. T. Oliver. 1973. Joint report of the Vth International Histocompatibility Workshop. II. HL-A and Hodgkin's disease. Pages 669–677 *in* J. Dausset and J. Colombani, eds. Histocompatibility Testing 1972. Munksgaard, Copenhagen.

Naito, S., N. Namerow, M. R. Mickey, and P. I. Terasaki. 1972. Multiple sclerosis: Association with HL-A3. *Tissue Antigens* **2**:1–4.

Nandi, S. 1967. The *H-2* locus and susceptibility to Bittner virus borne by red blood cells in mice. *Proc Natl Acad Sci USA* **58**:485–492.

Nandi, S., S. Haslam, and C. Helmich. 1971. Inheritance of susceptibility to erythrocyte-borne Bittner virus in mice. *Transplant Proc* **3**:1251–1257.

Nerup, J., P. Platz, O. O. Andersen, M. Christy, J. Lyngsøo, J. E. Poulsen, L. P. Ryder, M. Thomsen, L. Staub-Nielsen, and A. Svejgaard. 1974. HL-A antigens and diabetes mellitus. *Lancet* **2**:864–866.

Nyalassy, R. G., E. Svarová, and M. Buc. 1974. HL-A antigen in rheumatoid arthritis. *Lancet* **1**:450–451.

Ohno, S., K. Aoki, S. Sugiura, E. Nakayma, and M. Aizawa. 1973. HL-A5 and Behçet's disease. *Lancet* **2**:1383–1384.

Olstone, M. B. A., F. J. Dixon, G. F. Mitchell, and H. O. McDevitt. 1973. Histocompatibility-linked genetic control of disease susceptibility. Murine lymphocytic choriomeningitis virus infection. *J Exp Med* **137**:1201–1212.

Pirskanen, R. A., A. Tiilikainen, and E. Hokkenen. 1972. Histocompatibility antigens associated with myasthenia gravis. *Ann Clin Res* **4**:304–306.

Platz, P., L. Ryder, L. Nielsen, A. Svejgaard, M. Thomsen, J. Nerup, and M. Christy. 1974. HL-A idiopathic Addison's disease. *Lancet* **2**:289.

Rapaport, F. T., and F. H. Bach. 1973. Genetic studies of cell-surface determinants in human developmental anomalies. A preliminary report. *Transplant Proc* **5**:1139–1143.

Rapaport, F. T., and R. M. Chase. 1964. Homograft sensitivity induction by group A streptococci. *Science* **145**:407–408.

Rogentine, G. N., R. J. Trapani, R. A. Yankee, and E. S. Menderson. 1973. HL-A antigens and acute lymphocytic leukemia: The nature of the HL-A2 association. *Tissue Antigens* **3**:470–476.

Russell, T. J., L. M. Schultes, and D. J. Kuban. 1972. Histocompatibility (HL-A) antigens associated with psoriasis. *N Engl J Med* **287**:738–739.

Ryder, L. P., L. Staub-Nielsen, and A. Svejgaard. 1974. Association between HL-A histocompatibility antigens and non malignant diseases. *Humangenetik* **25**:251–264.

Schlosstein, L., P. I. Terasaki, R. Bluestone, and C. M. Pearson. 1973. High association of an HL-A antigen, W27, with ankylosing spondylitis. *N Engl J Med* **288**:704–706.

Schweitzer, M., C. J. M. Melief, and J. E. Ploem. 1973. Chronic lymphocytic leukemia in five siblings. *Scand J Haematol* **11**:97–105.

Seignalet, J., J. Clot, J. Sany, and H. Serre. 1972. HL-A antigens in rheumatoid arthritis. *Vox Sang* **23**:468–471.

Seignalet, J., J. Clot, J. J. Guilhou, F. Duntze, J. Meynadier, and M. Robinet-Levy. 1974. HL-A antigens and some immunological parameters in psoriasis. *Tissue Antigens* **4**:59–68.

Shearer, G. M. 1974. Cell-mediated cytotoxicity to trinitrophenyl-modified syngeneic lymphocytes. *Eur J Immunol* **4**:527–533.

Simons, M. J., N. E. Day, G. B. Wee, K. Shanmugaratnam, H. C. Ho, S. H. Wong, T. K. Ti, N. K. Yong, S. Darmalingham, and G. DeThé. 1974. Nasopharingeal carcinoma. V. Immunogenetic studies on southeast Asian ethnic groups with high and low risk for the tumor. *Cancer Res* **34**:1192–1195.

Simon, M., Y. Pawlotsky, M. Bourel, R. Fauchet and B. Genetet. 1975. Hémochromatose idiopathique. Maladie associée à l'antigène tissulaire HLA-3. *Nouv Presse Med* **4**:1432.

Stiffel, C., D. Mouton, Y. Bouthillier, A. M. Heumann, C. Decreusefond, J. C. Mevel, and G. Biozzi. 1974. Polygenic regulation of general antibody synthesis in the mouse. *In* L. Brent and J. Holborrow eds. Progress in Immunology II, Vol. 2. North-Holland Publ., Amsterdam.

Stokes, P. L., P. Asquith, G. K. T. Holmes, P. Mackintosh, and W. T. Cooke. 1972. Histocompatibility antigens associated with adult coeliac disease. *Lancet* **2**:162–164.

Strosberg, J. M., E. D. Harris, J. J. Calabro, and F. H. Allen. 1973. Ankylosing spondylitis: Clinical and genetic studies of a kindred. *Arthritis Rheum* **16**:774.

Svejgaard, A., C. Jersild, L. Staub-Nielsen, and W. F. Bodmer. 1974. HL-A antigens and disease. Statistical and genetical consideration. *Tissue Antigens* **4**:95–105.

Svejgaard, A., P. Platz, L. P. Ryder, L. Staub-Nielsen, and M. Thomsen. 1975. HL-A and disease associations. A survey. *Transplant Rev* **22**:3–43.

Takasugi, M., P. I. Terasaki, B. Henderson, M. R. Mickey, H. Menck, and R. W. Thompson. 1973. HL-A antigens in solid tumors. *Cancer Res* **33**:648–650.

Tennant, J. R., and G. D. Snell. 1965. Some experimental evidence for the influence of genetic factors on viral leukemogenesis. *Natl Cancer Inst Monogr* **22**:61–72.

Thomsen, M., P. Platz, O. O. Andersen, M. Christy, J. Lyngsoe, J. Nerup, K. Rasmussen, L. P. Ryder, L. Staub-Nielsen, and A. Svejgaard. 1975. MLC typing in juvenile diabetes mellitus and idiopathic Addison's disease. *Transplant Rev* **22**:125–147.

Van Rood, J. J., A. Van Leeuwen, A. Termijtelen, and J. J. Keuning. 1976. The genetics of the Major Histocompatibility Complex in man, HLA. *In* D. H. Katz and B. Benacerraf eds. The role of the products of the histocompatibility gene complex in immune responses. Academic Press, New York.

Vladutiu, A. O., and N. R. Rose. 1971. Autoimmune murine thyroiditis relation to histocompatibility (*H-2*) type. *Science* **174**:1137–1139.

Walford, R. L. 1966. Increased incidence of lymphoma after injections of mice with cells differing at weak histocompatibility loci. *Science* **152**:78–79.

Walford, R. L., S. Rinkelstein, R. Neerhout, P. Konrad, and E. Shanbrom. 1970. Acute childhood leukaemia in relation to the HL-A human transplantation genes. *Nature (Lond)* **225**:461–462.

Walford, R. L., G. S. Smith, and H. Walters. 1971. Histocompatibility systems and disease states with particular reference to cancer. *Transplant Rev* **7**:78–111.

Walford, R. L., H. Waters, G. S. Smith, and P. Sturgeon. 1973. Anomalous reactivity of certain HL-A typing sera with leukemic lymphocytes. *Tissue Antigens* **3**:222–234.

White, S. H., V. D. Newcomer, M. R. Mickey, and P. I. Terasaki. 1972. Disturbance of HL-A antigen frequency in psoriasis. *N Engl J Med* **287**:740–743.

Wiener, A. 1970. Blood groups and disease. *Am J Hum Genet* **22**:476–483.

Winchester, R. J., G. Ebers, S. M. Fu, L. Espinosa, J. Zabriskie, and H. G. Kunkel. 1975. B-cell alloantigen Ag-7a in multiple sclerosis. *Lancet* **2**:814.

Woolf, B. 1955. On estimating the relation between blood group and disease. *Ann Hum Genet* **19**:251–253.

Zinkernagel, R. M., and P. C. Doherty. 1974. Restriction of *in vitro T* cell-mediated cytotoxicity in lymphocytic chorio-meningitis within a syngeneic or semi-allogeneic system. *Nature (Lond)* **248**:701–702.

Zittoun, R., J. Zittoun, J. Seignalet, and J. Dausset. 1975. HLA and pernicious anemia. *N Engl J Med* **293**:1324.

CHAPTER 13

# THE ALLOGENEIC RESPONSE



The rejection of allografts is determined by two major components: (1) an allogeneic disparity between graft and host and (2) the response to this disparity by the host. In this chapter we first briefly review and attempt to interpret some aspects of component (1) and then concentrate on component (2).

Encounters with allogeneic cells may occur in nature under three circumstances: (1) pregnancy, except pregnancy within inbred strains;

(2) mutation- or virus-induced changes in cell surface antigens; (3) infection with venereal tumors, e.g., the well-known venereal tumor of dogs. It will be advantageous to the host not to mount a rejection response in case (1), but, in cases (2) and (3), and especially in case (2), if cell surface changes play a role in development of the cancer cell as they probably do, to respond aggressively. We may therefore expect to find in mammals mechanisms of response to alloantigens, but perhaps mechanisms of a contradictory nature.

Although allogeneic encounter probably occurs normally in many animals, the allograft is a strictly artificial experience. In all probability, the host draws as much or more on the mechanisms of defense against infectious organisms as on any mechanisms concerned with naturally occurring allogeneic encounters. This means that the allogeneic response may involve not only any possible mechanism concerned with fetus protection and immune surveillance against tumors but also the whole vast array of defenses against infection.

The allograft reaction thus could well be, and in fact probably is, an extraordinarily complex phenomenon. The literature with some degree of pertinance is enormous. To bring the subject within bounds we shall assume a knowledge of antibodies [reviews will be found in Hildemann (1970) and Nossal and Ada (1971)], review only the most relevant of the established facts of cellular immunity, and select from the less established areas of cellular immunity and from the vast literature on allografts only those portions that, in our personal judgments, contribute the most to an understanding of the allogeneic response. Our interpretations will, in varying degrees, be speculative.

## I. Alloantigens: The Stimulus

It is generally assumed that alloantigens are components of the cell membrane. In the case of the major histocompatibility complex (MHC) antigens, the human blood group substances, and alloantigens that, when exposed to antibody, show capping or modulation, there is definite experimental evidence for this (see, e.g., Chapter 11, Section II). The assumption is justified in the case of other alloantigens because it seems unlikely that antibodies or immune cells could easily destroy their targets via intracellular components.

If alloantigens are plasma membrane structures, cell membrane research and alloantigen immunogenetics should have significant and increasing relevance for each other. At present, we know little concerning the structural and functional relationships of alloantigens to the cell surface. We believe, however, that a few plausible assumptions can be made which should be testable and which may contribute to our understanding of the alloimmune response. However, we must first briefly review theories of cell membrane structure.

## A. Cell Membrane Structure

Singer and Nicolson (1972) have proposed a fluid mosaic model of the cell membrane. This is illustrated in Fig. 13.1. According to this model, the plasma membrane has two major components—a lipid bilayer and globular proteins embedded in the bilayer but free to move laterally within it. Studies of the protein component point to a great diversity of protein molecules. Polypeptides and proteins varying in molecular weight from 5000 to 670,000 have been reported. On the basis of their degree of integration into the membrane, two classes of proteins can be distinguished: peripheral proteins, easily dissociable from the membrane, and integral proteins that are firmly embedded in the membrane.

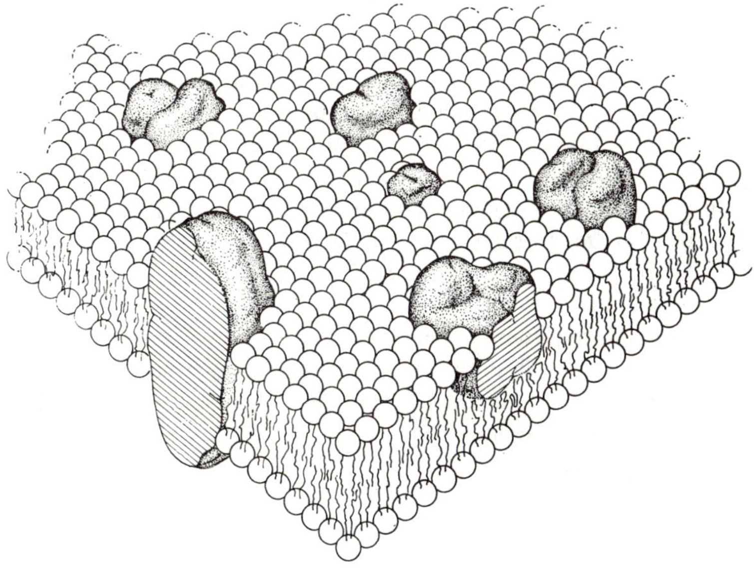

Fig. 13.1. The lipid–globular protein mosaic model of the plasma membrane (the fluid mosaic model). The phospholipids are arranged in a discontinuous bilayer with their ionic and polar heads in contact with water. The solid bodies with stippled surfaces represent the globular integral proteins. These may be either randomly distributed or may form specific aggregates (two aggregates are shown). (From Singer and Nicolson 1972. *Science* **175**:720–731. Copyright 1972 by the American Association for the Advancement of Science.)

Presumably alloantigens, which seem to be relatively constant features of the cell membrane, fall in the latter category. Only this category is shown in Fig. 13.1. The integral proteins may or may not entirely penetrate the bilayer. Also, as indicated in the figure, they may protrude above the bilayer to different degrees. (See, e.g., Kiehn and Holland, 1968; Laico *et al.*, 1970; Pardee, 1968.)

In addition to the lipid and protein cell boundary, cells possess, in widely varying degrees, an outermost layer of glycoprotein. This has been referred to as the *glycocalyx* (Rambourg *et al.*, 1966).

## B. Cell Membrane Function

The plasma membrane serves many functions. There are two functions which must be of major importance: (1) *transport* through the membrane of a great variety of molecules, and (2) the regulation of *cell interactions.* The cell interaction function can operate via direct cell contact or via hormones or other secreted cell products that deliver their message by binding to an appropriate and probably highly specific *receptor.*

The responsible agents in both these functions, except perhaps for some cell interaction substances, are presumably integral constituents of the membrane. A great many proteins, each with its own special properties, must play a role in each function. There is evidence, for example, that transport proteins are quite specific in their transport of substrate molecules through the membrane (Boyse, 1971; Pardee, 1968). One of the few membrane proteins (perhaps peripheral rather than integral) with a known structure and an identifiable function is cell-bound immunoglobulin. Clearly, this belongs in our second category.

The functional requirement that there be a diversity of membrane proteins is fully compatible with both the evidence from cell membrane chemistry and the immunogenetic evidence concerning the number of cell membrane alloantigen determining (CMAD) loci presented in earlier chapters of this book.

## C. Speculations

There is almost no firm evidence that ties together our knowledge of cell membrane alloantigens (as revealed by immunogenetics) and our knowledge of the morphological and physiological properties of the membrane. Perhaps, however, some ground for suggesting significant associations can be found.

Cell interaction proteins, by their very nature, should be so exposed on the cell surface as to readily encounter their appropriate counterparts on other cells. Transport proteins, on the other hand, need only be in contact with the substrate from which the cell derives its nourishment.

Cell membrane alloantigens can be rather clearly divided into antigens readily demonstrable by antibody (e.g., H-2, Ea, and Ly antigens), and H antigens readily demonstrable only by histogenetic techniques. Is it possible that ease of demonstration by antibody is associated with exposure of a substantial part of the molecule above the lipid bilayer, and this in turn with the cell interaction function, and that difficulty of demonstration by antibody is associated with immersion in the lipid bilayer and this in turn with the transport function? There is reason to believe that much of H-2, the prototype of the antibody-demonstrated alloantigen, is outside the bilayer, and similar evidence is turning up for a few other antibody-demonstrated antigens (Chapter 11). The antigens that have been characterized as differentiation antigens, and which therefore, presumably, are involved in cell interactions, all engender good antibody responses.

Even if these postulates are valid in a general way, there are certain to be exceptions. And of course, also, there must be membrane components that do not fit into our simple classification. Thus the glycocalyx is probably concerned neither with transport nor cell interactions, unless perhaps in a protective capacity. It will be interesting to see, however, how the postulates fit with the facts that we shall develop in this chapter.

## II. Lymphoid Cells: The Responders

We have already identified the major classes of lymphocytes (Chapter 5, Section II,A) and summarized information concerning the recently reported M cell (Chapter 8, Section II,D,2). We shall not elaborate further concerning the B lymphocyte or discuss the important contributions of macrophages to the immune response. However, because T cells are, as each new discovery emphasizes, both complex and a major agent in graft rejection, more details concerning these cells are necessary. We shall also describe reports of cells that resemble and may be the same as M cells.

The standard marker in mice for T cells is the Thy-1 or $\theta$ antigen. T cells are also distinguished by the absence of easily demonstrable surface immunoglobulin, although this can be demonstrated by appropriate methods. Whether immunoglobulin is the T cell receptor for interactions with antigen has been the subject of much debate. Possibly it is the receptor on only one or two of the several categories of T cells.

Circulating T cells pass from blood to lymph by two routes. Some leave the capillaries in the skin and other peripheral organs, and, after a brief residence in the tissues, return to the blood via the afferent lymph and the lymph nodes. A much larger circulation occurs directly in the lymph nodes, via the postcapillary venules. According to one study, the lymphocytes following these two routes are functionally different. (Marchesi and Gowans, 1964; Scollay and Lafferty, 1975.)

There are probably at least four classes of T cells. One of them is distinguished by the presence of both the Ly-1 and Ly-2,3 alloantigens. This class makes up about 50% of the T cells in the nodes and spleen of adult B6 mice. It disappears rapidly after adult thymectomy and, hence, is presumably short-lived. The other three, the T helper cell, the T effector cell, and the T suppressor cell, we shall consider in more detail.

### A. T Helper Cells

Functionally, the *T helper cells* are defined as thymus-derived lymphocytes that collaborate with B cells in the production of antibody. They are also distinguished by the presence of the Ly-1 alloantigen and the absence of Ly-2,3. They appear somewhat after the cells bearing Ly-1 plus Ly-2,3, and may be derived from them. They make up about 33% of the T cell population of nodes and spleen in contrast to only about 6–8% for effector cells (Cantor and Boyse, 1975).

T helper cells, of all lymphocytes, probably play the most important role in initial recognition of antigen. Like policemen on patrol, they are out looking for trouble. About 70% of the lymphocytes in the blood and 80% of those in thoracic duct lymph are T cells. Whether these are divided between helpers and effectors in the same proportions as are T cells in nodes and spleen has not yet been determined. It is also not clear whether the T helper cell circulation pattern is the same as or different from that of the T effector cell.

### B. T Effector Cells

There are several classes of lymphoid or lymphoid-derived *cytotoxic effector cells* that destroy their targets via cell contact. In one form of cytotoxicity, a lymphoid cell, acting nonspecifically, destroys targets coated with specific antibody. Monocytes and macrophages, perhaps again with the assistance of antibody, engage in a form of cytotoxicity requiring only cell contact, not phagocytosis. (Grant *et al.*, 1973; and others.) Here we consider cytotoxicity due to the *T effector cell.*

The T effector cell can be defined in two ways. Antigenically, according to recent evidence, it is characterized by the presence of the Ly-2,3 alloantigen. Functionally, it is characterized as the Thy-1 bearing cell that, following an appropriate period of encounter with allogeneic targets, either *in vivo* or *in vitro,* will kill the same or cross-reacting targets *in vitro.* At least some cytotoxic T cells make up part of the recirculating pool.

### C. T Suppressor Cells

The two phenomena of tolerance and immunological enhancement play an important role in the allogeneic response, and particularly in the response to successful allografts. Because we shall have occasions in this chapter to refer to them, and because they must be understood for an understanding of T suppressor cells, this is an appropriate place to describe them. Our summary will be greatly condensed; reviews will be found in Brent and French (1973) and Katz and Benacerraf (1974).

#### *1. Immunological Unresponsiveness*

Tolerance and immunological enhancement are both phenomena that lead to partial or total specific unresponsiveness to allografts. Both, like immunity, are induced by prior exposure to antigen. *Tolerance* is typically induced by prenatal or neonatal exposure (Billingham *et al.*, 1953). It was originally conceived as being due to the deletion of all clones of lymphocytes with the capacity to respond to the specific antigen introduced. The capacity to respond to other antigens remained, but the capacity to respond to the tolerizing antigen was lost. We shall use the term tolerance to apply to unresponsiveness due to this mechanism. *Immunological enhancement* can be induced by exposure to alloantigen at any age. It often exists in a delicate balance with its opposite, immunity. It is due to some form or forms of antibody, perhaps complexed in some cases with antigen, and, in typical cases, can be transferred with serum (Kaliss *et al.*, 1953; Bansal *et al.*, 1973). The serum factors probably operate by a variety of mechanisms; one of the major mechanisms is an interference by humoral antibody with the development of cell-mediated immunity (Snell *et al.*, 1960).

As we shall see later, there are circumstances in which antibody can be cytotoxic rather than enhancing. There are also cells other than T effector cells that can participate in the destruction of allografts.

While we have outlined only tolerance and enhancement of allografts, which presumably act via T cells, there are B cell counterparts that are manifest as suppression of antibody production. The basic mechanisms are probably not very different. A good, brief review of various forms of immune blockade attributable to antibody will be found in Hildemann and Mullen (1973).

### 2. *Cells That Induce Unresponsiveness*

An important contribution to the understanding of the mechanism of immunological unresponsiveness was the discovery of lymphocytes that suppress the immune capacity of other lymphocytes. The active cells are sensitive to anti-Thy-1 and hence probably are T lymphocytes. They have been shown to suppress antibody production and hence to act, directly or indirectly, on B cells, but they also suppress the mixed lymphocyte reaction (MLR) and delayed hypersensitivity which are manifestations of T cell activity.

The existence of these populations of T lymphocytes, with the capacity to suppress, usually specifically but in some cases also apparently nonspecifically, the activity of other lymphocytes is well established. Characterization of the other properties of these cells is still very incomplete. If they should be found to act by the release of antibody-like substances or of antigen–antibody complexes, this would constitute an important extension of our concept of immunological enhancement. (Basten *et al.*, 1974; Gershon, 1974; Rich and Rich, 1975; Zembala and Asherson, 1973; and others.)

## D. M Cells and Other Possibly Related Cells of Uncertain Classification

In Chapter 8, Section II,D,2 we summarized reports by Bennett and co-workers of a lymphocyte, originating in bone marrow but found also in spleen and lymph nodes, which does not have the properties of a B cell, and which is active in resistance of $F_1$'s receiving parental marrow grafts (hybrid resistance) and in resistance to Friend virus leukemia. This has been called the M cell. There have been other reports of a lymphocyte that is neither a T nor a B cell, usually found either in marrow or spleen. While the tests systems used by the different investigators of this cell are so different that they could be studying different cell types, we shall briefly summarize some of the observations on the assumption that all observers are perhaps dealing with one cell type and that this cell type corresponds to the M cell.

The M cells lack Thy-1, the standard marker for T cells, and surface immunoglobulin, the standard marker for B cells. They are present in athymic mice. They cause rapid cytolysis of leukemias induced by the Moloney virus. In one allogeneic test system, thymus cells showed a synergistic effect on marrow cells, and transferred sensitized marrow cells caused skin graft rejection in either irradiated or nonirradiated mice. (Strobo *et al.*, 1973; von Bohmer, 1974; Kiessling *et al.*, 1975; Dyminski and Argyris, 1972.)

## III. The Allogeneic Reaction

The reaction of a host to an allograft can be divided into three phases: a recognition phase, an immunization phase, and an effector phase. In discussing these, we shall attempt to interpret the observations recorded in this and previous sections. In a brief and speculative treatment of a complex phenomenon, some oversimplification is inevitable and some error altogether possible.

### A. The Recognition Phase

#### *1. Peripheral Recognition versus Central Recognition*

The initial recognition of foreignness by the lymphoid system of the host—presumably in most cases by T helper cells—may occur either *peripherally* in the graft or *centrally* in a lymphoid organ. There is reason to believe that recognition in these two different locales may lead to somewhat different outcomes.

In the graft, the complement of host cells concerned in the immune response is less complete than in the nodes or spleen. Macrophages that are competent to digest antigen and dendritic cells that probably display the antigen on their surfaces in forms appropriate for lymphocyte stimulation may be infrequent or lacking (Guttman and Weissman, 1972). Also, while there may be a considerable influx of lymphocytes into the graft, there is not the very active circulation of these cells that occurs in the nodes and spleen. It is possible, therefore, that peripheral recognition is a less complex process than central recognition. We suggest that it is the *in vivo* counterpart of the *in vitro* mixed lymphocyte reaction (MLR). When there are differences in the allograft reaction and the MLR, as for example in the somewhat lower order of uniqueness of the rcle played by the MHC in the former, this may be due to contributions that can be made *in vivo* by the more complex recognition processes that occur centrally in the nodes and spleen.

Another possible source of difference resulting from peripheral as compared with central recognition is the site of subsequent interaction of the stimulated T helper cell with other cell types. A stimulated T helper cell is programmed to cooperate with B cells in IgG production. Perhaps such cells acquire the potential to migrate to B cell-dependent areas of the nodes and spleen where they can initiate antibody production. In so far as initial recognition by T helper cells occurs centrally, it would occur in T cell-dependent areas where immediate contact would be primarily with T effector cells.

### 2. *Organ Grafts versus Tissue Grafts*

Organ allografts are generally less rigid in their histocompatibility requirements than skin allografts. Kidneys or hearts, for example, when transplanted across multiple minor *H* locus barriers, will sometimes show prolonged survival, whereas skin grafts are rapidly rejected. This is not due to differences in antigen content. In preimmunized hosts, kidneys with only minor *H* locus disparities are strongly rejected. Also neonatal heart tissue grafted in a manner resembling a skin graft is rejected like skin. (White and Hildemann, 1969; Fabre and Morris, 1975; Warren *et al.*, 1973; and others.)

One difference between organ and skin grafts that may explain differences in host response concerns the way in which the blood supply is reestablished. In organ transplants, where the blood vessels of the graft are anastomosed to those of the host, circulation is restored immediately. Host lymphocytes thus promptly enter the graft, and throughout their passage are in contact with donor vascular endothelium. The first encounter of most of these lymphocytes with a lymphoid organ will be with the spleen, although some may migrate from the capillaries and pass to the draining lymph node. We shall see that this distinction between immunization via the spleen as contrasted with immunization via the nodes can be quite important. In skin grafts, it is about 3 days before a blood supply is reestablished, and circulation may be sluggish for several additional days. When circulation does begin, the cells encountered in the capillaries are of host origin, since in the healing process there is replacement of the vascular endothelium of the graft with ingrowing cells from the host (Converse and Ballantyne, 1962).

While skin grafts, during the first few days following placement, cannot immunize via the blood–spleen route, they can immunize almost immediately via the lymphatic-lymph node route owing to the escape of passenger lymphocytes, cellular debris. or phagocytized necrotic tissue. As we shall show later, passenger lymphocytes may play a particularly important role.

There are a number of studies that bear quite directly on the occurrence of peripheral recognition in organ grafts. We saw in Chapter 8, Section I,D,1 that the cells of the vascular endothelium are effective stimulators in the mixed lymphocyte reaction (MLR). If the MLR is, as we have suggested, the *in vitro* counterpart of peripheral recognition, then we should expect recognition to occur in the capillaries of organ grafts, and, indeed, there is evidence that it does.

Strober and Gowens (1965) perfused the kidneys of rats to remove donor cells, and then perfused the kidneys with allogeneic blood, either *in vitro* or by anastomosis to an allogeneic host. The lymphocytes of the passaged blood were then tested for immunity by adoptive transfer to isogeneic hosts bearing a skin graft of the same genotype as the kidney. Immunization was demonstrated, but it took 5 to 12 hours of attachment to an allogeneic host for immunization to develop. Immunization due to *in vitro* perfusion developed in 1 hour.

If, instead of remaining in the blood stream, host lymphocytes pass into the tissues of the graft, the course of events is somewhat different. Hamburger *et al.* (1971) collected lymph from human kidney allografts and studied the cell content. The number of lymphocytes and the percent of total lymphocytes showing stimulation (blast transformation and thymidine incorporation) rose steadily for the first 5 days. The changes were typical of those seen in MLR. Similar results have been reported in a study of kidney transplantation in sheep (Pederson *et al.*, 1975).

Just where, in the case of these tissue-passage lymphocytes, the initial recognition event occurred is not clear. It could have been prior to the exit from the blood. Kidney and heart tissue, except probably the vascular endothelium, lack the Ia antigen. Lindquist *et al.* (1971) believe that recognition occurs as a result of contact with passenger lymphocytes carried over in the graft. Whatever the exact site of the triggering, these studies indicate that sensitized lymphocytes ultimately reach the lymph nodes as well as the spleen.

### 3. *The Role of Passenger Lymphocytes*

Central recognition could occur as the result of passage to the nodes or spleen of cellular debris, of phagocytized necrotic tissue, or of donor lymphocytes carried over as passengers in the graft. There is considerable evidence that passenger lymphocytes are the major agents in central recognition and the major inducers of cellular immunity. That they are an effective source of central immunization is not surprising, since lymphocytes are rich in alloantigens, stimulate effectively in the MLR, and show homing tendencies for the lymph nodes or spleen. They are also usually present in some abundance not only in any blood carried over in the graft but also in the tissues themselves.

The clearest evidence concerning their role in allograft immunity comes from studies with skin grafts. To ensure the absence of donor-genotype lymphocytes not only in the blood vessels (these could be removed by simple perfusion) but also from the tissues themselves, investigators have made use of chimeras. Such chimeras can be produced by heavy irradiation followed by restoration of the hemopoietic and lymphoid systems with allogeneic marrow and spleen. In these animals, the skin itself is of one genotype and the passenger cells of another type. With donors thus derived, two types of test can be performed; grafts can be put on recipients that are isogeneic with the skin itself but allogeneic to the passenger cells, or grafts can be put on recipients where the situation is reversed. If the allogeneic element is the passenger cells, the graft is accepted, but a second graft matching the cells shows accelerated rejection. If the allogeneic element is the skin itself, its immunizing capacity depends on how long it is left in place. Immunization is tested by removing the graft and replacing it with a second graft of the same donor strain. During the first 48 hours of residence, no immunity is induced, although if allogeneic lymphocytes are present, this is ample time to induce immunity. However, if the graft is left in place 7 days, sensitization is induced. The significance of the 7 day interval is probably that this is about the time required to restore active circulation and to allow the passage of host lymphocytes into the tissues, thus creating the conditions necessary for *peripheral* sensitization. (Snell, 1957; Steinmuller and Hart, 1971; Kyger and Salyer, 1973.)

Studies on the immunizing role of passenger lymphocytes in organ transplants usually have not given as unequivocal results as the studies with skin grafts, but in general they confirm the importance of this role. Survival seems to be related to the completeness of passenger lymphocyte elimination. A study with heart transplants failed to reveal an effect of removal of passenger lymphocytes, but the methods used left appreciable numbers of lymphocytes still present. (Guttman *et al.*, 1969; Lameijer *et al.*, 1972; Nielsen *et al.*, 1975; and others.)

One study of the role of passenger lymphocytes in immunization against cardiac allografts has unusual features and deserves special note. Dittmer and Bennett (1975) transplanted hearts into lethally irradiated, Rt *H-1*-incompatible rats and reconstituted the hematopoietic and lymphoid systems of the hosts with an isogeneic cell infusion. Rt *H-1* is the rat homolog of the mouse *H-2*. If the infusion was given immediately after the graft, typical rejection occurred. If the infusion was given 2 days after the graft, the transplanted heart survived indefinitely. The authors interpret their results in terms of the radiation-resistant allogeneic lymphocyte rejection that we have described in Chapter 8, Section II. During the 2 days that the host, as the result of the irradiation, was incompetent to become sensitized to or attack the heart itself, it still was able, through the agency of its radiation-resistant M cells, to attack the passenger lymphocytes present in the heart. Presumably the passenger lymphocytes were killed and thereby rendered nonimmunogenic, or perhaps they lost their capacity to induce cellular immunity but retained a capacity to induce enhancing antibody. There is some evidence that there is such a distinction in the immunizing role of dead as compared to living cells. In any case, this experiment points to a very striking role of passenger lymphocytes, although, in view of the complexities of the method used, any interpretation must be regarded as tentative. One interesting implication of this study is that M cells circulate in the blood and can pass from the capillaries into the tissues.

#### 4. *The Role of Mucoprotein*

A structural feature that is important in the survival of certain types of allografts including, probably, the fetal trophoblast and placenta and hence, indirectly, the fetus itself, is the presence of a protective coat of mucoprotein. The most obvious example is cartilage, which may survive indefinitely, even when transplanted across the major *H* barrier. (Currie and Bagshawe, 1968; and others.)

Whether protective coats of mucoproteins are more effective in blocking the recognition phase or the rejection phase of the immune response is not entirely clear. Cartilage grafts do immunize weakly. One possibility that might be considered is that protective mucoprotein, perhaps particularly on the trophoblast, favors the escape of antigen in molecular forms that would tend to be enhancing.

### B. The Immunization Phase

The generation, in the lymph nodes and spleen, of antibody and of effector lymphocytes is a complex process. The events that occur following recognition of antigen by helper T cells may include the release of messenger compounds (lymphokines) or "arming factors," the trapping of antigen by macrophages or dendritic cells, a process in which cytophilic antibody or arming factors may play a part; sometimes the digestion of antigen by macrophages; the display of antigen in appropriate matrices on the macrophage surface; complex collaborative interactions involving helper cells and either T effector or B cells and macrophages; and perhaps in some cases the recruitment of potential effector cells from the circulation. These processes are common to all immune reactions and have received relatively little study in the specific context of the allogeneic response. It would be inappropriate to try to describe them here. A review covering work up to 1971 will be found in Nossal and Ada (1971).

We know relatively little about what happens to peripherally sensitized lymphocytes after they reach the nodes or spleen, and we shall not attempt to explore this subject. We shall see, however, that it can make a substantial difference in which of the two organs they settle.

### 1. *Influence of Type of Drainage*

Antigen or peripherally sensitized lymphocytes can pass from a graft to the lymphoid organs by either of two routes: (1) the lymphatics, in which case the immune response will occur predominantly in the lymph nodes, or (2) the bloodstream, in which case the response will occur predominantly in the spleen. The effect of immunization via these two routes is quite different. Immunization via the lymph nodes is favorable to the development of cellular immunity; immunization via the blood stream is favorable to the development of antibody and may lead to enhancement.

The clearest evidence for this comes from studies with rats in which skin grafts or cell inocula were placed in the anterior chamber of the eye (Kaplan and Streilein, 1974: Kaplan and Stevens, 1975; Kaplan *et al.*, 1975). The anterior chamber has long been recognized as a *privileged site* in which grafts show prolonged or permanent survival, and this was evident in these studies. Intraocular skin grafts with an Rt *H-1* disparity survived 25.2 ± 1.4 days as compared with 8.4 ± 1.1 days for orthotopic controls. Intraocular grafts with multiple Rt non-*H-1* disparities survived >84 days (1 exception) as compared with 11.0 ± 1.2 days for the controls. Appropriate experiments showed that, for both types of disparity, the intraocular grafts both generated cellular immunity and were susceptible to it. Hence the prolonged survival was not due to defects in either the afferent or efferent limbs of the immune process.

Results such as these have been observed by other authors using a variety of transplants, but there has been uncertainty as to the reason for this. The results of Kaplan and co-workers point to the development in the spleen of enhancing antibody as the causative agent in the prolonged survival. The anterior chamber of the eye has no lymphatic drainage, but cells do pass via the bloodstream to the spleen, and some cells are trapped there. Several experiments showed that this leads to the development of enhancing antibody. Thus when rats were given intraocular injections of Rt *H-1* disparate lymphocytes, hemagglutinating antibodies developed rapidly, but subsequent skin grafts from the same donor strain showed prolonged survival. In splenectomized animals, the enhancing effect of intraocular grafts was eliminated. This marked development of enhancing antibody was the unique feature of the intraocular grafts. Allogeneic skin grafts placed orthotopically or allogeneic cell inocula made into a foot pad generated effective cellular immunity but little or no enhancing antibody. With such transplants, passenger lymphocytes or other forms of antigen pass via the lymphatics to the draining node, where highly effective trapping of antigen occurs. Probably only very little antigen (at least in the case of MHC disparities) reaches the spleen. The result is the generation of effective cellular immunity.

The striking difference in the outcome of immunization via the spleen as compared with the nodes is at least partly explained by lymphocyte population statistics. In the nodes the ratio of T cells to B cells is about 2 to 1, in the spleen the ratio is reversed (see, e.g., Raff and Owen, 1971). It may also be that the spleen is particularly rich in T suppressor cells.

Most grafts have both lymphatic and venous drainage, but the degree of circulation via the two may show characteristic differences. The skin is extraordinarily rich in lymphatics; Hudack and McMaster (1933) have emphasized this in the statement that: "Every intradermal injection is an intralymphatic one." Skin grafts artifically deprived of lymphatics may show greatly prolonged survival and evidence of immunological enhancement. Alymphatic kidney grafts are rejected; this is an apparent exception to which we shall return later. (Barker and Billingham, 1968; Vetto and Lawson, 1967.)

### 2. *The Development of Cellular Immunity*

The generation of effector lymphocytes in response to an allogeneic stimulus can be measured quantitatively by harvesting lymphocytes from the lymphoid organs and assaying their cytotoxic potential against appropriate target cells. In a study of this type, Canty and Wunderlich (1971) examined the generation of cytotoxic activity in mice in response to skin grafted across multiple *H* barriers, including *H*-2. Immune cells were abundant in the draining nodes from days 3 to 7, but had largely disappeared by day 12. In view of the time required to generate cytotoxic effector cells *in vitro*, antigen (presumably in the form of passenger lymphocytes) must have reached the nodes almost immediately after the graft was placed. The appearance of immunity in the spleen lagged behind its appearance in the draining nodes by several days (Fig. 13.2). The source of immunity in the spleen is not entirely clear. Probably some of it was due to the trapping of donor lymphocytes that had escaped the draining nodes. There is also transmission of information between different lymphoid organs by activated lymphocytes (memory cells?) and possibly some transfer of ingested antigen. The response in the spleen thus may have been due to the interaction of multiple agencies. The mesenteric nodes behaved like the spleen.

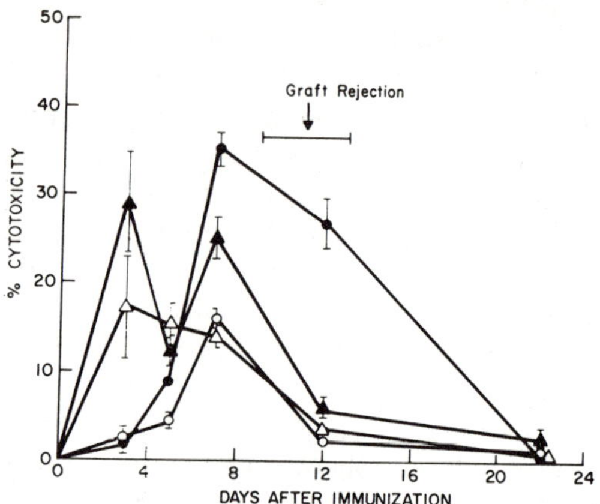


Fig. 13.2. Variation with time of the cellular immunity generated in the dfferent lymphoid organs of C mice following a B6 skin graft. Immunity was measured as the percentage of maximal $^{51}$Cr release after 4 hours of incubation of immune lymphoid cells with target cells in the ratio 100:1. ●, spleen; ○, mesenteric node; ▲, axillary node; △, inguinal node. (From Canty and Wunderlich, 1971. *Transplantation* **11**:111.)

## C. The Effector Phase

The end result of the immunization phase of the allogeneic response is the generation in the nodes and spleen of anti-graft antibodies of several immunoglobulin classes and of anti-graft effector T cells. We now turn to a consideration of how these destroy the graft.

### *1. Cell-Mediated Cytotoxicity*

The subject of cell-mediated immunity has been well reviewed by Cerottini and Brunner (1974). The activated T effector cell appears to be a physiologically active cell that incorporates thymidine and shows increased migratory tendencies. Its appearance in the blood and lymph coincides with or slightly precedes signs of graft rejection. Thus, in studies of patients with kidney or heart transplants, the appearance of increased numbers of thymidine-incorporating lymphoblasts in the peripheral blood was found to coincide with rejection episodes. (Cochran *et al.*, 1971; Hersh *et al.*, 1971; Rouse and Wagner, 1973.)

While early reports were conflicting, there now appears to be substantial evidence that activated lymphocytes from immunized animals specifically localize in the immunizing graft, or in grafts of the same genotype on secondary hosts to which they have been adaptively transferred. Thus Lance and Cooper (1972) found that $^{145}$IUdR labeled splenic or lymph node lymphocytes from skin allografted mice were not distributed at random. They localized in grafts from the original donor to a much greater degree than in isografts or third party grafts. $^{145}$IUdR is a compound which is incorporated preferentially in dividing cells. Cells tagged with $^{51}$Cr, which labels both dividing and non-dividing cells, showed no specific localization in the graft.

While the sensitized T effector cell appears to be the major agent in graft rejection, there are other cell types that can participate independently or collaboratively in the rejection process. The multiple and complex pathways to rejection are still poorly understood, but at least a partial picture has emerged.

As we have already indicated (Section II), there are several cell types in addition to the T effector cell that are capable of cytotoxic activity. These include the M cell, antibody-dependent cytotoxic lymphocytes, and monocytes and macrophages. There is evidence that, at least in some cases, one or more of these other cytotoxic cells may play an essential accessory role in rejection by T effector cells. In the most typical situation, the T cells may provide the specificity, and the other cells may provide the necessary amplifying action.

Gelfand and Steinberg (1974) have found evidence that three types of lymphoid cells present in lymph nodes and spleen play an essential role in allograft rejection. Two of these are anti-Thy-1 sensitive and are therefore T cells. Presumably, they can be equated with the T helper cell and the T effector cell. The third cell type is removed by treatment with anti-$\gamma$-globulin and therefore appears to be a B cell.

Kongshavn and Lapp (1973) have also reported a requirement in graft rejection for the collaboration of a cell of bone marrow origin, but the cell revealed by their tests did not have the properties of a typical B cell. It was present only in bone marrow, not in nodes or spleen. It was also sensitive to rabbit anti-mouse lymphocyte serum (ALS), which is supposed to suppress T rather than B cells. The authors suggest that the cell may belong to the monocyte–macrophage lineage.

A clue to the different accessory cell requirements revealed in these two studies can perhaps be found in a difference in the genetics of the two systems employed. Gelfand and Steinberg used mice with multiple histoincompatibilities, including *H-2;* Kongshavn and Lapp used congenic mice with an *H-1* difference. Antibody would appear early in a system involving an *H-2* disparity, and very minute amounts of MHC antibody are sufficient to activate antibody-dependent lymphocyte-mediated cytotoxicity (Hersey *et al.*, 1973). The active cells are of marrow origin but have the properties neither of monocytes nor typical B cells (MacLennan, 1972). It would be interesting to know if either of these accessory cell types is the same as the M cell of Mayhew and Bennett

(1971), but there does not appear to be sufficient evidence to determine this.

At least one of the mechanisms by which effector cells kill their targets is the release of a *lymphotoxin.* In humans, this is a proteinaceous molecule with a molecular weight of about 90,000. It is nonspecific in its action (Hessinger *et al.*, 1973).

### 2. *Antibody-Mediated Cytotoxicity*

While the principal agent in graft rejection is cell-mediated immunity, there are circumstances in which antibody can play the predominant role. This is a complex subject, but there are three simple rules that are usually valid guides to the conditions of antibody cytotoxicity. (1) Complement is necessary. (2) Cells with a high concentration of cell surface alloantigen—lymphocytes are the typical example—are more readily subject to cytotoxicity than are cells with a low concentration of alloantigen. (3) IgM formed in the primary response tends to be cytotoxic, and at least some of the classes of IgG formed in the secondary response may be enhancing. According to Harris and Harris (1975), $IgG_1$ is both late to appear and is blocking rather than cytotoxic because it is non-complement-fixing. While this rule seems to be supported by most studies, there may be substantial exceptions (see, e.g., Carpenter, 1976).

There is some reason to believe that conditions (2) and (3) are likely to be met only in the case of MHC disparities. The finding of several authors that minor H antigens tend to induce enhancing rather than cytotoxic antibodies and the findings of Miller and DeWitt (1973, 1974) in rats with IgM is not produced in response to the minor H antigens would both suggest that only major disparities are likely to induce cytotoxic antibodies. Also only major disparities may lead to the necessary concentration of antigen. The HLA and ABO alloantigens have both been shown to be abundant on the vascular endothelium of kidneys, and kidneys, at least in some species, are one of the organs particularly susceptible to cytotoxic antibody (Linscott, 1970; Sybesma *et al.*, 1974; Szulman, 1960).

## IV. MHC versus Minor *H* Locus Incompatibilities

An important question concerning the allogeneic response is why the antigens of the major histocompatibility complex (MHC) induce rapid rejection, while all other H antigens induce a slower rejection—a rejection, indeed, that in the limiting cases is so slow and weak as to be barely detectable. There is substantial immunological evidence bearing on this problem, but before we turn to this we need to examine a characteristic property of weak rejections which is revealed by transplantation data.

### A. Variability in Graft Survival

Whereas rejections determined by MHC disparities occur within a rather uniform interval, usually of the order of 10 or 12 days, rejections determined by weak histoincompatibilities not only are slower, but also more variable. The spread in the rejection times, moreover, and the chance of some grafts surviving permanently increase as the median survival time increases. This fact is noted as one of the laws of transplantation (Chapter 3, Section III).

Lengerová and Matousek (1968) showed that this variability in survival times is due to variation in the host and not in the graft. Skin grafts were made from multiple donors to one host and from one donor to multiple hosts, across non-*H-2* histocompatibility gaps. For any one histoincompatibility, graft survival time was almost entirely contingent on the host. Grafts from different donors on the same host were rejected together, grafts from the same donor on different hosts showed a wide range of survival times. The delayed rejection shown by some hosts was not due to a generalized weakness of that host's immunocompetence, since when single hosts received grafts with different non-*H-2* disparities, rejection times could be very different. Thus an *H-1* graft might be rejected in 27 days and an *H-3 H-13* graft on the same host in 44 days, whereas on another host the survival times might be reversed.

There are at least two possible explanations of this variation in the host reaction: (1) If the many lymphocyte classes in each individual's immune armament are generated in part by some mutational process, as is now rather generally supposed, then different individuals, even within an inbred strain, will have different batteries of reactive cells. One individual might have several clones particularly suitable for reacting with a particular graft, another individual might lack such clones. It is well established that different mice of the same inbred strains may produce quite different antibodies to the same antigen, a strong argument for clonal diversity (Mattioli *et al.*, 1968). (2) Because recognition is a clonal phenomenon, and because clones capable of reacting with a particular antigen are a small fraction of the total, there may be an *encounter lag* in the case of weak alloantigens. Whatever the nature of allogeneic weakness—and we have no firm knowledge as to what it is—it is not unreasonable to suppose that the time required for an encounter competent to trigger the immune response to a particular alloantigen is inversely related to the strength of that alloantigen. Whether encounter lag, in the case of weak alloantigens, can extend for a matter of days or weeks, and hence fully explain prolonged survival, is a separate question.

Bailey (1971) has pointed out that the rejection of a graft bearing two, weak incompatibilities might, as a matter of chance, be due to the host's reaction to either one of the incompatibilities. The earliest response would prevail. This would result in a shorter median rejection time for the double incompatibility than for either incompatibility acting alone. Bailey suggests that this can account for the cumulation effect of multiple incompatibilities reported by Graff *et al.* (1966). It should be noted that the two hypotheses here suggested to account for variability in rejection intervals are not mutually exclusive; both factors may be at work.

## B. Immunity Induced by Minor *H* Locus Disparities

It will be convenient to divide our examination of investigations of immunity induced by minor *H* locus disparities into two parts: (1) studies of cellular immunity and of morphological changes in the lymphoid organs perhaps indicative of cellular immunity, and (2) studies of humoral immunity. To permit comparisons, some *H-2* results will be described.

### *1. Cellular Immunity: Morphological Indications of Immunity*

In studying non-*H-2* disparities, considerable use has been made of the congenic strain pair B10 and B10.LP, which provided the original identification of the *H-3* locus. We now know that, besides the originally recognized *H-3* and *A* (agouti) differences, these strains also differ at *H-13, Ly-4,* and *Ir-2.* Tests made with these strains are not testing a single CMAD locus, but perhaps this is fortunate. If comparisons are drawn, they are between the *H-2* complex and what we might call the *H-3* complex.

Studies with this strain pair and an *H-2* congenic pair, also on a B10 background, have revealed the following. In mice immunized with $5 \times 10^5$ spleen and tested for immunity by challenge with a skin graft, H-2 immunity peaked between 2 and 8 days, had substantially weakened by 32 days, and had disappeared by 64 days. H-3 immunity did not appear till 8 days, peaked at 16 days, and did not disappear until 128 days. An attempt to assay, in harvested lymphocytes, the immunity generated by skin grafts, emphasized both the weakness and tardiness of H-3 as compared to H-2 immunity. Only in the draining nodes could H-3 immunity be demonstrated. Whereas H-2 immunity was already strong at 7 days, H-3 immunity did not appear until 10 days or peak until about 24 days. (McKhann and Berrian, 1961; McKhann, 1964.) However, additional studies reveal surprising complexities concerning the presumed "weakness" of non-*H*-2 disparities.

McKhann and Berrian (1961) tested the interval required for induction of H-2 and H-3 immunity by removing a primary skin graft at various intervals and then challenging with a second graft. It was found that across both barriers, 4 days residence of a graft served to induce immunity, but it required a longer interval subsequent to graft removal for the H-3 immunity to become demonstrable. If recognition was peripheral, the H-3 lag must have been in the inductive phase. The test is uninstructive in regard to central recognition.

A somewhat similar situation has been found when draining nodes have been weighed or sectioned at various intervals after skin grafting. In the study based on node weight, the first slight increase in the draining nodes was apparent at day 7 for transplants across both *H-2* and *H-3* barriers. But whereas the *H-2* disparity engendered a peak at 10 days, the *H-3* disparity engendered a peak at 20 days. The *H*-3 peak, surprisingly, was the higher. The contralateral nodes, not directly draining the graft, showed little weight increase. This emphasizes the widely recognized capacity of the draining nodes to recognize and trap any foreign material (see, e.g., Widdicombe *et al.*, 1955), even when the foreignness is only that of a weak histocompatibility alloantigen. We should note, however, that the lymphoid organ most likely to trap antigen escaping the draining nodes would be the spleen. (McKhann, 1961.)

A study based on counting germinal centers (unfortunately made with noncongenic lines) gave somewhat similar results. Germinal centers in excess of the control were present on day 1 across both sets of multiple disparities, that with and that without an *H-2* differences. The count was substantially higher for the non-H-2 group (Mariani e*t al.*, 1973). Unfortunately interpretation is complicated by the presence of different *Ly* disparities and different genetic backgrounds in the two test pairs. Male to female grafts, where the only disparity would be at *H-Y*, caused a doubling in the number of germinal centers on day 1, but this was a smaller increase than was noted in either of the other combinations.

### 2. *Humoral Immunity Induced by Minor H Locus Disparities*

One of the most striking differences between H-2 and non-H-2 antigens is the ease with which anti-H-2 antibody is produced and demonstrated and the difficulty of producing, or at least of detecting, anti-non-H-2 antibodies. The difficulty of demonstrating non-H-2 antibodies can be illustrated by studies with strains B6 and C. Bailey has identified 25 *H* loci by which these strains differ. Congenic resistant (CR) lines have been produced for each locus, and recombinant inbred (RI) strain distribution patterns established (see Chapter 3). The information thus provided, and particularly the information concerning the RI strain distribution patterns, furnishes a background that should make it easy to associate any of these 25 loci with hemagglutinating or lymphocytotoxic antibodies that their respective antigens are competent to engender. Attempts have been made to produce such antibodies in 23 appropriate recipient–donor combinations (M. Cherry and G. D. Snell, unpublished). Either B6 or some CR or RI derivative of B6, was used as recipient or one parent of the recipient or donor, and C or some derivative thereof was used in the reverse position. Hybrid recipients were used in nearly all cases; this increases the chance that favorable immune response genes will be present. All combinations were chosen so that anti-H-2 would not be produced. Anti-Ly-1, anti-Ly-2,3, and anti-Thy-1 were also ruled out, because B6 and C carry identical forms of these three antigens.

Most of the combinations yielded detectable hemagglutinating and/or cytotoxic antibodies. None, however, had titers comparable to anti-H-2, and the only workable titers in most of them were attributable to a group of three or four cytotoxic antibodies and two or three hemagglutinating antibodies identifiable by their RI strain distribution patterns. Anti-Ea-4.1, anti-Ea-4.2, anti-Ly-4.1, anti-Ly-4.2, anti-Ly-6, and anti-Ly-7 recurred frequently. A weak anti-Ea-6 may have been present in some antisera. Anti-Ly-4 has an RI pattern identical to that of *H-3;* the loci are possibly the same. *Ly-6* and *Ly-7* are distinct from any known *H* loci (Chapter 5, Section I,F). While not all antisera are fully analyzed, it is apparent that few additional RI strain distribution patterns will be established. Thus rather extensive (although not fully completed) tests have turned up only one antibody that could be attributed to the 24 non-*H-2* loci known to distinguish B6 from C. One cautionary note should be added. It is possible that, despite the use of hybrid recipients, the absence of favorable immune response alleles was a significant limiting factor in the variety of antibodies produced.

Despite this evidence that non-*H-2* histocompatibility locus disparities rarely engender workable hemagglutinating or cytotoxic antibodies, there is evidence that they can lead to antibody formation. Some reports point to weak hemagglutinating or cytotoxic antibodies, but the antibody usually indicated is an enhancing and in some cases non-complement-fixing antibody.

Hildemann and Mullen (1973) have studied enhancing antibody formation in rats with Rt *H-1* and minor *H* locus disparities. Purified IgM and IgG fractions were prepared and tested for their ability to prolong the survival of skin and kidney allografts from the same strain as the antigen donor. Kidney allografts enhance more easily than skin grafts; the kidney test system was thus relatively sensitive. The IgM fraction, in all cases where tested, shortened graft survival; the IgG fraction prolonged it. The degree of prolongation, moreover, was inversely proportional to the strength of the histocompatibility barrier. The authors propose a new genetic rule of transplantation: the weaker the histoincompatibility, the greater the effectiveness of specific immunoblocking antibodies.

Cantrell *et al.* (1974) have extended, and in general confirmed, the results of Hildemann and Mullen with three graded non-*H-2* incompatibilities in mice. The strongest was a combined *H-1* and *H-3* incompatibility. Skin grafts provided the test system. Two kinds of antisera were used: antisera from mice rendered tolerant by neonatal injections of spleen and hyperimmune sera induced by multiple grafts and cell injections. Because of the difficulty of enhancing skin grafts, radiation was combined with serum treatment in some experiments. The authors found that enhancement could be produced across all three barriers by an appropriate combination of treatments, but, in confirmation of Hildemann and Mullen, enhancement was easiest across the weakest barrier. The results also confirmed the induction of enhancing products, presumably antibodies or antigen–antibody complexes, in response to non-*H-2* incompatibilities. The antiserum from "tolerant" mice had enhancing activity, but less than the hyperimmune serum prepared in adults. Other studies with mice disparate at known minor *H* loci confirm the appearance of enhancing antibodies (Baldwin and Cohen, 1973; Nemec and Nouza, 1974). Miller and DeWitt (1973, 1974) used, as did Hildemann and Mullen, Rt *H-1* and multiple non-Rt *H-1* disparities in the rat, but used as their test for humoral or cell-mediated cytotoxicity, the *in vitro* lysis of lymphocytes or embryonic fibroblasts. Enhancing activity was not tested directly, but the antisera were examined for the presence of antibodies that could block the cytotoxic activity of other antibodies or of immune cells. Again, a preferential induction of noncytotoxic antibodies by non-Rt *H-1* disparities was noted. Cytotoxic antibodies showing high titers but low maximum lysis were induced by these disparities, but these resembled, and probably were, homologues of the anti-Ly antibodies of mice. Attempts to absorb the antisera suggested the presence of high titered blocking (non-complement-fixing) antibodies, and the antisera, indeed, protected target fibroblasts from cytolytic action of immune lymphocytes. The Rt H-1 antisera showed no such blocking activity.

An unusual finding of this study concerned the relation of Rt *H-1* and non-Rt *H-1* disparities and of T cells, to the induction of IgM and IgG antibodies. T lymphocytes (presumably T helper cells) were found to be necessary for IgG antibody production across both major and minor barriers. The secondary response to both Rt H-1 and non-Rt H-1 antigens was thus T-cell-dependent. But T-deprived rats, while they produced anti-Rt H-1 IgM, produced no anti-minor *H* locus IgM. This apparent failure of IgM induction in rats by weak H antigens would partly account for the enhancing potential of antisera against these antigens. The most potent cytotoxins would be absent. Hildeman and Mullen report no comparable observation. However, while their tables show that they obtained an anti-Rt H-1 IgM, they do not list any anti-minor *H* locus IgM.

In partial confirmation of the Miller and DeWitt study, Klein *et al.* (1974) have shown that in mice with *H-2* disparities, the IgM response is thymus-independent, and the IgG response is thymus-dependent. Klein *et al.* did not test non-*H-2* disparities.

### 3. *Interpretation*

Why are histocompatibility (H) antigens so different in their immunogenic properties from Ly and Ea antigens? And why, within the H antigen family, are H-2 and other MHC antigens so different from non-H-2 antigens? Firm answers to these questions are as yet impossible, but it will be interesting to try to piece together, from the facts that we have assembled, some possible interpretations. We should point out that available facts come from tests with only a few of the many H antigens.

While murine non-H-2 and rat non-Rt H-1 antigens are traditionally considered as, in varying degrees, "weak" antigens, we have found evidence that they can induce substantial manifestations of immunity. They induce more readily demonstrated enhancing antibody than does H-2; they induce a greater enlargement of the draining nodes, although with a longer interval to the peak response; and they, perhaps, induce the formation of more germinal centers in the draining nodes.

There are, of course, such things as genuinely weak antigens. Some amino acid substitutions, for example, are substantially less immunogenic than others. Doubtless some of the variation in the rejection times engendered by different H antigens traces to such causes. However, it is possible that much of the "weakness" of this group of alloantigens is due, directly or indirectly, not to their inherent lack of antigenicity but to their relative inaccessibility to antibodes and cytotoxic cells. We have suggested in Section I,C that H antigens may, in a disproportional number of cases, function as transport components of the plasma membrane rather than as cell interaction components, and that this function may be associated with the immersion of much the greater part of the antigen in the lipid bilayer. H antigens, so to speak, have a low profile. This could make them relatively inaccessible to the recognition structures of lymphocytes and thus obstruct, although not necessarily prevent, the induction and/or expression of immunity.

One study offers at least some support for this suggestion. Staines (1974) has reported that some non-MHC membrane components that induce weak xenoantibodies when still in the membrane behave as strong xenoantigens when separated. This suggests that chemical structure may be less important than some feature of membrane association. It should be noted, however, that the use in this study of xenoimmunization, and of papain solubilization that cleaves the molecule, perhaps at the membrane surface, make interpretations difficult.

By way of compairson, there is, of course, substantial evidence that much of the structure of H-2 molecules is outside the lipid bilayer (Chapter 11). The postulated shielded position of non-H-2 alloantigens could have a variety of consequences. Recognition might be delayed, effective reaction might occur with only the most avid of the potentially reactive T and B cell clones, an exaggerated production of effector cells might be necessary to effect rejection, and macrophage processing might be an important facilitating step in the immune response or even an absolutely necessary one. All these deflections of the immune process are compatible with what we know of the non-H-2 antigen alloimmune response.

One apparently well-established feature of the non-H-2 response is the relative potency of the enhancing antibody that is engendered. Can this be explained by the postulated properties of non-H-2 antigens? If a relatively high proportion of any one of these antigens were recognized and processed in the spleen rather than the nodes, this could account, at least in part, for their tendency to induce enhancing antibody. We have seen (Section III,B,1), that immunization via the spleen is strikingly favorable to enhancement. For most types of transplants, the original drainage of non-H-2 antigens (or passenger lymphocytes), no less than that of H-2 antigens, occurs certainly almost exclusively to the nodes. Blood remaining in the blood vessels of an organ graft would be an exception. However, it may well be that trapping within the nodes of non-H-2 antigens is of a lower order than that occurring with H-2. This would be quite in keeping with our postulated properties.

Passenger lymphocytes escaping the draining nodes would, in the great majority of cases, pass through the spleen next rather than some other node. Even if only a fraction were trapped, some induction of enhancement could result.

There has been no study directly concerned with the degree of trapping within the draining nodes of passenger lymphocytes borne within a graft, but there is some relevant evidence. While this is not entirely consistent, it does suggest that there may be differences in the degree of trapping dependent on the histoincompatibility. We have already mentioned studies that emphasize the remarkable efficiency of the nodes as filters. This might be taken to mean that few lymphocytes from the afferent lymph, even if marked by only non-*H-2* disparities, would escape. However, Snell *et al.* (1961) found that some labeled allogeneic thymocytes with multiple incompatibilities, including *H-2,* injected subcutaneously were picked up in the spleen. This study provides no comparison of *H-2* and non-*H-2,* but Zatz *et al.* (1972) have compared the trapping of lymph node cells with *H-2, Ly-1, Ly-2, Thy-1, Ea-2,* and *Mls* disparities. No cells from specifically non-*H-2* congenic lines were used, but weak *H* loci are closely associated with *Ly-1* and *Ly-2* (Chapter 3). Unfortunately, for our purposes, the cells were injected in the tail vein, so that the first lymphoid organ encountered would probably be the spleen. There was much trapping in the liver. But *H-2* trapping was different from non-H-2 trapping, even by 90 minutes after injection. The difference showed up in greater H-2 trapping in the liver and less in the nodes.

Despite the imperfections in the evidence, the postulate does seem warranted that presence of only non-*H-2* disparities on passenger lymphocytes carried over in a graft might lead to proportionally high spleen trapping, and hence to a proportionally high production of enhancing antibody. It should be noted that if passenger lymphocytes bear *H-2* as well as non-*H-2* disparities, extensive node trapping would presumably occur. What sort of a non-H-2 response this would lead to is a separate problem.

There may be other properties of non-H-2 alloantigens besides a propensity to spleen trapping that would influence the immunologic outcome of their presence in a graft. In the case of T cell-dependent antigens, antibody production is presumed to be contingent on the possession by the antigen of two reactive sites. One of these functions as a carrier and reacts with T helper cells; the other functions as a hapten and reacts with B cells. The antigenically complex H-2 molecule probably has more than one alloantigenic site and can, therefore, meet the requirements for this type of antibody induction. We have no evidence as to the antigenic complexity of the various non-H-2 molecules, but if they had only one reactive site, it is quite possible that they would induce an immune response quite different from that induced by H-2. Our postulate that non-H-2 antigens tend to be largely buried in the lipid bilayer is in keeping with the assumption that the exposed part, at least, is antigenically simple. Pearson and Raffel (1971) have stated that small antigens, or larger antigens only partially recognized as foreign by the responder, tend to invoke cellular immunity (typically expressed in this kind of study as delayed hypersensitivity). If, as the foregoing discussion might suggest, these studies are applicable to non-H-2 alloantigens, then cellular immunity might be the outcome of exposure to these antigens also.

We arrive at the same conclusion from a somewhat different approach. If we are correct in our postulate that non-H-2 antigens are largely buried within the lipid bilayer, a lipophilic chemistry is implied. This could influence their immunogenic properties. Dailey and Hunter (1974) have reported that lipophilic antigens tend to localize in the paracortical area of the lymph nodes, in close proximity to thymus-derived cells, and that they are strong inducers of delayed-type hypersensitivity. Since delayed hypersensitivity is a manifestation of a cellular immune response, we are led by this line of reasoning also to the conclusion that non-H-2 alloantigens should invoke a cellular immune response.

But the induction of cellular immunity, and cellular immunity alone, would not account for the very delayed rejection of some non-H-2 allografts. As we have noted, evidence such as the weight of the draining lymph nodes, suggests that at least some non-H-2 antigens do engender a strong, although perhaps somewhat delayed, cellular immune response. Their delayed rejection is not due to the lack of cellular immunity but to the concomitant development of strong immunological enhancement with little accompanying production of cytotoxic antibody. Such an outcome is not necessarily incompatible with the findings of Pearson and Raffel (1971) and Dailey and Hunter (1974) especially when considered together with the major differences in the nature of the response occurring in the spleen as contrasted with the nodes (Section III,B,1). Either the simple or the lipophilic nature of non-MHC alloantigens might conceivably account for the failure, noted by Miller and DeWitt (1973, 1974), of these alloantigens to induce IgM production. There is no clue to associate a lipophilic surface with the production of blocking (enhancing) antibodies, but since suppressor cells are T cells, localization of non-H-2 antigen in the T cell-dependent areas of the spleen could very well favor graft survival by the induction of such cells. Enhancing antibody has been sought for and found in the recipients of non-

MHC grafts, but so far as we know, no one has looked for supressor cells.

The long survival of non-H-2 skin grafts, often accompanied by episodes of partial rejection, is in keeping with the simultaneous presence in the host of cellular immunity and blocking antibody. Their fate is contingent on the direction in which a delicate balance between opposing forces is finally tipped. Manickavel and Cohen (1975) have specifically suggested that the chronic type of rejection seen with non-MHC grafts is due in part to autoenhancement.

Other factors that probably contribute to the prolonged survival of non-H-2 grafts are recognition lag and the inaccessibility of the antigen to effector cells or antibody.

## V. Organ Grafts versus Tissue Grafts: Conclusions

The evidence herein assembled permits a reasonable interpretation of the substantial differences in host response to organ as compared with tissue allografts. Despite the large number of non-MHC disparities in the typical organ graft, they play a minor role in the rejection process; they play a major role, cumulatively, in the rejection of skin or other tissue grafts.

We suggest that this can be explained by differences in the immunogenic pathway. Organ grafts, with their retained vasculature, sensitize promptly via the spleen. Passenger lymphocytes, if present, also lead to a response in the draining nodes, but one that, at least with respect to non-MHC antigens, is subordinate. The result is, for these antigens, a preponderance of enhancement over cellular immunity. With tissue grafts the situation is reversed. They have an abundant lymphatic drainage but, during the first few days, no functional vasculature. and when the vasculature is restored, it is of host origin, and hence noninductive. Initial immunization is almost exclusively via the nodes, and with respect to both MHC and non-MHC antigens is favorable to rejection rather than enhancement.

Another difference between organ and skin grafts is that at least some organ grafts are relatively sensitive to the cytotoxic action of anti-MHC antibody. This is perhaps less true of heart than of kidney grafts and of mice and rats than of some larger mammals. Where antibody sensitivity is present, the elimination of node immunization need not prevent rejection by spleen-produced antibody if an MHC disparity is present.

These same principles can explain the results of various experimental modifications of the usual graft situation. Alymphatic organ grafts are rejected because of their special sensitivity to spleen-engendered anti-

MHC. The heart allografts in Dittmar and Bennett's (1975) experiment, with their passenger lymphocytes destroyed by host M cells, and hence with node immunization inhibited, might have been expected to behave similarly, but they did not. They survived permanently. Perhaps this is because rat hearts are relatively insensitive to MHC antibody. These are probably oversimplified interpretations, particularly in the case of the complex Dittmar–Bennett experiment, but they perhaps point to some of the major trends that determine the diverse outcome of different types of grafts.

## REFERENCES


Bailey, D. W. 1971. Cumulative effect or independent effect? *Transplantation* **11**:419–422.

Baldwin, W. M., III, and N. Cohen. 1973. Immune serum implements either accelerated rejection or prolonged survival of murine skin grafts. *Transplantation* **15**:633–637.

Bansal, S. C., K. E. Hellström, I. Hellström, and H. O. Sjögren. 1973. Cell-mediated immunity and blocking serum activity to tolerated allografts in rats. *J Exp Med* **137**:590–602.

Barker, C. F., and R. E. Billingham. 1968. The role of afferent lymphatics in the rejection of skin homografts. *J Exp Med* **128**:197–221.

Basten, A., J. F. A. P. Miller, J. Sprent, and C. Cheers. 1974. Cell to cell interactions in the immune response. X. T-cell-dependent suppression in tolerant mice. *J Exp Med* **140**:199–217.

Billingham, R. E., L. Brent, and P. B. Medawar. 1953. "Actively acquired tolerance" of foreign cells. *Nature (Lond)* **172**:603–606.

Boyse, E. A. 1971. Organization and modulation of cell membrane receptors. Pages 5–30 *in* R. T. Smith and M. Landy, eds. Immune surveillance. Academic Press, New York.

Brent, L., and M. E. French. 1973. Workshop on mechanisms of tolerance and enhancement. *Transplant Proc* **5**:1001–1010.

Cantor, H., and E. A. Boyse. 1975. Functional subclasses of T lymphocytes bearing different Ly antigens. I. The generation of functionally distinct T cell subclasses in a differentiation process independent of antigen. *J Exp Med* **141**:1376–1389.

Cantrell, J. L., N. Kaliss, and W. H. Hildemann. 1974. Characteristics of histocompatibility barriers in congenic strains of mice. III. Passive enhancement of skin allografts in X-irradiated hosts. *Transplantation* **19**:95–101.

Canty, T. G., and J. R. Wunderlich. 1971. Quantitative assessment of cellular and humoral responses to skin and tumor allografts. *Transplantation* **11**:111–116.

Carpenter, C. B. 1976. The role of antibodies in the rejection and enhancement of rat organ allografts. *Transplant Proc,* in press.

Cerottini, J.-C., and K. T. Brunner. 1974. Cell-mediated cytotoxicity, allograft rejection, and tumor immunity. *Adv Immunol* **18**:67–132.

Cochran, A. J., E. Klein, and G. Petranyi. 1971. Migration of lymph node cells during the primary immune response. *Transplantation* **12**:523–525.

Converse, J. M., and D. L. Ballantyne, Jr. 1962. Distribution of diphosphopyridine nucleotide diaphorase in rat skin autografts and homografts. *Plast Reconstr Surg* **30**:415–425.

Currie, G. A., and K. D. Bagshawe. 1968. The antigenicity of normal and malignant trophoblast: Some implications. *Adv Transplant* **6**:523–530.

Dailey, M. O., and R. L. Hunter. 1974. The role of lipid in the induction of hapten-specific delayed hypersensitivity and contact sensitivity. *J Immunol* **112**:1526–1534.

Dittmar, J., and M. Bennett. 1975. Long-term survival of cardiac allografts in lethally irradiated rats repopulated with syngeneic hemopoietic cells. *Transplantation* **19**:295–301.

Dyminski, J. W., and B. F. Argyris. 1972. *In vitro* sensitization to transplantation antigens. III. Thymus-bone marrow cooperation. *Transplantation* **13**:234–238.

Fabre, J. W., and P. J. Morris. 1975. Studies on the specific suppression of renal allograft rejection in presensitized rats. *Transplantation* **19**:121–133.

Gelfand, M. C., and A. D. Steinberg. 1974. Cooperation of three lymphoid cells in allograft rejection. *Cell Immunol* **11**:221–230.

Gershon, R. K. 1974. Lack of activity of contra-suppressor T cells as a mechanism of tolerance. Pages 441–469 *in* D. H. Katz and B. Benacerraf, eds. Immunological tolerance. Academic Press, New York.

Graff, R. J., W. K. Silvers, R. E. Billingham, W. H. Hildemann, and G. D. Snell. 1966. The cumulative effect of histocompatibility antigens. *Transplantation* **4**:605–617.

Grant, C. K., R. Evans, and P. Alexander. 1973. Multiple effector roles of lymphocytes in allograft immunity. *Cell Immunol* **8**:136–146.

Guttman, G., and I. L. Weissman. 1972. Lymphoid tissue architecture. Experimental analysis of the origin and distribution of T cells and B cells. *Immunology* **23**:465–479.

Guttmann, R. D., R. R. Lindquist, and S. A. Ockner. 1969. Renal transplantation in the inbred rat. IX. Hematopoietic origin of an immunogenic stimulus of rejection. *Transplantation* **8**:472–484.

Hamburger, J., A. Dimitriu, L. Bankir, M. Debray-Sachs, and J. Auvert. 1971. Collection of lymph from kidneys homotransplanted in man: Cell transformation in vivo. *Nature (Lond)* **232**:633–634.

Harris, T. N., and S. Harris. 1975. Shifts from $IgG_2$ to $IgG_1$ class in CBA and C3H anti-BALB/c antibody. *Transplantation* **19**:318–325.

Hersey, P., P. Cullen, and I. C. M. MacLennan. 1973. Lymphocyte-dependent cytotoxic antibody activity against human transplantation antigens. *Transplantation* **16**:9–16.

Hersh, E. M., W. T. Butler, R. D. Rossen, R. O. Morgen, and W. Suki. 1971. Lymphocyte activation during allograft rejection. *Transplant Proc* **3**:457–460.

Hessinger, D. A., R. A. Daynes, and G. A. Granger. 1973. Binding of human lymphotoxin to target-cell membranes and its relation to cell-mediated cytodestruction. *Proc Natl Acad Sci USA* **70**:3082–3086.

Hildemann, W. H. 1970. Immunogenetics. Holden-Day, San Francisco, California.

Hildemann, W. H., and Y. Mullen. 1973. The weaker the histoincompatibility, the greater the effectiveness of specific immunoblocking antibodies. *Transplantation* **15**:231–237.

Hudack, S. S., and P. D. McMaster. 1933. The lymphatic participation in human cutaneous phenomena. A study of the minute lymphatics of the living skin. *J Exp Med* **57**:751–774.

Kaliss, N., N. Molomut, J. L. Harriss, and S. D. Gault. 1953. Effect of previously injected immune serum and tissue on the survival of tumor grafts in mice. *J Natl Cancer Inst* **13**:847–850.

Kaplan, H. J., and T. R. Stevens. 1975. A reconsideration of immunological privilege within the anterior chamber of the eye. *Transplantation* **19**:302–309.

Kaplan, H. J., and J. W. Streilein. 1974. Do immunologically privileged sites require a functioning spleen? *Nature (Lond)* **251**:553–554.

Kaplan, H. J., J. W. Streilein, and R. E. Billingham. 1975. Splenic influence on cellular interactions in allograft immunity. *Fed Proc* **34**(3):989 (abstr.)

Katz, D. H., and B. Benacerraf, eds. 1974. Immunological tolerance. Mechanisms and potential therapeutic applications. Academic Press, New York.

Kiehn, E. D., and J. J. Holland. 1968. Multiple protein components of mammalian cell membranes. *Proc Natl Acad Sci USA* **61**:1370–1377.

Kiessling, R., E. Klein, H. Pross, and H. Wigzell. 1975. "Natural" killer cells in the mouse. II. Cytotoxic cells with specificity for mouse Moloney leukemia cells. Characteristics of the killer cell. *Eur J Immunol* **5**:117–121.

Klein, J., S. Livnat, V. Hauptfeld, L. Jeřábek, and I. Weissman. 1974. Production of anti-H-2 antibodies in thymectomized mice. *Eur J Immunol* **4**:41–44.

Kongshavn, P. A. L., and W. S. Lapp. 1973. Bone marrow origin of nonsensitized effector cells in skin allograft rejection. *Transplantation* **16**:382–385.

Kyger, E. R., III, and K. E. Salyer. 1973. The role of donor passenger leukocytes in rat skin allograft rejection. *Transplantation* **16**:537–543.

Laico, M. T., E. I. Ruoslahti, D. S. Papermaster, and W. J. Dreyer. 1970. Isolation of the fundamental polypeptide subunits of biological membranes. *Proc Natl Acad Sci USA* **67**:120–127.

Lameijer, L. D. F., J. Smith, and J. F. Mowbray. 1972. Effect of kidney perfusion on renal allograft survival in azathioprine treated rats. *Br J Exp Pathol* **53**:130–137.

Lance, E. M., and S. Cooper. 1972. Homing of specifically sensitized lymphocytes to allografts of skin. *Cell Immunol* **5**:66–73.

Lengerová, A., and V. Matoušek. 1968. Analysis of the background of graft rejection time variation in weak histocompatibilty systems. *Folia Biol (Praha)* **14**:1–8.

Lindquist, R. R., R. D. Buttmann, and J. P. Merrill. 1971. Renal transplantation in the inbred rat. VI. Electron microscopic study of the mononuclear cells accumulating in rejecting renal allografts. *Transplantation* **12**:1–10.

Linscott, W. D. 1970. Effect of cell surface antigen density on immunological enhancement. *Nature (Lond)* **228**:824–827.

McKhann, C. F. 1961. Regional lymph node response to skin grafts between strains of mice differing by strong and weak histocompatibility genes. *J Surg Res* **1**:294–298.

McKhann, C. F. 1964. Transplantation studies of strong and weak histocompatibility barriers in mice. I. Immunization. *Transplantation* **2**:613–619.

McKhann, C. F., and J. H. Berrian. 1961. Immunologic properties of weak histocompatibility genes. *J Immunol* **86**:170–176.

MacLeenan, I. C. M. 1972. Antibody in the induction and inhibition of lymphocyte cytotoxicity. *Transplant Rev* **13**:67–90.

Manickavel, V., and M. Cohen. 1975. Does chronic rejection elicited by weak H-antigens in mice and salamander result from active enhancement? *Transplant Proc* **7**:451–453.

Marchesi, V. T., and J. L. Gowans. 1964. The migration of lymphocytes through the endothelium of venules in lymph nodes: An electron microscope study. *Proc Roy Soc, Lond* [*Biol*] **159**:283–290.

Mariani, T., J. Demhof, and R. A. Good. 1973. Germinal center formation in response to skin grafted across weak and strong histocompatibility barriers. *Adv Exp Med Biol* **29**:597–602.

Mattioli, C. A., Y. Yagi, and D. Pressman. 1968. Production and properties of mouse anti-hapten antibodies. *J Immunol* **101**:939–948.

Mayhew, E., and M. Bennett. 1971. An in vitro reaction between lymphoid cells and target fibroblastic cells: A possible model for *in vivo* rejection of haemopoietic allografts. *Immunology* **21**:123–136.

Miller, C. L., and C. W. DeWitt. 1973. Cellular and humoral responses to major and minor histocompatibility antigens. *Transplant Proc* **5**:303–305.

Miller, C. L., and C. W. DeWitt. 1974. The effect of neonatal thymectomy on antibody responses to histocompatibility antigens in the rat. *Cell Immunol* **13**:278–287.

Nemec, N., and K. Nouza. 1974. Possible role of serum factors in non-H-2 allograft response in mice. *Folia Biol* (*Praha*) **20**:75–78.

Nielsen, H. E., I. Heron, and C. Koch. 1975. Passenger cells in rat heart allografts. No effect of removal. *Transplantation* **19**:360–362.

Nossal, G. J. V., and G. L. Ada. 1971. Antigens, lymphoid cells, and the immune response. Academic Press, New York.

Pardee, A. B. 1968. Membrane transport proteins. *Science* **126**:632–637.

Pearson, M. N., and S. Raffel. 1971. Macrophage-digested antigen as inducer of delayed hypersensitivity. *J Exp Med* **133**:494–505.

Pederson, N. C., E. P. Adams, and B. Morris. 1975. The response of the lymphoid system to renal allografts in sheep. *Transplantation* **19**:400–409.

Raff, M. C., and J. J. T. Owen. 1971. Thymus-derived lymphocytes: Their distribution and role in the development of peripheral lymphoid tissues of the mouse. *Eur J Immunol* **1**:27–30.

Rambourg, A., M. Neutra, and C. P. Leblond. 1966. Presence of a "cell coat" rich in carbohydrate at the surface of cells in the rat. *Anat Rec* **154**:41–72.

Rich, S. S., and R. R. Rich. 1975. Regulatory mechanisms in cell-mediated immune responses. I. Regulation of mixed lymphocyte reactions by alloantigen-activated thymus-derived lymphocytes. *J Exp Med* **140**:1588–1603.

Rouse, B. T., and H. Wagner. 1973. The in vivo activity of *in vitro* immunized mouse thymocytes. *Transplantation* **16**:161–170.

Scollay, R., and K. Lafferty. 1975. Differences in the graft-versus-host reaction of cells migrating through nonlymphoid tissue or lymph nodes. *Transplantation* **19**:170–176.

Singer, S. J., and G. L. Nicolson. 1972. The fluid mosaic model of the structure of cell membranes. *Science* **175**:720–731.

Snell, G. D. 1957. The homograft reaction. *Annu Rev Microbiol* **11**:439–458.

Snell, G. D., H. J. Winn, J. H. Stimpfling, and S. J. Parker. 1960. Depression by antibody of the immune response to homografts and its role in immunological enhancement. *J Exp Med* **112**:293–314.

Snell, G. D., H. J. Winn, and A. A. Kandutsch. 1961. A quantitative study of cellular immunity. *J Immunol* **87**:1–17.

Staines, N. A. 1974. Relative immunogenicity of H-2 and other membrane components in xenoimmunization. *Transplantation* **17**:470–476.

Steinmuller D., and E. A. Hart. 1971. Passenger leukocytes and induction of allograft immunity. *Transplant Proc* **3**:673–675.

Stobo, J. D., A. S. Rosenthal, and W. E. Paul. 1973. Functional heterogeneity of murine lymphoid cells. V. Lymphocytes lacking detectable surface $\theta$ or immunoglobulin determinants. *J Exp Med* **138**:71–88.

Strober, S., and J. L. Gowans. 1965. The role of lymphocytes in the sensitization of rats to renal homografts. *J Exp Med* **122**:347–360.

Sybesma, J. P., L. Kater, E. Borst-Eilers, B. A. de Planque, T. van Soelen, and G. Tuit. 1974. HL-A antigens in kidney tissue. Localisation by means of an immunofluorescence technique. *Transplantation* **17**:576–583.

Szulman, A. E. 1960. The histological distribution of blood group substances A and B in man. *J Exp Med* **111**:785–800.

Vetto, R. M., and R. K. Lawson. 1967. The role of vascular endothelium in the afferent pathway as suggested by the alymphatic renal homotransplant. *Transplantation* **5**:1537–1539.

von Boehmer, H. 1974. Separation of T and B lymphocytes and their role in the mixed lymphocyte reaction. *J Immunol* **112**:70–78.

Warren, R. P., J. S. Lofgreen, and D. Steinmuller. 1973. Factors responsible for the differential survival of heart and skin allografts in inbred rats. *Transplantation* **16**:458–465.

White, E., and W. H. Hildemann. 1969. Kidney versus skin allograft reaction in normal adult rats of inbred strains. *Transplant Proc* **1**:395–399.

Widdicombe, J. G., R. Hughes, and A. J. May. 1955. The efficiency of filtration by the popliteal lymph node of the rabbit. *Brit J Exp Pathol* **36**:473–478.

Zatz, M. M., R. Gingrich, and E. M. Lance. 1972. The effect of histocompatibility antigens on lymphocyte migration in the mouse. *Immunology* **23**:665–675.

Zembala, M., and G. L. Asherson. 1973. Depression of the T cell phenomenon of contact sensitivity by T cells from unresponsive mice. *Nature* (*Lond*) **244**:227–228.

# INDEX

## I

## T



## U

V



X



Y



A 6
B 7
C 8
D 9
E 0
F 1
G 2
H 3
I 4
J 5